THE ANTIBODY
ENIGMA

THE ANTIBODY ENIGMA

THOMAS J. KINDT

National Institute of Allergy and Infectious Diseases
National Institutes of Health
Bethesda, Maryland

AND

J. DONALD CAPRA

University of Texas Health Science Center
Dallas, Texas

PLENUM PRESS • NEW YORK AND LONDON

Library of Congress Cataloging in Publication Data

Kindt, Thomas J., 1939–
  The antibody enigma.

  Includes bibliographical references and index.
    1. Antibody diversity. I. Capra, J. Donald, 1937–   . II. Title. [DNLM: 1. Antibody diversity. QW 575 K51a]
QR186.7.K56 1984   599′.0293   84-4761
ISBN-13: 978-1-4684-4678-4   e-ISBN-13: 978-1-4684-4676-0
DOI: 10.1007/978-1-4684-4676-0

©1984 Plenum Press, New York
Softcover reprint of the hardcover 1st edition 1984

A Division of Plenum Publishing Corporation
233 Spring Street, New York, N.Y. 10013

This book is dedicated to our teachers, H. Edward Conrad, Charles Todd, Richard Krause, Thomas B. Tomasi, Jr., Alan Peterkofsky, and Henry Kunkel, and to our many graduate students and postdoctoral fellows. Both groups have been a continuous source of inspiration and ideas.

The empirical basis of objective science has thus nothing "absolute" about it. Science does not rest upon solid bedrock. The bold structure of its theories rises, as it were, above swamp. It is like a building erected on piles. The piles are driven down from above into the swamp, but not down to any natural or "given" base; and if we stop driving the piles deeper, it is not because we have reached firm ground. We simply stop when we are satisfied that the piles are firm enough to carry the structure, at least for the time being.

—KARL POPPER *(The Logic of Scientific Discovery)*

PREFACE

The Antibody Enigma is a somewhat personal view of the antibody diversity question from two investigators who have spent the past 18 years trying to penetrate the enigma. It is not and was not meant to be an all-embracing comprehensively referenced review of the subject of antibody diversity. Because of the subjective viewpoint, there are undoubtedly omissions of data that others consider to be seminal, and if we have offended anyone by omitting their own contribution we sincerely apologize.

We have lived with "The Enigma" on and off for the past two years. It has been both hard work and good fun but, above all, it has been a learning experience. There were several difficult decisions to make in putting together the final text, but perhaps the most difficult was deciding upon a stopping point. The field of antibody diversity is presently enjoying an unparalleled expansion of information, and because of this it was very tempting to await further developments in hopes of tying up as many loose ends as possible. This was decided against for several reasons; the major factor was that the project was growing burdensome for both of us. From a more objective point of view this appears to be a reasonable time to stop our exposition. The questions that began to take shape in the mid-1950s with the first serious genetic studies have been answered and a new set of rules for antibody diversity generation has been defined. New and different questions have replaced the old, and while some of these will be answered by studies in progress, there are other questions that will be with us for a much longer time. Although we have not written solely from an historic point of view there is emphasis in this volume on the development of concepts related to our subject. It is our opinion that an understanding of this development will help investigators to better understand what is happening today and what may happen tomorrow in this field.

Another difficult decision concerned determination of the audience to which the book is directed. Related to this decision was the choice of a title that would reach this intended group. In this respect we must admit defeat. It has been impossible for us to say exactly for whom the book is intended and perhaps this uncertainty is further reflected in our choice of a title. Certainly it remains impossible to write a book entitled *The Solution to the Question of Antibody Diversity*. Numerous title formulations were tried and rejected on the basis of being either too amorphous or too indicative that the problem has been solved.

There have been a number of persons who have put much time and effort into this project. First of all, Richard Wasserman, Lisa Steiner, and Edward Max deserve special mention for reading the draft of the text, finding errors and inconsistencies, and pointing these out to us. The enormous job of typing, correcting, and retyping was faithfully carried out by Kathy van Egmond in Dallas and Virginia Shaw and Lynette White in Bethesda. Their patience is to be commended. It was a pleasure to work with the staff of Plenum Press, and we wish to thank Kirk Jensen for his enormous contributions to this text. If all of the abbreviations are finally consistent and all *thats* and *whichs* properly sorted out, it is certainly due to the efforts of Jane Woolsey. We thank numerous colleagues for prepublication information in various forms. Finally we wish to thank our families for suffering with us through the birth of this work.

T. J. Kindt

J. D. Capra

CONTENTS

THE ANTIBODY
ENIGMA

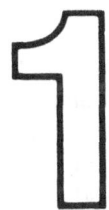

THE NATURE OF THE PROBLEM

> *This is in essence the oldest of biological problems—the classic struggle between the Lamarckians and the Darwinians on the nature of adaptation in evolution. It is a theme that has been played on in an infinity of variations over the last 100 years, and I can only hope that in the present treatment there are scattered elements of novelty, either in regard to example or approach, which will make up for the inevitable inclusion of much that is trite and familiar.*
>
> —Sir Macfarlane Burnet

1.1. INTRODUCTION

The immune system can be viewed as a device that plays sentry over a continuous onslaught of stimuli and negotiates with each appropriately for the preservation of the organism. As a receptor, processor, and interpreter of information, this organ system is rivaled by none in sophistication and sensitivity save possibly the nervous system.

The immune and nervous systems, in fact, share many features. Both must respond to a vast array of external stimuli. Both are composed of cells that penetrate virtually all other organ systems and tissues of the body. Consequently, with their responsibility of preserving the entire organism, both can be conceptualized as consisting of afferent and efferent modes; that is, the cells of both systems not only receive information but transmit it as well. Critically, both are also modulated by a balance of positive and negative regulatory mechanisms: excitation and inhibition, depolarization and polarization in the case of nerves, help and suppression in the control of lymphocytes. In a sense, the immune system has an additional level of complexity over that of the nervous system, although this very complexity also affords immunologists an experimental advantage over neuroscientists. Although the nervous system is well moored in the body in a static webb of axons, dendrites, and synapses, the elements of the immune system are in a continuously mobile phase incessantly scouring over and percolating through the body tissues, returning through an intricate system of lymphatic channels, and then blending again in the blood. This dynamism is relieved only by scattered concentrations called lymphoid organs.

In large part because of the accessibility of the immunoglobulin molecule and the ease of manipulation of a cellular system unencumbered by any rigid organ matrix, the immune system has served as a forerunner providing a model for differentiation in the storage and expression of information in a complex biological system. More than most other systems, it is amenable to detailed cellular and molecular analysis.

1.2. ANTIBODY SYNTHESIS

A major function of the immune system is to synthesize molecules capable of binding foreign substances and rendering them harmless to the host organism. These molecules are called *antibodies* and the bound materials are called *antigens*. The synthesis of an antibody in response to the administration of an antigen is an adaptive phenomenon capable of exacting, yet wide-ranging specificity. For over fifty years it has been known that antibodies are globular proteins of varying size, the majority of which are associated with the gamma fraction of the serum proteins. The term immunoglobulin is of more recent origin and serves to emphasize the basic unit of structure and function underlying the varied forms of reactivity and seemingly endless variety of antibodies.

Immunoglobulins derive from lymphoid cells, generally from those terminally differentiated lymphoid cells called plasma cells. These cells, once sensitized by antigen, become "committed" and are referred to as immunocytes. Lymphocytes are divided into two types, one concerned with cell-mediated immunity (T lymphocytes) and the other with humoral immunity (B lymphocytes). In general, for antibody production to take place, both B and T lymphocytes are required. Early lymphocytes of the B-lymphocyte lineage contain immunoglobulin on their cell surface. These immunocytes are not normally secreting cells, but undergo differentiation to plasma cells—cells specialized for secretion of antibodies. Antibodies are largely made in the lymphoid organs of the body, particularly those that contain large concentrations of B lymphocytes, the spleen, and lymph nodes (Fig. 1.1). The secretory immune system, which is primarily concentrated beneath endothelial surfaces such as along the respiratory and gastrointestinal tracts, represents almost a separate immune system in that the mode of antigen presentation, the class, and composition of the antibody molecule itself (secretory IgA) as well as its local transport into the gut and respiratory "tubes" are unique. However, from the point of view of this volume, the secretory immune

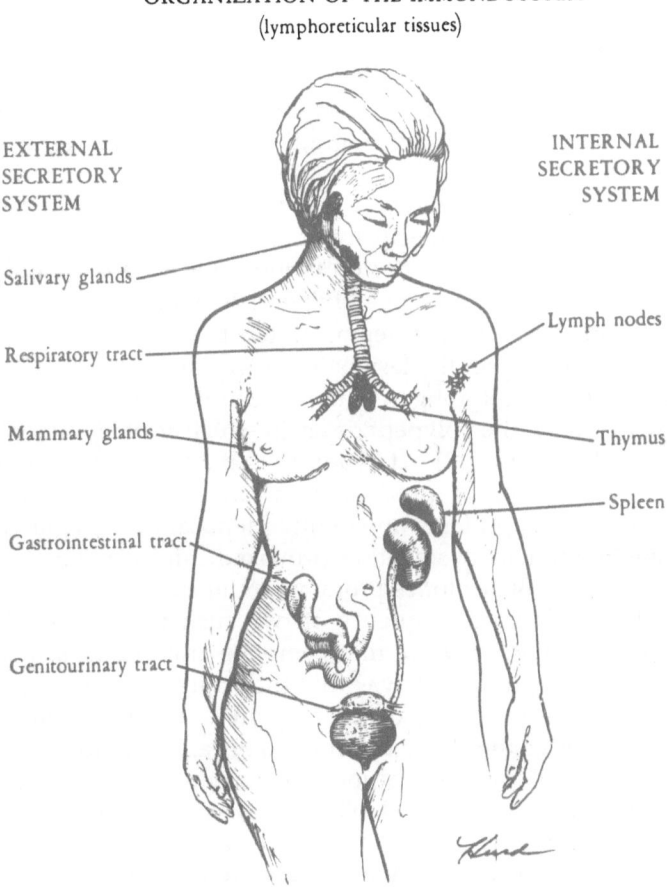

Figure 1.1. Schematic representation of the lymphoid system. Reproduced from Bellanti (1979).

system must still cope with an identical problem; that is, the antigen-binding problem must still be solved by the genetic apparatus of the individual. Thus, although the secretory immune system as well as those other specialized forms of immunity such as immediate hypersensitivity (mediated by the immunoglobulin class IgE) will be dealt with briefly in further chapters, the major focus of this volume is on the antigen-binding function of immunoglobulin molecules.

To account for the extremely diverse range of antigens against which antibodies can be elicited, the *instructive or template theory* of antibody formation was put forward in 1930. In this theory an antibody molecule is synthesized in the presence of the antigen that acts as a template. In the 1940s this theory was extended to include the notion that all the antibody molecules of a given organism had an identical primary structure, but differed from each other in the conformation of their polypeptide chains. This view was initially supported by the finding that various antibodies had an almost identical amino acid composition. In the early 1950s however, partition chromatography indicated that gammaglobulin was a complex mixture of similar components.

This and other considerations led to the *subcellular selection theory*, which proposed that the specificity of each antibody molecule was determined by a unique sequence of amino acids, and that antibody diversity arose from a high degree of spontaneous mutation.

In the late 1950s, it was demonstrated that immunoglobulins had two subunits, subsequently designated heavy and light chains (both of which were needed for antigen binding). Studies on these subunits led to the elucidation of the polypeptide chain structure of immunoglobulins in the early 1960s (Fig. 1.2). At about the same time, it was shown that the Bence Jones proteins, products of a cancer of the lymphoid cells, were homogeneous proteins apparently identical to the light chains of immunoglobulin. This observation provoked intensive amino acid sequence studies on Bence Jones proteins culminating in a comparison of the complete amino acid sequence of two such proteins in 1965. The most striking feature of these first complete amino acid sequences of immunoglobulin light chains was that the entire carboxy terminal half was identical in both chains [constant region (C)], the considerable variance between the chains being confined to the amino terminal half (variable region (V)]. These observations led to one of the most radical of ideas ever to emerge in modern biology: *two noncontiguous structural genes encode each polypeptide chain.*

As more amino acid sequence data were accumulated, immunologists were faced with a striking fact: almost every immunoglobulin chain

S-S

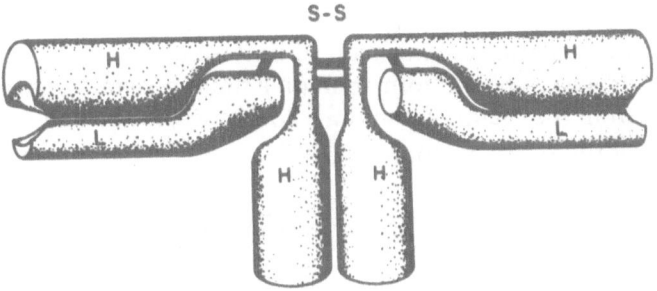

Figure 1.2. An early model of an immunoglobulin molecule.

studied had a unique amino acid sequence. The origin of the sequence diversity became the central arena of confrontation in the field of immunology and remained so for 15 years. Two camps emerged relatively early. In one camp were those who held the view that there were relatively few genes in the germline and that these were acted on by a series of somatic processes, each of which contributed to immunoglobulin diversity, whereas the other camp held that the diversity existed totally in the germline and had been acted on through evolution; that for every "new" amino acid sequence that was deduced, a new germline gene had to be invoked. Using this construct, the number of genes required from the amino acid sequence data began approaching 1000 in the inbred BALB/c mouse. It became increasingly clear that neither theory could explain the observed facts. The ultimate resolution of the dilemma awaited experimental approaches to the DNA itself.

The story of this polemic, the arguments for each position, and the crucial experiments that swayed opinions in one direction or the other are the subject of this book.

1.3. HISTORICAL ROOTS

The unequivocal linking of immunity with substances contained in the blood emerged from the findings of Von Behring and Kitasato in 1890 that sera from animals immunized with bacterial toxins protected other animals, on passive transfer, from the otherwise lethal effects of the toxin. Elaborate extensions of these observations were made by Bordet at the turn of the century who demonstrated that antibodies appeared in sera after the injection of innocuous materials. These observations placed antibody formation on a more general basis, removing it strictly from the realm of immunity to disease, a function with which it was until then exclusively associated.

1.3.1. Introduction of the Germline Concept of Immunologic Specificity

After the discovery of antibodies in serum, Paul Ehrlich in 1900 was among the first to consider in detail the problem of immunologic specificity. He envisioned immunocytes as pluripotential, each equipped with a diversity of "side chain groups" exposed to the environment of the cell surface (Fig. 1.3). Antigens, on introduction into the organism, were then viewed as interacting in a complementary way with one or more side chain constituents, resulting in the release of that side chain(s) in complex with antigen from the immunocyte cell surface. This release triggered the synthesis of more of that side chain group in the corresponding cell. This construct constituted the first *selective theory* of antibody diversity suggesting that the role of antigen was to select a complimentary antibody and amplify that antibody with a selective immune response. The ability of an antibody to discriminate between the homologous antigen and other substances results from the complementary nature of the two reacting surfaces. In Ehrlich's words "the groups . . . must be adapted to one another e.g., . . . as lock and key," echoing precisely Emil Fisher's earlier sentiment regarding enzymes (Ehrlich, 1906). Implicit in the concept of preformation of antibodies in Ehrlich's theory is an assumption of the origin of antibody diversity. The problem of antibody diversity reduces to the question of where and how in the antibody lineage antibody diversity is actually introduced. The germline hypothesis supposes that it arises in the germline and that it is propagated or discarded by natural selection in proportion to the extent that the germline gene contributes to the overall fitness of the individual. It would follow then that the genetic information for the entire range of antibody specificities that an individual can produce is encoded in the DNA of its zygote, and that diverse structural genes for different antibodies are present in the genome. Thus, since Ehrlich proposed that the antibody repertoire is predetermined, it is to the germline hypothesis of antibody diversity to which Ehrlich's theory implicitly subscribed, spawning the first of the two major camps into which the controversy of the origin of antibody diversity divided.

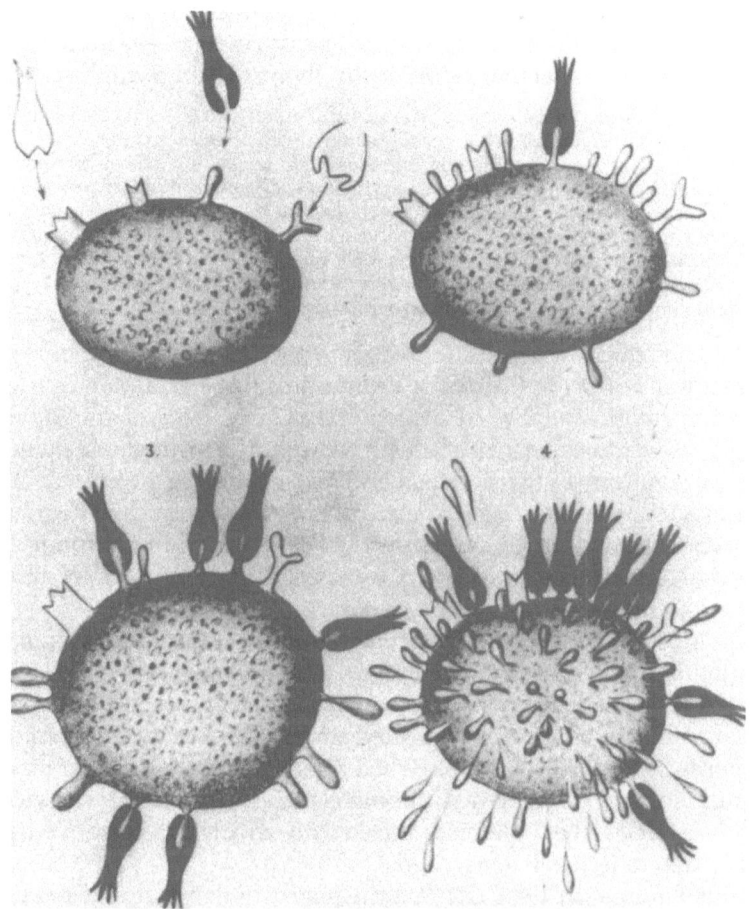

Figure 1.3. Diagrammatic representation of Ehrlich's "side-chain" theory. Taken from his Croonian lecture of 1906. The antigen (black) combined with its corresponding "side-chain" or receptor, resulting in the excess regeneration of the specific receptor.

1.3.2. Introduction of the Somatic Concept of Immunologic Specificity

Elements of Ehrlich's model fell from favor in the 1920s and 1930s as this period brought with it an expansion and characterization of the notion of immune specificity, particularly through the work of Landsteiner (1947) which demonstrated that the immune system had an exquisite specificity and a near global range of responses. Haurowitz in 1930 countered the selective theory by applying the following reasoning:

> The unlikelihood of any direct action of the antigen in the organism led Ehrlich to the conclusion that small quantities of antibodies are preformed in the organism and that the injection of antigen merely increases the level of normal antibody synthesis. . . . this hypothesis could be satisfactory as long as only a few natural antigens were known. Since the work of Landsteiner and his co-workers, however, an almost unlimited number of artificial antigens . . . can be produced which have never appeared in nature. It is unimaginable that an animal routinely produces predetermined antibodies against thousands of such synthetic substances.

Rather, it seemed more reasonable to the theorists of the time that antigen must *instruct* the immune system in some fashion and provide its own information for the construction and synthesis of antibody molecules. These features highlight the essence of the instructionist theories. This must further be regarded as a singular development in theoretical immunology as it encouraged speculation about alternative theories of diversity predicated on the apparent limitlessness of the immune repertoire. This construct sought to circumvent the traditional line of natural selection operating on germline genes.

This primordial age of ideas fomented the second major camp in the antibody diversity issue, collectively constituting the *somatic hypothesis* that proposed that antibody diversity arises separately in each individual. Albeit in continually updated forms, the somatic and germline hypotheses of the 1930s have survived major explosions of information in immunology, particularly at the molecular level, and have endured to the present as the polemic scaffolds on which the controversy of antibody diversity has been waged.

Linus Pauling, in 1940, defined the instructionalists' interpretations in molecular terms by proposing that antigens served as a template that permitted the antibody polypeptide chain to fold around it in a complementary fashion and thus mold itself into a specificity for that antigen. By this interpretation, antibody diversity arises by the variety of three-dimensional configurations that these molecules could assume under the influence of antigens. This theory had immediate difficulty with certain known properties of the immune response such as immunologic memory, and it required the persistence of antigen in the cell for very long periods of time. Leaping ahead from this historical juncture and using contemporary hindsight, the template theory can be discounted as untenable. We know that antibodies, like other proteins, are synthesized from amino acids using mRNA, not antigen, as the template.

Studies by Anfinsen and others in the early 1960s indicated that the primary amino acid sequence of proteins determines their three-dimensional configuration, rendering any instructionalist theory at the level of the polypeptide chain unlikely. Haber and then Tanford in the mid 1960s vitiated the remnants of the theory by extending the concept directly to antibodies. They chemically unfolded antibodies of known specificity in certain denaturing solvents and cleaved the disulfide linkages to remove all possible structural information except that of the primary amino acid sequence, then renatured the molecules in physiological medium in the absence of antigen to find restoration of the original antigen-binding specificity. This result has been reconfirmed several times and the concept has been amply reinforced by amino acid sequence studies of immunoglobulins.

1.4. CLONAL SELECTION

A theory to replace antigen template models was present long before template theories proved to be inadequate. The first form of a modern selectionist theory of antibody diversity was probably Jerne's, who in 1955 postulated the presence of antibodies of all potential specificities in the serum of each individual. Antigen, when introduced, complexed with its complementary antibody and this complex was subsequently recognized by an immunocyte, which by an unknown mechanism, stimulated the synthesis of that antibody (Fig. 1.4). The seminal elements of this theory were soon expanded into the prototype modern selection theory by Burnet (1957) and by Talmage (1957) as the *clonal selection*

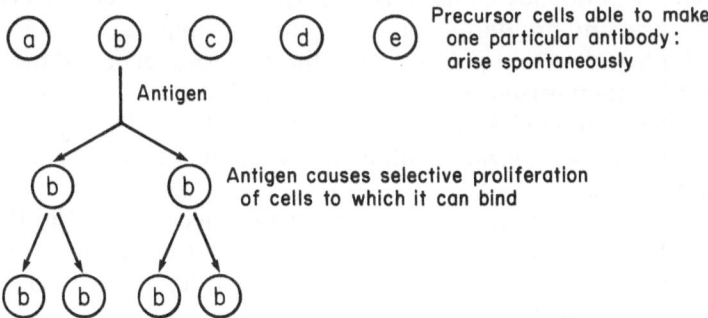

Figure 1.4. A simplified version of clonal selection by antigen.

hypothesis that has so permeated the field that it is difficult to think of immunology outside of its framework.

The power of the clonal selection theory emanates from its clear, economical, and uncontrived explanation of the major problems of the immune system: the specificity of antibody production, the secondary response, and tolerance to self-antigens. The basic premise of the theory borrows from bacterial genetics. Both bacterial variation that results from random mutation and by analogy antibody diversity are preadaptive; that is, the capability to respond to an environmental agent is present before that agent is introduced. Burnet (1957) proposed that antibody structural genes accumulate random somatic mutations in the course of cell proliferation during the development of the immune apparatus. Each antibody variant (a modern phrasing would be V-region variant) thus arises in a single cell and is carried indefinitely in the progeny of that cell or clone of cells. Although somatic mutation was the assumed origin of antibody diversity, it is not a necessary element of the clonal selection theory. Those clones committed to the production of antibody variants reactive with self-antigens are purged, at or shortly after birth, thus eliminating inappropriate clones and explaining self-tolerance. Exogenous antigen on the other hand would influence cells with an antibody reactive to it in a positive fashion resulting in stimulation, proliferation, and production of that antibody. This accounts for the specificity of antibody produced on immunization. The accelerated and enhanced antibody response that is produced in a memory response results from a prior contact with antigen and expansion of these specific cell clones in the history of the individual's immune system. These, in turn, should respond in greater force and numbers on secondary challenge. At least three major postulates are implicit in this theory of heritable cellular commitment: (1) the antigen receptor site, presumably on the cell surface, and the antibody combining site whose synthesis that cell controls are identical and are derived at least partially from the same structural gene; (2) the condition guaranteeing the correspondence of the immunoglobulin synthesized with the antigen is that they are limited to the same cell, i.e., the cell is specialized for the synthesis of a *single* antibody; and (3) the cell specialization stipulated in number two is inherited and, therefore, clonal.

Sporatic refutations of these postulates have occurred in the literature but the great bulk of evidence is supportive of the clonal selection theory. The theory's sheer eloquence, however, has probably been most responsible for its dominant role in immunologic thought and its acceptance as dogma since the early 1960s.

1.5. EFFECTOR FUNCTIONS

Binding antigen is not the sole function of the antibody molecule. Subsequent to binding, an effector action generally takes place that rids the organism of the invader. It is important to appreciate that immunoglobulins are polyfunctional molecules. The most thoroughly studied and currently best understood of the numerous functions of this protein family is antigen binding, the subject of this volume. However, various other functions are collectively referred to as the "biological properties" or "effector functions" of antibodies. These properties are mediated by the constant regions of the heavy chains of the various immunoglobulin molecules. In fact, most of the properties recognized at present have been associated with that carboxyterminal subcomponent of the heavy chain constant region referred to as the Fc segment or fragment.

A considerable number of biological properties of immunoglobulins have been recognized and studied to varying degrees up to the present. Such properties are listed in Table 1.1. There is every reason to believe that future research may uncover additional presently unappreciated properties that have definite physiologic significance. In addition, it seems likely on the basis of contemporary analyses of previous evolutionary trends that future evolutionary developments such as the appearance of additional subclasses of immunoglobulins through heavy chain C-region gene duplication and divergence will be due at least in part to favorable selection pressures for still other immunoglobulin bi-

Table 1.1. Currently Known Biological Properties (Effector Functions) of Immunoglobulin Molecules

Antigen-dependent properties
    Complement fixation (classical pathway)
    Complement fixation (alternative pathway)
    Opsonic activity (neutrophils and monocytes)
Antigen-independent properties
    Attachment to mast cells and basophils
    Macrophage-binding
    Lymphocyte-binding
    Placental-passage regulation
    Intestinal-passage regulation
    Immunoglobulin-metabolism regulation
    Passive cutaneous anaphylaxis (PCA)
    Interaction with protein A of *Staphylococcus aureus*
    Antigenic target for rheumatoid factor

ological properties, the exact nature of which we can perceive only dimly at present.

In a general sense the biologic properties of immunoglobulins play two major functional roles. They come into play after the antibody has bound antigen, and serve to amplify or extend the physiologic consequence of antigen binding. A prototypic function of this sort is complement fixation by the classical pathway. Alternatively, the ability of an antibody to carry out a biologic function might assure that the molecule is available in a particular site to provide for a subsequent encounter with some antigen with which its variable region is able to interact. Examples of this type of property would be regulated passage across a membrane such as the placenta, or the specific attachment to a cell that is likely to encounter antigen, such as a macrophage or mast cell. Certain other biological properties such as the interaction of antigenic determinants in the Fc segment with rheumatoid factors may simply represent pathologic or even incidental consequences of certain structural attributes of the heavy chain C region.

Given the multiplicity of biologic properties characteristic of the immunoglobulin family, it is not always clear exactly what teleological significance any particular function has in a given situation. Certainly the Fc fragment is subjected to a wide variety of distinct selection pressures that are doubtless mutually contradictory on some occasions. For example, a protein structure ideal for complement fixation may be quite inappropriate for the mediation of the passage of this very molecule across a placental membrane. A unique pressure on the Fc region of many immunoglobulins is thus to provide for the *simultaneous* presence of a number of functional capabilities that may be required on different occasions. All attempts to relate structure to function for this region of the antibody molecule must take this into account. It seems clear that this kind of selection pressure has been an important element in the appearance of the numerous classes and subclasses of immunoglobulins that have been observed to date among the various species.

1.6. THE EXTENT OF DIVERSITY—THE PROBLEM IN A NUTSHELL

It has been known for many years that the most striking feature about an immune serum is the specific nature of its interaction with antigen. For example, an immune serum can distinguish between two proteins having as little as a single amino acid difference between them.

It can also discriminate between two chemical compounds differing in a single functional group, between D and L amino acids, and between many other closely related compounds. The principles of immunological specificity were formulated by Landsteiner and the concept has been one of the hallmarks of immunological thinking for 50 years.

Determinations of the extent of diversity have been approached both experimentally and theoretically by a number of investigators. One of the most widely quoted studies is that of Kreth and Williamson, who in 1973 investigated the antihapten immune potential of individual mice immunized with carriers to which the hapten o-nitro-p-iodophenyl (NIP) had been conjugated. They developed a clone dilution transfer technique by which they were able to transfer single clones of cells producing antibodies to NIP to irradiated mice. The individual NIP-binding immunoglobulins produced by these clones could then be identified by the pattern they exhibited after resolution by isoelectric focusing (IEF). The reasoning was that if one counted the total number of clones transferred and then identified from the IEF pattern how many identical or "repeating" clones were in that number, it would be possible to infer from statistical considerations how many different anti-NIP clones a single mouse could produce. After considerable analysis, a repeat of only five clones out of 234 transferred was found. From this, it was calculated that there may exist between 8000 and 15,000 individual clones in a mouse capable of forming antibodies to this hapten.

If the simple hapten, NIP, can elicit in the neighborhood of 10,000 different antibody molecules, then the repertoire must be astronomical. Investigators over the years have quoted the often stated notion that a vertebrate immune response represents well over 10 million different specificities; that is, 10 million different antibody molecules. It is extremely difficult to pinpoint the place and time at which this 10 million number of specificities emerged into immunological thinking. It can be found in the writings of the 1940s and 1950s, and by the 1960s and 1970s it became part of the collective wisdom of the discipline. Early on, it was appreciated that a repertoire of 10 million antibody genes was likely an impossibility in a strict germline sense. Since by the early 1960s it was appreciated that both chains were needed for antigen binding, there emerged the so-called $p \times q$ hypothesis that assumed that every light chain could combine with every heavy chain in a relatively random manner. It is important to appreciate that the hypothesis did not specify that antigen selection would not deviate the immune response such that the majority of molecules might not show a random distribution of heavy and light chains, but only that every combination was possible. Thus, the $p \times q$ hypothesis allowed, for example, 3000 heavy chains to combine with 3000 light chains to provide the appropriate 3000 × 3000 or 10,000,000 specificities requiring but 6000 genes.

Thus, the problem in a nutshell reduces to "How can 10 million antibodies arise in a single organism?"

1.7. SCOPE OF THE BOOK

This book will deal primarily with the antibody molecule and the genetic basis for its diversity. The several approaches to the problem of antibody diversity will be discussed and the respective contributions of each approach will be noted. Because this volume is about antibody diversity, certain other topics relevant to antibodies will not be discussed. Despite its direct relationship to the antibody molecule, the complement system will not be covered. The self/non-self problem will not be further considered because by its very definition this nonreactivity cannot be genetically encoded. We will also not deal further with questions concerning the cellular nature of antibody synthesis. Rather, it is the question of antibody diversity—the accounting of the myriad of specificities—that this volume will address.

1.8. PRECIS

The basic theory of evolution, all life from pre-existing life, has as its molecular counterpart, all DNA from pre-existing DNA. It is then a direct logical consequence that biological information has descended from a small amount of ancestral information and is related to it by a multiplicity of ordered divergences, each of which in essence represents the replication of a DNA molecule. These ordered divergencies are what allow the progression of alteration in DNA information to be represented as a genealogical tree. The diversity of this information arises as small discrete steps (mutations), each of which occurs in a single molecule. The endless proliferation of information is offset by the constant attrition of information contained in organisms not selected for reproduction.

In multicellular organisms, the overwhelming preponderance of the organism is invested in somatic cells, and consequently, most of the divergences in an organism arise during cell division during the life of the individual organism. These divergences or mutations are called *somatic* and are only transmitted to some of the cells of the individual in which they arise. Additionally, any further manipulation superimposed on the pre-existing DNA or its products, whether they occur before, during, or after transcriptional events, is also designated somatic. A few of the divergences occur in the germ cells. All of the variations accumulated therein are referred to as *germline*. Mutations occurring in the germline can be inherited by the descendants of the individuals in which they occur. It is between the concepts encompassed by the terms *somatic* and *germline* that immunological thought has traditionally meandered. The central question of antibody diversity has largely been the relative contributions of each of these concepts to the antibody problem: How do the specificities arise? The next two chapters will detail the problem as approached by the serologist and the biochemist.

REFERENCES AND BIBLIOGRAPHY

Bellanti, J. A., 1979, *Immunology: Basic Processes*, W. B. Saunders, New York, p. 27.

Breinl, F., and Haurowitz, F., 1930, Chemische Untersuchung des Precipitates aus Hämoglobin und Anti-hämoglobulin-serum und Bemerkungen über die Natur der Antikorper, *Z. Phys. Chem.* **192**:45.

Burnet, F. M., 1957, A modification of Jerne's theory of antibody production using the concept of clonal selection, *Aust. J. Sci.* **20**:67.

Burnet, F. M., 1959, *The Clonal Selection Theory of Acquired Immunity*, Cambridge University Press, Cambridge.

Edelman, G. M., and Gally, J. A., 1964, A model for the 7S antibody molecule, *Proc. Natl. Acad. Sci. U.S.A.* **51**:846.

Ehrlich, P., 1906, On immunity with special reference to cell life, *Proc. R. Soc. Lond. (Biol.)* **66**:424.

Haber, E., 1964, Recovery of antigenic specificity after denaturation and complete reduction of disulfides in a papain fragment of antibody, *Proc. Natl. Acad. Sci. U.S.A.* **52**:1099.

Jerne, N. K., 1955, The natural selection theory of antibody formation, *Proc. Natl. Acad. Sci. U.S.A.* **41**:849.

Kreth, H. W., and Williamson, A. R., 1973, The extent of diversity of anti-hapten antibodies in inbred mice, *Eur. J. Immunol.* **3**:141.

Landsteiner, K., 1947, *The Specificity of Serological Reactions*, Harvard University Press, Cambridge, Massachusetts.

Pauling, L., 1940, A theory of the structure and process of the formation of antibody, *J. Am. Chem. Soc.* **62**:2643.

Talmage, D., 1957, Allergy and immunology, *Ann. Rev. Med.* **8**:239.

Von Behring, E. A., and Kitasato, S., 1890, Uber das zustandekommen der diphterieimunitat bei thierek, *Dtsch. Med. Wochenshr.* **16**:1113.

2

THE SEROLOGIST'S APPROACH TO THE PROBLEM

To every thing there is a season and a time for every purpose under heaven. . . .

—ECCLESIASTES 3:1

2.1. INTRODUCTION

The problem of antibody diversity was of great concern to immunologists, and therefore it was appropriate that they study this problem with the serologic methods with which they were familiar. In retrospect, this was a fortuitous circumstance that allowed a rapid initial burst of information on this subject. At the time these serologic studies were begun, techniques for protein structure determination were not sufficiently developed to handle large complex molecules, nor were there available procedures for protein isolation suitable for the mixtures of molecules contained in most antibody populations. Indeed, the concept that a single molecule might have multiple, disulfide-linked subunits was years away. Even more remote was the idea of directly studying the genes encoding antibodies. Serology, on the other hand, was highly developed by the early 1950s. The fact that antibodies with exquisite specificity could be produced by immunization was fully appreciated. An impressive list of scientific pioneers including Pasteur, Koch, Von Behring, Erhlich, and Landsteiner had already contributed to this area.

As mentioned in Chapter 1, synthetic chemicals as well as naturally occurring substances could be fully discriminated by appropriate antibodies. Antibodies could distinguish galactose from glucose and even the alpha and beta anomers of either sugar. What then, was to stop immunologists from using these highly discriminatory techniques to study the complexity of the antibody universe? First of all, there was the pervasive notion that the corresponding proteins of individuals within a species were identical. Although variations in the blood group antigens in various species had been found, it was known that these were carbohydrate and not protein in nature. Allograft rejection had been investigated, but the nature of the reacting antigen was not clear. Furthermore, there was a tendency among physical scientists to consider serologic data inferior. The biochemists' attitude toward serology could be summarized by the comments of a famous molecular immunologist discussing idiotypy in a lecture given around 1970: "That's the classic immunologist's dream, an unbroken circle of immunization with antibodies and immunization with antibodies against these antibodies and so on." Although this comment represents an extreme opinion of serology, the use of immunologic techniques to provide solutions to the problem of antibody diversity did not enjoy high regard in most scientific circles. Even today, the fact that many of the obvious questions concerning antibody genes were formulated and refined using serologic techniques is not generally appreciated.

The year 1955 marked the serologist's initial serious confrontation with the problem of antibody diversity. Studies on the antigenicity of immunoglobulins began at about the same time in three different countries, and in each case the approach used was different. This simultaneous realization that antibodies could be differentiated by other antibodies was an indication that the time for this idea had come. In Paris, Oudin (1956a) immunized rabbits with other rabbit antibodies and assessed the specificity of the anti-antibodies formed; in Lund (Sweden), Grubb (1956) studied the specificity of human rheumatoid factors; and in New York, Kunkel (Slater et al., 1955) investigated the antigenicity of myeloma proteins. From these three separate endeavors would spring information and ideas that paved the way to our eventual understanding that antibodies were encoded by genes that have unique features.

2.2. RABBIT ALLOTYPES

2.2.1. Discovery

The 1956 paper by Oudin in *Compte Rendu* entitled "Réaction de précipitation spécifique entre des sérums d'animaux de même espèce" (specific precipitation reactions among sera from animals of the same species) (Oudin, 1956a) and those that followed shortly thereafter gave to the immunology literature a new word and a new set of experimental procedures. The word allotypy is from the Greek and means "other types or forms."

In a systematic and irrefutable manner, Oudin demonstrated that antibody populations carry specific antigens that may be present or absent in the serum of individuals of the same species. The inheritance patterns of these intraspecies antigens present on antibodies suggested that antibodies were genetically determined. It was assumed that the antigenic differences reflected primary structural differences in the antibodies themselves that in turn reflected differences in the genes that encoded them. Accordingly, the genetic determinism of the antigens rather than the antigenicity itself was the major feature of interest. A quote taken from the introduction to a paper given by Oudin in 1966, ten years after his initial report on allotypy, reveals his deep understanding of the relevance of his findings:

> Every notion concerning the primary structure of the immunoglobulin is in some way related to their genetic determinism, the same is true for their antibody function and specificity, not only because of the role assigned by theories to genetic mechanisms involved in antibody formation but also because of the structural differences between antibodies and because of a hereditary factor in the ability of animals to make antibodies against one given antigen. Since the most convenient approach to the genetics of immunoglobulins is based on their antigenic specificity and since differences in antigenic specificity may, as a working hypothesis which is in agreement with many facts, be considered to reflect differences in the primary structure of immunoglobulins the scope of this paper will be limited to the genetic data related to antigenic specificity.

Before going on to extensions of Oudin's original findings, it may be useful to outline the experimental approach that led to his discovery. The system used by Oudin for the detection of allotypes involved preparation of a specific antibody, for example antiovalbumin, in a rabbit. Serum was taken from this rabbit (rabbit 1) and ovalbumin was added to the serum to the point of optimal precipitation (equivalence). The precipitate was then injected into a second rabbit. After several injections, the serum from rabbit 2 formed a precipitin line in agar gels with serum taken from rabbit 1. Surprisingly, the reaction also took place with serum samples taken from rabbit 1 even before immunization with ovalbumin. In addition, rabbit 2 serum would react not only with serum from rabbit 1, but also with serum samples from some, but not all, other rabbits. This observation indicated that differences in antibody populations could be detected antigenically and further that these differences did not relate solely to a specific (antiovalbumin) antibody. The presence of a given allotype in some but not all rabbits indicated that allotypes and therefore antibodies were under genetic control.

Because Oudin was a master of the technique of immunodiffusion, he was able to obtain quantitative information by application of these techniques to the allotypes (Fig. 2.1). Data concerning the serum concentration of individual allotypes helped him to develop the concept of heterozygosity of certain allotypes. By 1960, Oudin had developed the concept of allotypy to a point where a number of important conclusions

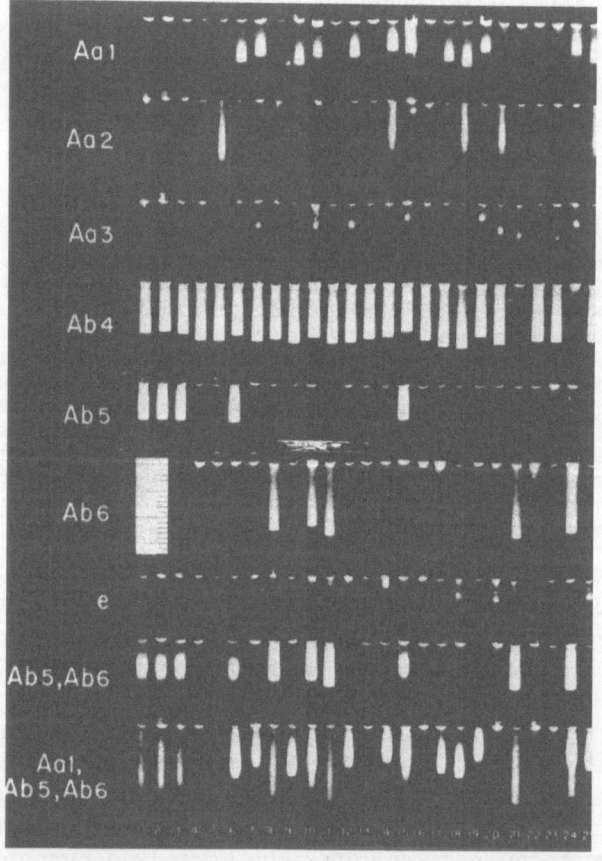

Figure 2.1. The single diffusion method was used by Oudin to determine rabbit allotypes. Each row contains a different antiallotype serum in a soft agar gel. The specificity against which the antiserum is directed is noted in the column to the left. The columns contain 25 different rabbit sera; a sample of each of these is added to the 9 antisera. The typing results are read directly by observation of precipitation in the various tubes. For example, serum sample 1 has allotypes a3/b4, b5 and serum 25 has allotypes a1,a2/b4. Note that the symbol A is usually omitted in writing the allotypes of the rabbit and may be used to separate unlinked allotypes. From Oudin (1966).

concerning the allotype genes could be easily drawn: (1) there were two independent groups of allotypes with three alleles in each group; and (2) any individual rabbit might have one or two but not three allotypes from either group. Extensive breeding experiments by Dubiski (1962) showed that the two allotype groups (a and b) were neither linked to one another nor to the X chromosome. The description of heavy and light chains by Porter and his colleagues (Fleischman *et al.*, 1962) led Stemke (1964) to demonstrate by immunochemical means that the group a allotypes were on the heavy chains and the group b allotypes were on light chains. These results along with similar studies of human allotypes indicated that the two chains of immunoglobulins were encoded at unlinked genetic loci.

The novelty of the finding that an antibody molecule was encoded by (at least) two unlinked loci was minor compared with the revolutionary nature of other findings for these proteins. The reports of Todd and of Feinstein in 1963 describing the presence of heavy chain allotypes (group a) on several different heavy chain classes (isotypes) of immunoglobulins challenged a basic genetic dogma: the one gene–one polypeptide chain theory. The observations of Todd and Feinstein would soon be followed by those of Pernis *et al.* (1965) and Weiler (1965) that a single antibody-producing cell from a heterozygous individual would produce only one of the two allelic products. Except for products of the X chromosome, both allelic proteins are always synthesized by a diploid cell. The impact of these discoveries along with independent data from other serologic and structural sources would provide fuel for the notion that antibody biosynthesis involved mechanisms that had not yet been considered. (A more extensive discussion of the two gene–one polypeptide chain hypothesis and the concept of allelic exclusion is given in Chapter 4.)

2.2.2. Variable-Region Allotypes

Although immunoglobulin allotypes have been described for a number of species, the majority of allotype studies have used markers of the human, the rabbit, and the mouse. Each of these allotypic systems has distinct advantages and disadvantages, and important contributions to our understanding of immunoglobulin genes have come from each. Although there were no inbred or congenic rabbit strains (as there were in mice) and although there were not myeloma proteins representing all classes of immunoglobulin (as in the human and the mouse), the rabbit allotype system had the advantage of multiple allotypes on the immunoglobulin molecule (Fig. 2.2). Included among these allotypes was a unique and valuable feature of the rabbit system, a variable (V) region allotype for the heavy chain.

The group a allotypes of the rabbit deserve special mention in their role as the first experimental system with the potential to yield data bearing directly on the question of antibody diversity. The constant (C)-region allotypes, although extremely useful, do not directly address the question that is most relevant to antibody diversity: how many V regions are encoded in an individual's genome? The group a allotypes of the rabbit provided a genetic marker located in the center of the controversy: the V region. There are a number of implications of an allelic marker in the V region. For example, if a group of V regions all bear the same marker, then they must be identical to the extent required by this shared marker but must be sufficiently different from one another to account for their different antigenic specificities. If all the information for the

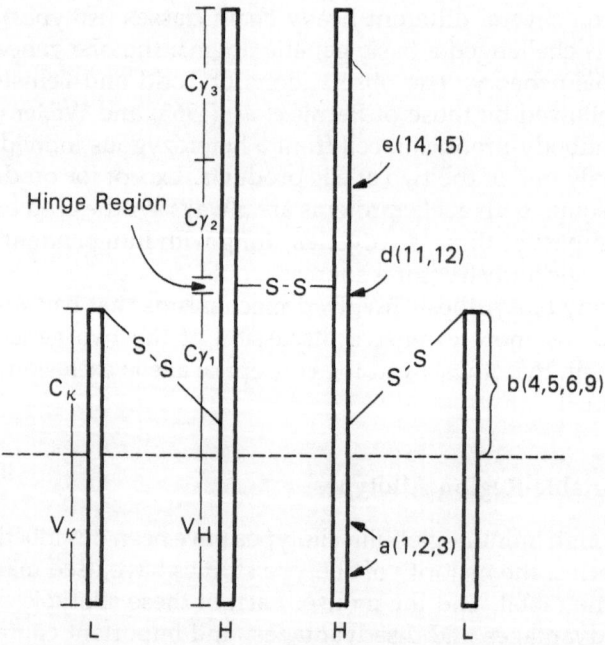

Figure 2.2. A schematic of rabbit IgG showing the locations on the molecule of the major allotypic groups. The numbers in parentheses indicate the major alleles for each group. A number of additional alleles for the group b allotypes have recently been described. The IgG molecules may have lambda rather than kappa chains; these express the group c allotypes (c7, c21). The V_H region may express allotypes of the x or y groups rather than the a group. Allotypes of the c, x, and y groups occur in relatively low concentrations in normal rabbit serum samples.

synthesis of antibody V regions is encoded in the germline, then the group a allotypes differentiate inherited sets or groups of V-region genes. The germline theory, however, could not easily explain how the mutations giving rise to the allotypically distinct sets could be spread over every member in each set. As will be discussed in subsequent chapters, a more reasonable explanation for rabbit V-region allotypes may be developed in the context of somatic theories in which relatively few genes are encoded in the germline with diversification in the soma to generate the antigen-binding information.

Rabbit V-region allotypes were an embarrassment to germline theories, and accordingly proponents of this theory did not initially accept the fact that the rabbit group a allotypes were truly markers for V regions. Consequently, the localization of these allotypes to the V region of the heavy chain was long a subject of controversy. (Structural evidence for their V-region location will be presented in later chapters.) It would be alleged that the true determinants of the allotypes were not in the V region but in the C region; however, even this maneuver did not totally solve the problem because group a allotypes were present on heavy chains of different classes each of which must somehow mutate to the appropriate allotype.

If one allowed that each member of a large set of V genes carried the same allotype marker (ignoring for the moment the question of how the mutation spread over the entire set), one faced the problem of maintenance of the genetic purity of the multigenic system. Unless some mechanism to suppress cross-over were operative, the allelic sets of V-region genes would soon become indistinguishable because of multiple cross-overs among the many different members (Fig. 2.3). The clear-cut patterns of Mendelian inheritance observed for the group a allotypes in laboratories all over the world argued strongly against the possibility that the V genes were being scrambled.

The nature and significance of the group a allotypes of the rabbit remained a point of controversy for a number of years. The problem was not lessened by structural information showing amino acid correlates for the a allotypes in framework residues of the heavy chain V region.

2.2.2.1. Allelic Selection of Allotypes

Relevant to the issue of allotypes as V-region markers was the experimental emphasis on quantitative analyses of immunoglobulin and antibody populations in order to determine what percentage of molecules carried a given marker. These studies indicated first that the majority of molecules in a sample of rabbit immunoglobulin carried group

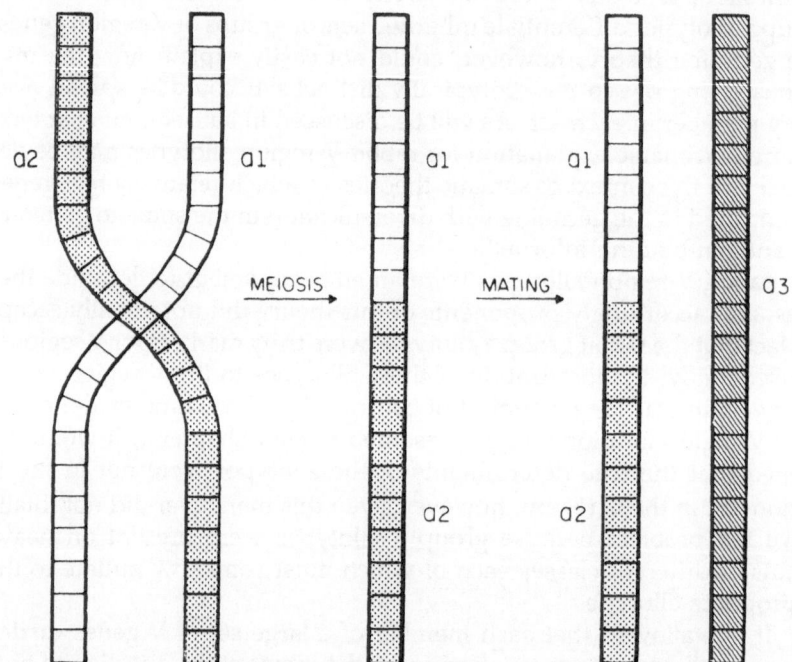

Figure 2.3. The problem of maintaining genetic purity in a polygenic system is depicted. The squares represent V_H region genes, each expressing a given group a allotype. Unless recombination is suppressed, the inheritance of group a allotypes could not be maintained in the simple Mendelian fashion that has been observed. From Todd (1972).

a markers. The population lacking the a allotypes was always less than 10% no matter what group a allotypes were present in homozygous or heterozygous rabbits. In extensions of these studies, rabbits were immunized using various protocols, specific antibodies were isolated, and their allotypes were quantified. In most of the early studies the ratio of allotypes in the antibody reflected those seen for the preimmune immunoglobulin sample. It was not possible to assign a specific antigen-binding function exclusively to antibodies bearing one allotype or to exclude this function from those bearing another. The antibody repertoire therefore appeared to contain binding sites reiterated for each of the V-region allotypes. These findings suggested that binding site information was contained in multiple copies in the genome.

Krause (1970) showed that certain antigens, such as streptococcal vaccines, could induce antibody responses of limited heterogeneity in the rabbit, some of which showed allotype exclusion. Antibodies from heterozygous rabbits giving high, homogeneous response to streptococcal vaccines often excluded allotypes but in a random rather than a predictable fashion. In some instances, the homogeneous antibody represented the group a allotype negative population that was a minor component of the normal preimmune IgG. Studies of such antistreptococcal antibodies indicated that this minor population contained information encoding functionally active antibodies; this finding argued for further duplication of V-region binding site information.

2.2.2.2. Subspecificities of Allotypes

Assays that measured binding to antiallotype antibodies were unable to differentiate the group a allotypes present on the homogeneous antibodies from the allotypes of normal IgG samples. However, when inhibition of binding reactions were used to compare the markers, a significant degree of heterogeneity was observed. For example, a group of allotype a3 positive homogeneous antibodies gave a spectrum of different patterns of inhibition of the binding between a pooled a3 IgG sample and anti-a3. This property of allotype subspecificities indicated that a given allotype comprised a spectrum of very similar but not identical structures. These sets, however, were sufficiently different one from another to preclude any significant confusion in the serologic determination of the a1, a2, and a3 specificities.

2.2.2.3. Allotype Suppression

Another type of experiment was used to explore the extent of the allotype repertoire. Antiallotype sera were used to suppress the in vivo synthesis of certain allotypes. Initial experiments by Dray (1962) were directed at suppression of paternal allotypes in neonates. The pups could be safely injected with antiallotype sera before they expressed detectable serum levels of the paternal allotype (Fig. 2.4). The alternative allele compensated for the suppressed allotype and the immunoglobulin in the animal bore a single allotype, just as if the animal were homozygous for that marker.

A somewhat more complex variation of this experiment aimed at suppression of allotypes in homozygous rabbits. An 8- to 16-cell embryo from the mating of allotype-matched homozygous rabbits was transferred to a pseudopregnant doe that had been previously immunized to make antiallotype antibodies directed against the group a allotype of

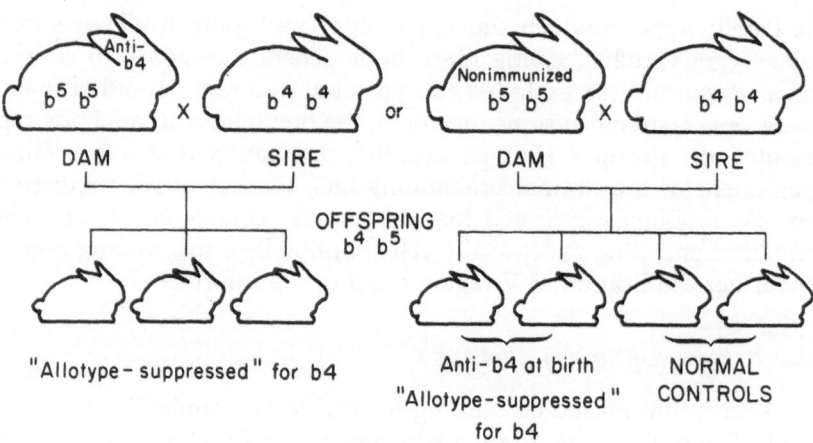

Figure 2.4. Heterozygous allotype suppression of the kappa chain allotype b4 by two different experimental approaches. The mother may produce antibody to the paternal type or the newborn rabbit may be injected at birth with antibody. From Mage (1967).

the implant. Although the offspring obtained in these experiments had normal levels of immunoglobulin, their sera contained none of the known group a allotypes. Therefore, an alternative set of V-region genes, presumably maintained in coupling with the group a allotype genes, contained at least enough genetic information to synthesize the antibodies to prevent these young rabbits from wasting and dying as would be expected if they were immunoglobulin deficient.

When homozygous allotype suppression experiments involved the group b allotypes of the kappa light chain C region, the offspring produced no kappa chains. Even though lambda chains made up only a few percent of the IgG molecules under usual conditions, these suppression experiments yielded animals that derived their entire antibody repertoire using molecules having *only* lambda chains.

The extent of the antibody repertoire was tested by the allotype suppression experiments. An obvious conclusion was that only a small segment of the total information carried was necessary for survival and protection (of the domestic animals under study). For example, the heavy chain V regions lacking group a allotypes (group a negative) that make up less than 10% of the total antibody population under normal conditions contain sufficient capacity for antigen binding appeared to serve the needs of the organism. Similarly, lambda chains that normally are associated with between 4% and 20% of the immunoglobulin molecules can carry the entire immune burden of the light chains if necessary.

2.3. HUMAN ALLOTYPES

2.3.1. Discovery

At about the same time that the allotypes of the rabbit were yielding data concerning antibody genes, the immunoglobulin allotypes of the human were undergoing similar investigations. The first mention of these markers was in a 1956 report by Grubb and Laurell. There were some significant differences between the reagents and techniques used for allotype detection in the human compared with the rabbit. The antisera used to detect human allotypes were not obtained from planned intraspecies immunizations as in the rabbit, but were sera from patients with rheumatoid arthritis; these sera were known to contain activities that would react with gamma globulins (rheumatoid factors). Sera were also obtained from patients with other diseases and from normal persons who were immunized as a result of pregnancy or multiple blood transfusions. Grubb's original observation was that rheumatoid factors had the ability to specifically agglutinate red blood cells coated with anti-Rh antibodies. The agglutinating systems could be inhibited by some human sera but not by others, and the inhibitory principle was found to be gamma globulin. The specificities were shown to be genetically transmitted.

An additional significant difference between the human and rabbit experimental systems involved the availability of myeloma proteins for the human. In addition to their irreplaceable value in the determination of structure (see Chapter 3), myeloma proteins would serve a critical role in answering certain questions involved in allotypy.

Because a large number of myeloma proteins were collected and studied, structural correlates and the locations of the determinants of human allotypes were quickly obtained. These allotypes were localized to specific domains of the heavy chain of the human immunoglobulin molecule. These allotypes have been described for IgG1, IgG2, IgG3, IgG4, and one of the two IgA subclasses. Table 2.1 lists some of the human allotypes and gives their location on the immunoglobulin molecules.

The nomenclature used for human allotypes is not uniform and this may cause some confusion. Early studies used a variety of symbols, and attempts have been made to give numbered designations to all of the allotypes. For example, the allotype Gm (a) is now called Gm (1). In order to designate which subclass is involved in the allotype, some authors will write these as G3m (16) and G1m (17) indicating that the 16

Table 2.1. Designations of Selected Human
Allotypes That Are Found on Only One Heavy
Chain Subclass or Light Chain Type

Nomenclature		Heavy chain
Current	Original	subclass
Gm antigens		
1	a	G1
2	x	G1
4	f	G1
17	z	G1
10	ba	G3
11	bo	G3
14	b4	G3
21	g	G3
23	n	G2
Am antigens		
1	1 or +	A2
Km antigens		Light chain type
1	Inv 1	K
2	Inv a	K
3	Inv b	K

allotype is on the IgG3 subclass and the 17 allotype is on the IgG1
subclass, respectively. Unfortunately this uniform nomenclature is not
widely used.

2.3.2. Allotypes and Isotypes

The concept of isotypy and its relationship to allotypy was recognized by Oudin and this relationship was utilized in the experiments of
Todd (1963) and of Feinstein (1963) who showed that group a allotypes
were present on IgM and IgA, respectively, as well as on IgG. Refinement of the concept of isotypy, as well as a more complete enumeration
of subclasses, required the human myeloma proteins. Subclasses of human IgG were originally defined using precipitation techniques by Gray
and Kunkel and Terry and Fahey in 1964 (reviewed in Mage *et al.*, 1973).
IgG subclasses have been found for the mouse which has four (IgG1,
IgG2a, IgG2b, IgG3) but none have been observed in the rabbit.

It was found that the subclass distribution of the myeloma proteins
tested mimicked the distribution in IgG from normal adult humans. IgG1
is the most abundant and composes approximately 66% of IgG; this is

followed by IgG2 at 28%, IgG3 at 7%, and IgG4 at 4%. Allotype studies on the available myeloma proteins of known subclass allowed assignment of allotypes to specific subclasses rather than just to IgG. In addition, availability of large amounts of these proteins permitted sophisticated immunochemical investigations regarding the location of the specific interchanges involved in the allotypes. These studies indicated that Gm markers were present in the C region of the heavy chain.

2.3.2.1. Nonmarkers

In the ordinary allotype situation, there are two or more allelic markers, one or two of which are found in any individual, for example, Gm (3) and its allele Gm (17). An alternative situation has been described for the human in which one marker is readily detected for a protein of a given subclass in some individuals, whereas the antithetic marker cannot be detected by conventional isoimmunization procedures. An example of this is the Gm (1) marker of IgG1; the antithetic marker (or nonmarker) is called Gm non (1). This situation results from the presence of the nonmarker on all molecules of another subclass. That is to say, the determinant that is allelic to Gm (1) on IgG1 is present on the IgG2 and IgG3 molecules in every individual. Non (1) is then an isotype (see Section 2.5.2), and because it is present in all members of the species it is not antigenic in that species. This puzzle was solved using heterologous immunizations with myeloma proteins and subjecting these antisera to appropriate adsorption. The Gm (1) marker was subsequently related to a peptide in the Fc region of IgG1, and it was shown that the non (1) peptide was present not only in non (1) IgG1 but also in all IgG2 and IgG3 proteins. The presence of nonmarkers argues for a common evolutionary origin of the IgG subclasses.

2.3.3. Haplogroups

The discovery of multiple Gm markers for various IgG isotypes of the human along with the Am markers for the IgA proteins allowed the first linkage studies of immunoglobulin heavy chain genes. Although certain informative groups of markers, which retrospectively indicated recombination and cross-over events, were found in typing studies, it was generally concluded from these initial genetic analyses that the heavy chain allotype genes were so closely linked that they were inherited as a unit. These close linkages, called haplotypes, are more prevalent in some populations than in others, and can be used in studies on the migrations of populations and in other anthropologic enterprises.

The close linkage of markers led to the notion that there was a *gene complex* encoding antibodies. These complexes were not split by crossovers among the C-region genes except in rare instances.

2.3.3.1. Light Chain Allotypes in the Human

The Inv (now called Km) markers were first described in 1961 by Ropartz *et al.*, and were shown to be present on light chains of the kappa type. Originally two alleles were reported and later a third was described. These allelic forms of the kappa light chain in the human were later correlated with amino acid interchanges occurring at positions 191 and 154 in the C region. Using the Gm and Km markers in the human, independent assortment of heavy and light chains was demonstrated and, in fact, the description of these two unlinked loci for heavy and light chains in the human predates the observation for the nonlinkage of rabbit group a (heavy chain) and group b (light chain) allotypes.

Of equal importance to the allotype findings was the observation that yet another locus for light chains was present in the human, that encoding the so-called lambda light chains. Although structural studies were required to clearly define the difference between lambda and kappa light chains, it was apparent from serologic studies that there were two very different types of light chain in the human.

2.4. ALLOTYPES OF THE MOUSE AND THE RAT

2.4.1. Mouse Allotypes

Approximately five years after the reports of allotypy in the human and in the rabbit, Kelus and Moor-Jankowski (1961) described the first murine allotypes. Although subsequent experiments would detail allotypes for a number of other species, the majority of immunoglobulin gene studies relevant to our topic have used those of the human, rabbit, and mouse.

Allotypy in the mouse was demonstrated by immunizing C57BL mice with antibody from BALB/c mice coated onto *Proteus vulgaris*. These antisera reacted with a determinant that was present in the sera of all BALB/c and certain other mouse strains, but was not present in the serum of any C57BL mouse. Early studies of murine allotypes were complicated by the fact that there were multiple IgG subclasses carrying different determinants. Initially, there were no characterized myeloma proteins, as in the human, to allow study of each of these subclasses individually. This limitation was soon circumvented, however, by the work of Potter and Lieberman (1970), who induced the equivalent of myeloma proteins in BALB/c mice by the injection of mineral oil. The mouse is an excellent subject for genetic studies because there are inbred strains and because the generation time is relatively short. Therefore, the murine allotype system became extremely valuable, especially in studies involving the linkage of allotypes and binding-site markers.

An extremely important contribution to our knowledge of C-region allotype genes came from studies of murine allotypes in which crosses between inbred strains of mice differing from each other by two or more genes in the heavy chain group were carried out. These heroic studies involved testing 1054 progeny from one breeding experiment and 1317 progeny from another for possible cross-overs between the two known C-region allotypes. In none of 2371 progeny tested was any cross-over detected. This result, confirmed by other investigators, argues strongly that the C-region genes for immunoglobulins in the mouse are closely linked and for most practical purposes could be considered to be inherited as a single gene. However, the existence in wild mice populations of allotype combinations that did not correspond to the linkage groups normally observed in the inbred strains suggested that cross-overs can and do occur among these closely linked genes. The IgC_H allotypes of some commonly used mouse strains are listed in Table 2.2.

Because the heavy chain gene cluster is inherited as if it were a single gene, it has been possible to construct congenic mouse strains that contain the complete heavy chain allotypic complement of one strain and the background genes of another. For example, the BALB/c allotype that is designated with the letter *a*, may be introduced onto a C57BL/6 background. Because selection is always for progeny carrying the desired gene, it is possible by a series of back-crosses followed by intercrosses to replace the normal b allotype of C57BL/6 with the BALB/c type.

Allotypes have been described for the IgM, IgD, IgG1, IgG2a, IgG2b,

Table 2.2. Distribution of IgCH Haplotypes in Selected Mouse Strains[a]

IgCH[a]	IgCH[b]	IgCH[c]	IgCH[d]	IgCH[e]	IgCH[f]	IgCH[g]	IgCH[h]	IgCH[j]
BALB/c	C57BL	DBA/2	AKR	A/J	CE/J	RIII	BDP/J	CBA/J
C3H	BAB14	DBA/1	AL/N	A/He	NHN	BSVS	P/J	PL/J
C57L/J	B10.D2		CAL20	NZB		DA/JU		SEC
C58/J								

[a]Adapted from Lieberman (1978).

and IgA classes of the mouse; all are localized in the C region. Data to be described later will indicate that the C-region allotype genes are linked to sets of V-region genes that are marked by different idiotypes. The serologic markers of mouse antibodies would provide valuable information on the genetics of antibody V regions.

2.4.2. Allotypes of the Rat

Two serologically detected allotypes of the rat kappa light chain have been reported. These variants are controlled by the RI-1 locus and segregate as codominant alleles that are designated a and b. These allotypes served as an example of complex allotypes in the initial definition of *simple* and *complex* allotypes. The differences between the chains controlled by the RI-1a and 1b loci were extensive when the amino acid sequences were compared (see Chapter 3). In the normal allelic situation, only one or two amino acid residues are different between the two products; however, in the case of complex allotypes as many as 20% or even 30% of the amino acids may differ from one allele to the next. It was argued that complex allotypes are not simple allelic products, but are simultaneously present in the genome and that their expression is controlled by regulator genes. The rat kappa light chain allotypes, which have now been described at the DNA level, played an important role in dispelling the notion that complex allotypes cannot be present as simple alleles.

2.5. INDIVIDUAL ANTIGENIC SPECIFICITY AND IDIOTYPY

Studies of isotypes and allotypes conclusively demonstrated that antibodies, like all proteins, are encoded by genes that are inherited in a simple Mendelian fashion. As mentioned above, these data indicated that there are three unlinked loci encoding immunoglobulins: the heavy chain locus, the lambda light chain locus, and the kappa light chain locus (Fig. 2.5). It was further shown that these are complex loci consisting of one or several genes for C regions and considerably more genes for the V regions. Most importantly, the allotype studies provided new experimental opportunities and laid a framework on which new genetic information could be placed. However, it should be emphasized that the valuable experimental tools of isotypy and allotypy did not provide a means to directly address the crucial question: how is antibody diversity generated? A tool to directly probe this question emerged from antigenic studies of antibodies; this tool was yet another marker des-

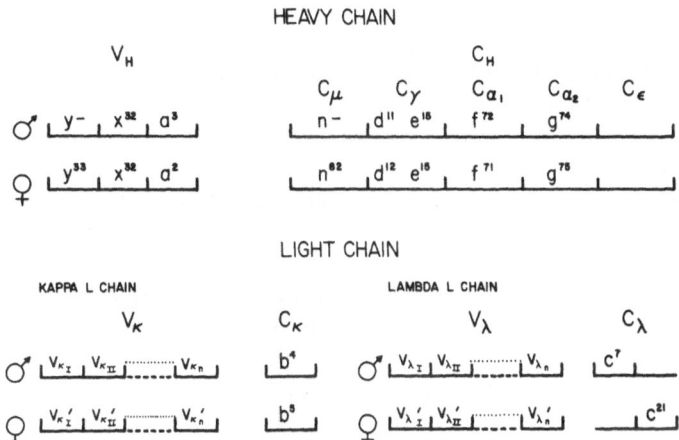

Figure 2.5. The three-locus model for immunoglobulin genes as determined by allotype markers. In the example of rabit immunoglobulin genes shown, the heavy chain V and C loci and the kappa and lambda loci are represented with maximum heterozygosity. The numbers of V_H genes within the a, x, or y groups are almost certainly greater than one.

ignated *individual antigenic specificity* or the *idiotype*, and it has proven invaluable in identifying specific V regions of immunoglobulins.

2.5.1. Idiotypes of Human Immunoglobulins

About the time Oudin and Grubb were carrying out their original studies with immunoglobulin allotypes, another antigenic marker was under investigation in Kunkel's laboratory at the Rockefeller University in New York. This marker called "individual antigenic specificity" (IAS) defined the unique features of an antibody molecule. In 1955, in a landmark paper entitled "Immunological Relationship Among the Myeloma Proteins," Slater *et al.* (1955) described studies in which sera from 21 patients with multiple myeloma were tested for their ability to react with a panel of absorbed antisera prepared against six human myeloma proteins. The variability of these proteins was indicated by their diverse mobilities in electrophoretic systems.

The major conclusion from the study was that every myeloma protein could be distinguished from all others by serologic reagents. Although the myeloma proteins with gamma mobility were related one to another, each was antigenically distinct. Likewise, the proteins with beta mobility were related one to another but again each had an individual reactivity. At that time there was no concept of the extent of class and subclass variation, different light chain types or even that immunoglobulins had a multichain structure. Nonetheless, this systematic study proved that each member of the diverse immunoglobulin family had distinct characteristics and these characteristics could be serologically defined by the IAS of that protein (Fig. 2.6).

The phenomenon of IAS was brought into the main stream of immunology when Kunkel reported in 1963 that human antibodies directed against the red blood cell group A antigen, as well as antibodies directed against the polysaccharides, dextran, or levan, could be shown to elicit antibodies directed against IAS determinants. The anti-A antibodies were made in rabbits and the rabbit anti-antibodies reacted only with the immunogen and not with sera from other individuals even though those sera also contained anti-A activity. Kunkel further demonstrated that antibodies directed against A substance and those directed against levan possessed different IAS, even though they were derived from the same individuals.

The IAS determinants were later localized to the Fab portion of the molecule, a finding consistent with the recently developed understanding that the Fab portion varied with antigen-binding specificity, whereas the Fc portion was common to all IgG molecules. The demonstration of IAS for antibodies showed unequivocally that the property of IAS was not an obscure phenomenon peculiar to the myeloma proteins but was

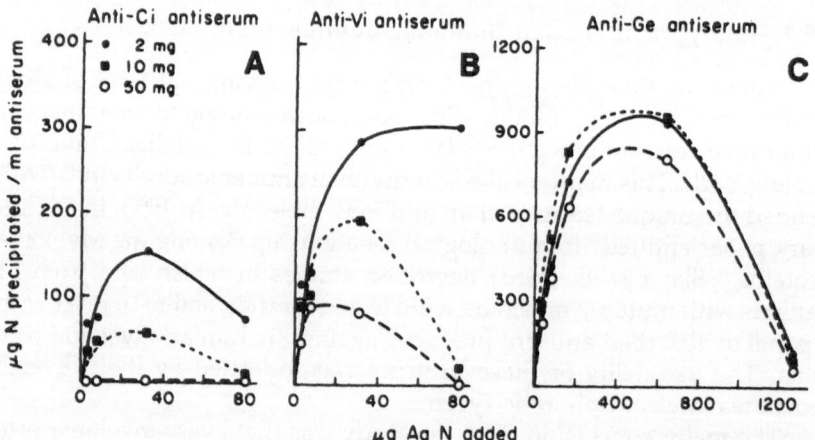

Figure 2.6. Antisera were prepared against human myeloma proteins in rabbits. These antisera were reacted with their homologous antigens after absorption with 2, 10, or 50 mg of human IgG; the precipitin curves are depicted here. In frame A, the antiserum is completely absorbed by the large excess of IgG. In B, some of the activity is removed but the individual antigenic specificity remains. In frame C, the antiserum shown is not affected in its reactivity by the absorption with normal IgG. From Natvig and Kunkel (1973).

indeed a property of functionally active antibodies. Realization of the generality of IAS determinants opened the possibility that each and every antibody had its own individual determinant. Expansion of the scope of IAS to include *all* antibodies and not just myeloma proteins could be likened to Bordet's demonstration that antibodies were not just anti pathogens but anti almost anything (Chapter 1).

A further advance stemmed from investigations of whether the determinants recognized by anti-IAS sera resided on the heavy chain or the light chain. Recall that the rabbit, mouse, and human allotypes had been localized to one chain or another. Experiments reported by Grey *et al.* in 1965, however, gave a different result for the IAS determinants of a number of myeloma proteins. Although it was possible in certain instances to localize IAS to a heavy or a light chain, the majority of the sera tested required both chains for reactivity. The specific heavy and the specific light chain of the immunogen were required for the molecule to be recognized by the anti-IAS and to form a precipitin line. Therefore, a strong link between IAS and the antigen-binding property of the antibody was forged: both properties were localized to the V region of the molecule and both required specific heavy-light chain pairs for their activity. This linkage of IAS to binding site along with the realization that IAS could mark specific antibodies in individuals gave strong indication of the future value of these markers.

2.5.2. Idiotypes of Rabbit Antibodies

By injecting specific antibodies from one rabbit into an allotypically matched rabbit, Oudin and Michel (1963) were able to show the presence of yet another antigenic determinant on rabbit antibodies. Similar to IAS, this marker had a very limited distribution and because of this was designated *idiotypy* (individual type). Oudin defined idiotypy as the marker for a given antibody in a single individual or group of individuals and further enunciated the principle of a hierarchy of antigens present on antibodies. These antigens are isotypes, allotypes, and idiotypes that were differentiated by their presence in all members of the species, some members of the species, and on certain antibodies from individual members of the species, respectively (see Table 2.3).

Idiotypy could be demonstrated by injection of antibody directed against a bacteria, such as *Salmonella typhi*, from a rabbit (rabbit 1) of known allotype into a second rabbit of the same allotype. The antiserum produced would react with anti-*S. typhi* from rabbit 1, but would not react with the preimmune serum of rabbit 1; it would further not react with anti-*S. typhi* from other rabbits of the same allotype, even those

Table 2.3. Antigenic Markers of Immunoglobulins

Designation	Occurrence	Method of detection	Examples
Isotype	All members of a species	Heterologous antiserum	IgG2 of the human; mouse kappa L chain
Allotype	Some but not all members of a species	Intraspecies immunization (alloantiserum)	a2 of rabbit H chain; Km1 of human kappa chain
Idiotype	Individual or member of related group	Antiserum prepared in same species as antibody donor animal or appropriately absorbed heterologous antiserum	Idiotype of rabbit anti-*S. typhi* antibody; idiotype of human antidextran antibody

closely related to the producer of the immunizing antibody. This animal model for idiotypy had as an advantage that extensive absorption was not necessary to render the antisera specific as in the human IAS studies, which used heterologous antisera.

An extensive study of idiotypic specificities was carried out in the 1960s by Gell and Kelus (1967) who immunized rabbits with complexes of *P. vulgaris* and antiproteus antibody from individual donor rabbits. The allotypes of the donor and recipient rabbit in each case were matched with respect to major specificities to minimize the possibility of elliciting antiallotype antibodies. Ten antiidiotype (anti-Id) antisera were prepared and tested for reactivity against 60 sera from rabbits immunized with *P. vulgaris*. These antisera showed specificity only for the antiproteus antibody of the donor; they would not react with the donor's preimmunization serum, nor with antiproteus antibodies from any of the large panel of immunized rabbits tested including close relatives of the donor. In each instance, when the antiproteus antibody was absorbed from the serum, the idiotypic reactive species was also removed. These experiments suggested that idiotypes were not inherited as Mendelian codominant alleles. It would require further work to discover why and how idiotypes differ from allotypes.

2.5.3. Presence of Idiotypes on IgG and IgM

Early studies had shown that myeloma proteins of the IgM type possessed individual antigenic specificities just as did those of the IgG type. Oudin and Michel (1969) demonstrated that IgG and IgM produced by a single rabbit and having the same specificity for antigen may have the same idiotype (Fig. 2.7). This observation of identical idiotypes on IgG and IgM antibodies strengthened the notion that antibodies differing in heavy chain class may have common V regions. The implications of identical idiotypes, and by extrapolation identical V regions, will be explored in later chapters.

The early studies of idiotypes emphasized their individuality. Antisera directed against an IAS of an IgM myeloma protein would react with that myeloma protein and not with other IgMs even though all were derived from patients with the same disease, Waldenström's macroglobulinemia. Similarly, the idiotype of anti-S. typhi from one rabbit, but not that of anti-S. typhi from littermates would be recognized by an anti-Id serum. Because of this individuality, it was reasoned that the IAS determinant was unique to a single antibody molecule and that this specificity could be used as a marker for a single antibody species in large mixtures such as the IgG fraction of an individual. Kunkel (1965) estimated that one molecule among 20 million could be detected by the sensitive inhibition of hemagglutination reactions used for the detection

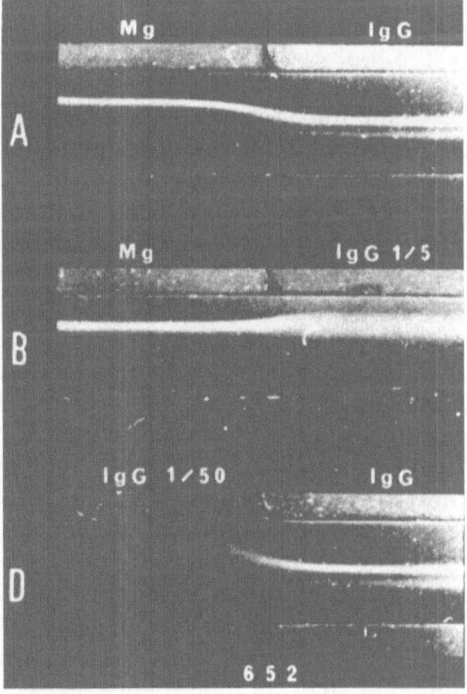

Figure 2.7. Reaction in three cells (double diffusion in agar) with the antiidiotypic serum of rabbit 6-52. A, A preparation of macroglobulin (Mg) and of IgG of S37 of rabbit 3-24; B, of the same macroglobulin preparation and a 1 : 5 dilution of the same IgG preparation as in A; D, of a 1 : 50 dilution of the same IgG preparation as in A and this IgG preparation, undiluted. It may be noticed that (1) that the precipitation zone is perfectly continuous in front of the macroglobulin (containing IgM) and IgG layers in A; (2) when the IgG preparation is diluted 1 : 5, the position of the precipitation zone in front of it is the same as in front of the macroglobulin layer, but that its appearance is definitely different; (3) when the IgG layer is diluted 1 : 50, there is definitely no precipitation zone in front of it, although the IgG content is still definitely larger in this dilution than in the macroglobulin layer. From Oudin and Michel (1969).

of IAS. When recurrent idiotypes were not found, the estimates of the number of different antibody molecules had to be reconsidered.

Thus a new and powerful serologic tool was available to aid in determination of how many antibodies were present in the individual repertoire. The speculations on the extent of the repertoire outlined in Chapter 1 were based on a completely different line of reasoning. Those estimates were based on the *number of antigens* that an individual might encounter and be required to bind. An increase in these numbers was required when it was shown that synthetic chemical haptens, presumably never encountered in the history of the species, would also give rise to highly specific antibodies. In a parallel fashion, idiotypy could be used to count the number of individual antibody molecules present in pools of immunoglobulin from different individuals. When sensitive inhibition of hemagglutination experiments failed to detect recurrence of idiotypes in antibody pools, the number of possible different antibody molecules was given a new and higher estimate. If idiotypes could be detected at the level of one molecule among 20 million and no recurrences were found, it was reasoned that there was a minimum of 20 million different molecules in the repertoire. Thus the estimated number of antibody molecules by this independent approach was similar to the estimate of needed binding sites given in Chapter 1.

2.5.4. Idiotype versus IAS

In the initial studies of idiotypes in rabbit families, the term used for the determinant under investigation was IAS, not idiotype, even though the rabbit was the subject of the study. The reason for use of this nomenclature was twofold. First, the antibodies used were purified to homogeneity and were presumably single molecules, as in myeloma proteins. Second, the antisera were prepared in a heterologous species (guinea pig) not in allotype-matched rabbits. Therefore, the system met the definition of IAS more closely than that of idiotypy.

The example of rabbit antibodies having a determinant that met the definition of IAS more closely than it fit that of idiotypy reflected a problem related to the dual terminology for the binding-site marker. There was no difficulty with terminology if either the system of Oudin (idiotypy) or the system of Kunkel (IAS) were followed exactly. However, most workers introduced variations of these systems and the terminologies became confused. For example, it was not clear which term to use when mouse myeloma proteins were used as the antigen. This was further complicated by the fact that the mouse protein could be injected into a heterologous species such as a rabbit or into the same or a different strain of inbred mice.

Much of the confusion relating to the dual terminology of idiotypy and IAS was resolved in 1971 at the First International Congress of Immunology. A workshop chaired by Kunkel and Potter recommended that the term IAS be put aside and that idiotypy be used to designate all of the individually specific antibody determinants. However, they urged that the term idiotypy be qualified by a prefix describing the animal system in which the idiotypic antisera were prepared. This prefix would be *heterologous, homogolous,* or *isologous.* Heterologous would refer to preparation of antisera in another species, homologous would refer to preparation in the same species, and isologous or autologous would refer to the use of either the same inbred strain of mice or, in the case of outbred animals like the rabbit, use of the same animal to produce the antiidiotype (Fig. 2.8).

Although the new terminology resolved some confusion concerning IAS and idiotypy, there are still a number of questions to be asked when data concerning an idiotype are reported. In addition to knowing the species in which the anti-Id was prepared, full evaluation of a system requires knowledge of the antibody preparation used to elicit the anti-Id. For example, was it a population of antibodies or was it a highly purified antibody or myeloma protein? It is also very helpful to know what specificity controls were used to establish that the idiotype is truly specific for a given antibody determinant and what absorptions, if necessary, were carried out on the antisera. The definition of an idiotype still relies heavily on functional criteria and two-Id reagents should not be considered equivalent unless data to substantiate their equivalency are shown.

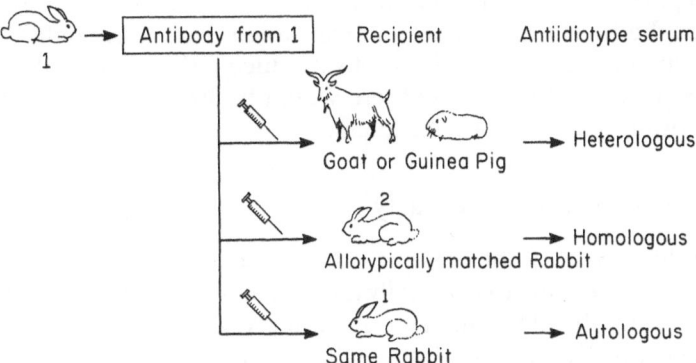

Figure 2.8. Antiidiotype serums are differentiated on the basis of the relationship between the antibody donor and the animal in which the antiidiotype serum is raised. In the example shown, heterologous, homologous, and isologous antiidiotype reagents are prepared against a rabbit antibody. From Sogn *et al.* (1977).

2.6. IDIOTYPES AS MARKERS FOR ANTIBODY-BINDING REGIONS

Studies of idiotypy soon developed in two important new directions. The relevance of these markers was greatly enhanced by findings indicating that idiotypes were markers for antibody-binding sites, and by findings that identical idiotypes were found in the sera of related individuals. These studies indicating that idiotypes could and did recur relieved some of the pressure to continually increase antibody numbers to account for the strict individuality of idiotypes. In addition, the value of idiotypy as an experimental tool was greatly enhanced by the new observations.

As long as the emphasis in idiotype studies focused on individuality, these markers had a rather limited appeal to immunologists. In addition, there was sufficient complexity in the experimental manipulation required to prepare and assay either anti-IAS or anti-Id sera to discourage many workers from studies in this arena. There was the further cloud of uncertainty concerning the exact definition of an idiotype. These factors led to disinterest in the idiotype as an investigative tool, and this persisted for several years.

Examination of the 1967 publication of the Cold Spring Harbor meeting on "Antibodies" reveals only one report of a major experiment that used idiotypes. The contribution of idiotypes to the study of antibodies filled less than one of the 600 pages in this volume. In the reported experiment, Pernis (1967) prepared an anti-Id antiserum against a human Bence Jones lambda chain. The activity of the antiserum was then monitored by fluorescent labeling of plasma cells. About 12 cells in one million gave a positive reaction with this light chain anti-Id. In his summary of the meeting, Jerne (1967) concluded from these data that the probability of two given plasma cells producing the same lambda chain must be 1 in 105. In this case there would be 100,000 different lambda chains produced in a normal human.

2.6.1. Idiotypic Cross-Specificity

Within a year of the meeting on antibodies at Cold Spring Harbor, a paper appeared that dramatically increased the potential of the idiotype by suggesting that it might be useful as a probe of the antibody-binding site. Williams, Kunkel, and Capra (1968) reported that human myeloma proteins with cold agglutinin activity might have similar individual antigenic specificities. Proteins were isolated from the sera of patients with cold agglutinin disease and were all of the IgM class. Highly purified samples of 20 of these myelomas were obtained by elution from red blood cell stroma and ten anti-Id sera were made against certain of these. After appropriate absorption, they found that three antisera gave cross-reactivity with as many as 12 of the cold agglutinins (Fig. 2.9). Although the reactions were not reactions of identity, they were clearly positive and *no* reactivity was found for any macroglobulins that did not have cold agglutinin activity. The authors introduced the term "cross idiotypic specificity" to describe these shared determinants. The cross idiotypes were private or individual in the sense of restriction to a small select group of antibodies, yet were different from idiotypes (as originally defined) in that nonidentical antigens were detected. It was also shown that anti-Id antibodies could block the reactivity of the cold agglutinins with the red blood cell antigens, an indication of binding site involvement of the Id determinant. The paper contains a cautious discussion of the findings:

> The major question raised by the above observation is whether the specific antigens characterizing cold agglutinins relate directly to the presumed antibody binding site of these proteins. A complete answer is not yet available, and the main evidence depends on simple correlation.

It would turn out that there was a relationship between idiotype and the binding site, and within a short time repeated demonstrations of this relationship would be reported for a number of different systems.

This first demonstration of recurrent idiotypes made possible a new series of experiments to probe the repertoire of antibodies. The conceptual link between an antigenic determinant and binding specificity had been made stronger. Correlation between idiotype and binding specificity was next observed by Cohn *et al.* (1969) for the products of BALB/c plasmacytomas. A myeloma protein with activity against the pneumococcal C carbohydrate was used for preparation of anti-Id serum. This

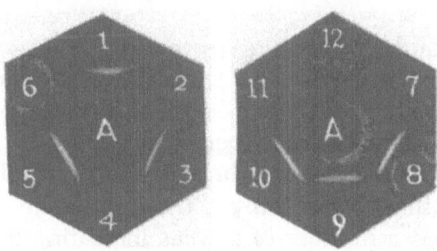

Figure 2.9. Ouchterlony analysis of cross-reactive idiotypes of cold agglutinin proteins. The central well (A) in each pattern contains anti-Id. The numbered wells contain the various cold agglutinins. From Williams *et al.* (1968).

antiserum was tested for reactivity with a panel of 160 murine plasma-cytoma proteins and only one gave a positive reaction. The single cross-reactive protein was a BALB/c myeloma that also had specificity for the pneumococcal C carbohydrate. This work was soon confirmed and extended by Potter who studied a group of eight proteins with C carbohydrate specificity and found five to possess indistinguishable idiotypes. These proteins, which react with the phosphorylcholine moiety of C carbohydrate and which carry the T15 idiotype (see below), would be put to good use in future studies on the chemical nature of the antigen-binding site and the precise relationship of an idiotype to the genes encoding antibodies. These studies of idiotypes in the human and the mouse suggested that antigenic determinants of the binding-site regions were recognized by anti-Id antibodies.

2.6.2. Antigen Inhibition of Idiotype Reactions

Direct experimental proof of the relationship between idiotype and antigen-binding site was provided by Brient and Nisonoff (1970) who showed inhibition of the precipitation reaction between rabbit antiar-sonate (anti-Ars) antibodies and anti-Id by various arsonate haptens. They observed that the hapten with the highest affinity for the antibody gave the best inhibition of the idiotype reaction. In one case, 69% of the binding between the anti-Ars and the anti-Id was inhibited. An important control was the demonstration that presence of the hapten did not interfere with binding of anti–group a or group b allotype antibodies to the anti-Ars antibodies. This finding demonstrated that determinants of group a allotypes are spatially distinct from the idiotypes, although both markers are present in the V region. Idiotypic determinants were therefore blocked or modified in some way as to prevent anti-Id binding, whereas the group a allotype determinants were recognized and bound by antiallotype despite the presence of hapten in the antigen-binding site.

The correlation between idiotypy and binding site was observed in a number of systems. Claflin and Davie (1974) extended the principle by preparation of site-specific anti-Id by elution with hapten of anti-Id antibodies from an immunoabsorbent consisting of a murine myeloma protein bound to Sepharose. This provided a means of obtaining a population of anti-Id that reacted only with binding-site components.

There followed a number of studies indicating that idiotypic reactions could be inhibited by haptenic determinants against which the antibodies were directed. A particularly thorough study was carried out by Carson and Weigert (1973) who studied the relationship between the idiotype and a combining site using mouse myeloma proteins with antidextran and antilevan activity. In each case the reaction between the antisera and the protein to which it was made was inhibited by appropriate oligosaccharides derived from the dextran or levan. The term "ligand-modifiable" idiotype was introduced to indicate an idiotypic reaction that is inhibited by the ligand or hapten against which the protein is directed. These authors stress, however, that although proteins demonstrating idiotypic cross-reactions generally have similar combining specificities, the converse need not be true. That is, all antibodies that bind a specific ligand will not necessarily show cross idiotypic specificity. However, if a ligand-modifiable idiotype is found, the correlation between this idiotype and the combining specificity of the antibodies that it will recognize is nearly perfect. It was further shown that the oligosaccharide ligands that most effectively inhibited the reaction between the antibody and the polysaccharide antigen also most effectively inhibited the reaction between the antibody and the anti-Id.

The localization of the idiotype to the V regions had been suggested by the demonstration that idiotypes were present on Fab fragments of human myeloma proteins. The most direct demonstration was provided by studies of the mouse myeloma protein MOPC-315, which has anti-2,4-dinitrophenyl activity. Givol and his co-workers (Wells *et al.*, 1973) found that the enzyme pepsin cleaved MOPC-315, producing a fragment smaller than the normal Fab fragment usually obtained in these experiments. It was established that little if any of the C_H1 domain of the heavy chain was present in the fragment nor were there any significant C_L region determinants. It was shown that this fragment, designated Fv, bound to the hapten antigen and contained the idiotypic determinant of 315.

All of these studies concerning the correlation of idiotype with antigen specificity and the inhibition of idiotypic reactions with haptens supported the notion that the idiotype was intimately involved in the binding site of the antibody. It has been implied that the binding specificity of an antibody resides in the V region; this point will be explored in depth in structural studies described in Chapter 3. However, even before structural confirmation, the idiotype had gained a new level of respectability; it was now a marker for antibody V regions.

2.6.3. Exceptions to the Correlation of Idiotypy and Binding Site

Although the majority of evidence suggested that there was a direct relationship between antibody-combining site and the idiotypic determinants, some disturbing exceptions were noted. Kelus and Gell (1967) in their studies of antiproteus antibodies observed that anti-Id antibodies would react with the antibody even when it was combined with the bacterium. Carson and Weigert (1973) noted that certain idiotypes were not ligand-modifiable and therefore represented determinants in portions of the V region other than the antibody-binding site.

The most systematic study of this phenomenon was carried out by Oudin and Cazenave (1972) who found that similar idiotypic specificities could be found in immunoglobulin fractions having different antibody function and even in fractions having no detectable antibody function! The study of idiotype identity among antibodies that differed in specificity was demonstrated using several nonrelated antigenic systems. It was noted that these observed idiotypic cross-reactions occurred only within the serum of single individuals. These exceptions to the correlation between idiotype and binding site later provided one of the cornerstones of the network theory that relates to the expression of antibodies under the control of anti-Id antibodies. However, for the present discussion, suffice it to say that the general rule of correlation between idiotype and binding site was sufficiently well documented to allow consideration of the idiotype as a binding-site marker.

2.7. THE INHERITANCE OF IDIOTYPES

Documentation of the correlation between idiotype and the antigen-binding site gave impetus to new lines of investigation using idiotypes. The most significant new area of research concerned the genetic control of antibody synthesis. A general understanding of antibody genes had been worked out from allotype studies, and a sketchy genetic map based on the few available hard facts had emerged. However, none of these facts (except perhaps the notion that the genes encoding the V and C regions may be separate in the genome) gave a clue to the questions of how the information for antibody diversity was encoded and utilized. In fact, the most uncertain feature of the map concerned the extent of the sets of V-region genes. The idiotype, if it truly marked the binding site of individual antibodies, had potential to increase our understanding of these genes.

If idiotypes were markers for antigen-binding sites, could they be used as experimental tools to follow the inheritance of specific antibody-binding sites through families of immunized animals? The original studies of Oudin and of Kelus on rabbit idiotypes in families had yielded negative results in this respect. The idiotype did not mimic the allotype's clear patterns of inheritance.

2.7.1. Discovery

It would require a special experimental system and probably a good ration of luck to demonstrate unequivocally that there was a familial element to the idiotype and by implication to the binding site. The experimental system was based on the observation of Krause (1970) that rabbits selectively bred for their highly restricted response to immunization with streptococcal vaccines produced antibody in serum concentrations as high as 50 mg/ml. Often, the majority of the response would consist of one or two antibodies. Electrophoretic studies of these rabbit sera gave patterns reminiscent of those obtained from humans with multiple myeloma. It was possible in this system to produce and purify sufficient amounts of homogeneous antibody to prepare reagents for idiotype studies.

The original report by Eichmann and Kindt in 1971 on the inheritance of idiotypes documented the recurrence of several antistreptococcal antibodies (directed against the group C carbohydrate) in members of a family of related rabbits. Four antibodies were purified to homogeneity by affinity chromatography and used to prepare anti-Id reagents in guinea pigs. The four anti-Id antisera against the streptococcal antibodies were shown to react with the antibodies used in their preparation (the proband antibodies), but not with preimmune sera from the rabbit producing the antibody or with pooled IgG or pools of antistreptococcal serum. The anti-Id sera were tested by immunodiffusion in agar for reactivity with hyperimmune sera from 42 members of the family from which the proband rabbits were taken. An additional 48 antisera from unrelated rabbits that contained antibodies directed against the same antigens were also tested. No reactivities were found for the unrelated group with any of the four antisera. One of the antisera gave no reactivity for any of the sera from related rabbits; two of the anti-Id reacted with three of the other sera and one reacted with serum samples of seven related rabbits. As seen in the pedigree (Fig. 2.10) the cross-reactions encompassed three generations of the family.

The antibodies showing cross-reactivity were studied in more detail, and it was found that certain of the antibody pairs were antigenically identical, whereas others were strongly cross-reactive but nonidentical (Fig. 2.11). Electrophoretic comparisons gave further evidence for identity of several pairs as did studies on binding affinity to immunoadsor-

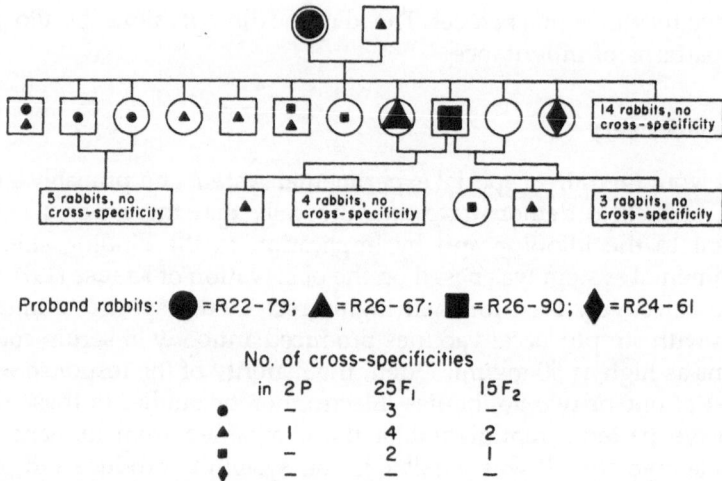

Figure 2.10. Pedigree of a rabbit family consisting of two parental, 25 F_1, and 15 F_2 generation rabbits. Large filled symbols indicate rabbits from which the proband antibodies were isolated. Small filled symbols designate rabbits which produced antibodies with precipitating cross-specificity for a proband antibody. Open squares, males; open circles, females. All rabbits were immunized with group C vaccine. From Eichmann and Kindt (1971).

bent columns and amino terminal sequence analysis. There was evidence to indicate that certain of the cross-reactive pairs were identical in their light chains but not in their heavy chains.

All antibodies that cross-reacted had the same group a and group b allotypes. It was further demonstrated that the precipitation reaction between the proband antibodies and the anti-IAS could be inhibited by large excesses of rabbit IgG. The most efficient inhibitor was the preimmune IgG from the proband rabbit or from a sibling that produced an antibody with a cross-specificity on immunization. The preimmune sera showing highest levels of inhibition were tested by a sensitive Farr assay for C carbohydrate antibody and none was found. Therefore, IgG devoid of antibody activity similar to that of the proband was reactive with the anti-IAS. These molecules were present at low concentrations in serum samples tested. This result was in agreement with findings of Kunkel (1965) that human IAS reactions were often inhibited by huge excesses of heterologous IgG.

This study on rabbit antibodies gave strong indication that identical antibodies (or in some cases heavy or light chains) could be expressed in related rabbits. Thus an idiotype could be considered an inherited gene product.

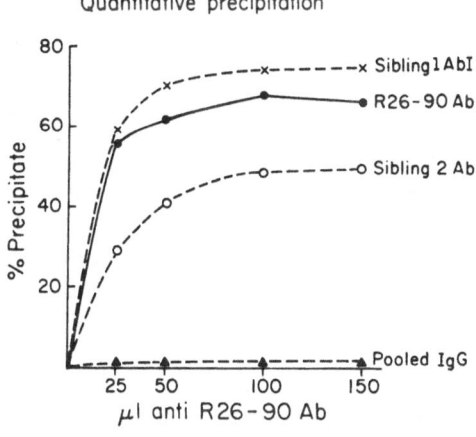

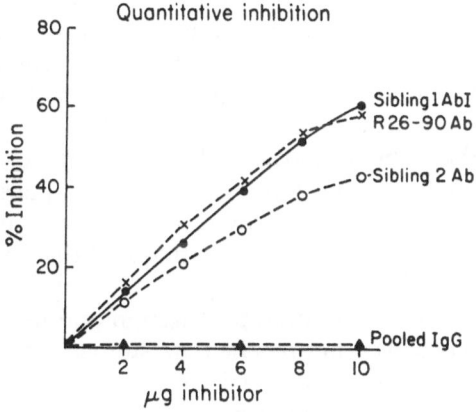

Figure 2.11. Top frame, quantitative radioprecipitin test performed with 5 μg radiolabeled R26-90Ab, sibling 1 antibody I, sibling 2 Ab, and pooled rabbit IgG, using increasing amounts of anti-R26-90Ab. Bottom frame, quantitative radioprecipitin inhibition test performed with 5 μg radiolabeled R26-90Ab and 25 μl anti-R26-90Ab. Increasing amounts of the cold antibodies were added as inhibitors. From Eichmann and Kindt (1971).

2.7.1.1. Are All Idiotypes Inherited?

The finding of idiotype inheritance in the rabbit was not confirmed for all systems studied. Haber and his co-workers (1976) used pneumococcal vaccine to elicit high and homogeneous responses in a system similar to that developed by Krause for streptococcal vaccine. Pneumococcal immunization was highly successful for preparing large amounts of homogeneous antibody. However, a study of idiotypes of the anti-pneumococcal antibodies failed to reveal occurrence of the proband idiotypes among related rabbits. By contrast, Braun and Jaton (1974) used the A-variant strain of streptococcus as antigen in rabbit families and found idiotypes that were inherited. In subsequent studies on idiotypes of antistreptococcal antibodies using homologous idiotype reagents, it was demonstrated that although certain antistreptococcal antibody idiotypes could be found in up to half of related rabbits, others were not elicited in any rabbit other than the proband. This variability in the genetic transmission of idiotypes of antibodies to these simple carbohydrate antigens raised difficult questions concerning mechanisms underlying the inheritance of idiotypes.

The question of why idiotype inheritance should be observed in some instances and not in others has some simple and some less than simple explanations. The variation in idiotype expression was also observed for idiotypes of inbred mice so it cannot be easily ascribed to degrees of relatedness among the different rabbit families studied. The most straightforward explanations involve the specificity of the anti-Id and the types of assay system used to detect cross-reactivity.

As mentioned above, certain idiotypes were present on isolated heavy or light chains, but the majority required the presence of a specific heavy–light (H-L) pair. This requirement demands the inheritance of two unlinked genes (or more accurately, gene complexes) and the simultaneous expression of two V regions from those inherited genes in the same antibody molecule. Estimates of the probability of recurrent idiotypes that require specific H-L pairs vary depending on the theoretical bias of the investigator; by any estimate, however, such events will be many times less frequent than occurrence of idiotypes marking only V_H or V_L regions.

The H-L idiotype question and its relevance to inheritance of idiotypes was approached in studies on light and heavy chain specific idiotypes in the rabbit antistreptococcal system. An anti-Id antiserum, prepared by injection of a purified antibody (4539Ab) into an allotype-matched rabbit, bound to the free light chains of the antibody. Antibodies binding to the light idiotype (LId) were purified by passing the antiserum over a column of isolated 4539Ab light chains bound to Sepharose and eluting the bound antibodies. This reagent was shown to be specific for the light chain of the proband antibody and was designated anti-LId. When serum samples of related rabbits were tested for inhibition of the reaction between anti-LId and the proband antibody, about half gave strong positive reactions. Other idiotypic antisera directed against 4539Ab lacking light chain binding reactivity and requiring the specific H-L pair detected *no* cross-reactions in the same samples. Therefore, the large number of cross-reactions observed for the LId can be ascribed to simplification of the reagent to detect only the specific V_L region.

A second example of a chain-specific idiotype in the rabbit furnished more convincing evidence of the generality of idiotype inheritance. A heavy-chain-specific reagent was deliberately prepared using an H-L recombinant molecule and the method depicted in Fig. 2.12. This antiserum (anti-HId) was used to screen for idiotypes in an extended rabbit family. It was found that 74% of the rabbits sharing the heavy chain allogroup of the proband were positive for the HId. Less than 6% of related rabbits lacking this heavy chain gene complex expressed the heavy chain marker, and most of these at very low levels. It is significant to note that rabbits having the a3 V_H allotype (the allotype of the proband) did not express HId unless they had the same complete allogroup as the proband. Therefore, it was possible to demonstrate idiotype inheritance linked to the a3 V_H genes in one given gene complex but not the a3 V_H genes in another.

The high frequency with which heavy- or light-chain-specific idiotypes occur in families as opposed to the low and variable expression of those requiring specific H-L pairs provides a partial answer to the question of why all idiotypes are not inherited in a simple pattern. Differences in the methods used in idiotype studies were an additional factor contributing to this complexity.

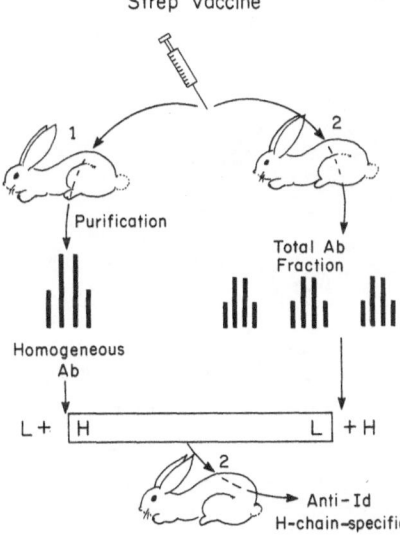

Figure 2.12. An anti-Id serum specific for the H chain of a homogeneous antibody was prepared by injecting H-L chain hybrid molecules containing the heavy chain from a homogeneous antibody and light chains from an allotypically matched donor back into the light chain donor. This reagent recognized an idiotype localized to the heavy chain of a homogeneous antibody. From Sogn *et al.* (1977).

2.7.1.2. Identical Idiotypes and Cross-Reactive Idiotypes

The concept of identical idiotypes (IdI) as opposed to very similar highly cross-reactive idiotypes (IdX) would be relevant to studies of binding regions. As structural data became available, the idea that the binding site was composed of sequences from discrete hypervariable segments within the V regions raised the possibility of partial identity based on identity of only certain elements of the binding site. Early findings of cross-reactivity among human cold agglutinin proteins that were recognized to be reactions of partial rather than complete identity were extended in the human system. The relevance of this classification to the binding site of the antibodies was made clear by further elucidation of the structure of the determinant recognized on the red blood cells. This determinant, designated I, was recognized by certain of the myeloma proteins and those proteins that could recognize the I determinant fell into one idiotypic cross-reactive group. Cold agglutinins with activity for an alternative specificity, Pr, formed a group of cross idiotypic specificities distinct from those proteins with I specificity. It was further shown in these studies that IgA and IgM cold agglutinins sharing the Pr specificity also had common cross idiotypic specificity.

Perhaps the best example of cross idiotypy is given by the studies of human myeloma proteins with activity for human immunoglobulin. Heterologous anti-Id reagents against two of a group of anti-gamma globulins were prepared in rabbits (Fig. 2.13). The anti-IgG myeloma proteins were coated onto red blood cells and each was tested for hem-

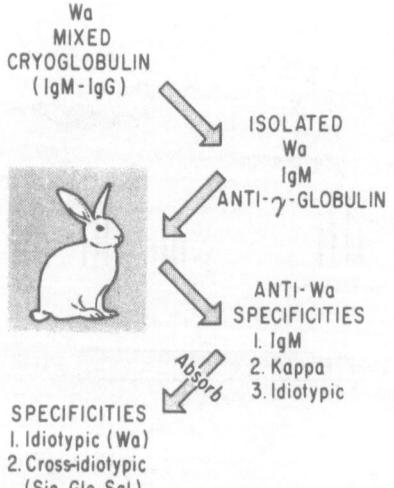

Wa
MIXED
CRYOGLOBULIN
(IgM-IgG)

ISOLATED
Wa
IgM
ANTI-γ-GLOBULIN

ANTI-Wa
SPECIFICITIES
1. IgM
2. Kappa
3. Idiotypic

Absorb

SPECIFICITIES
1. Idiotypic (Wa)
2. Cross-idiotypic
(Sie, Glo, Sal)

Figure 2.13. Preparation of an anti-Id reagent with cross-idiotypic specificity. From Capra and Kehoe (1975).

Table 2.4. Cross-Specificity of Isolated IgM Anti-γ-globulins[a]

	Inhibitor protein concentration (mg/ml)						
	1.0	0.25	0.06	0.015	0.004	0.001	0.0002
Ma[b]	0	0	0	0	0	0	1
Wa[b]	0	0	0	0	0	Tr	2
Bl[b]	0	0	0	0	0	2	2
Si[b]	0	0	0	0	0	1	2
Ea[b]	0	0	0	0	0	Tr	2
La[b]	Tr	2	2	2	2	2	2
Po[b]	1	2	2	2	2	2	2
Ga[c]	2	2	2	2	2	2	2
St[c]	Tr	1	2	2	2	2	2
Sz[c]	2	2	2	2	2	2	2
FrII	0	0	Tr	2	2	2	2

[a] Four of the six anti-γ-globulins inhibit the reaction whereas other macroglobulins do not (Wa system). Antiserum made against anti-γ-globulin Ma using the technique described in Fig. 2.13 red cells coated with protein Wa.
[b] IgM anti-γ-globulins.
[c] IgM proteins without anti-γ-globulin activity.

agglutination using the anti-Id sera. Several cross-reactions were noted by this test. However, when the myeloma proteins were tested for cross-reactivities by inhibition of hemagglutination, a different answer was found. In this case only the antibody used for preparation of the anti-Id inhibited the reaction. When the agglutination reaction between the anti-Id against one antibody and red blood cells coated with another cross-reactive anti-IgG (detected by the binding test) was used as the test system, there was inhibition by certain of the proteins (see Table 2.4). This test system allowed division of the anti-immunoglobulin myeloma proteins into three major cross-reactive groups. Similarities among the proteins in the different groups were later confirmed by a number of functional and structural criteria showing the discriminatory power of this classification. The differentiation of IdI and IdX was very useful, and examples will recur frequently in development of the ideas concerning antibody diversity.

2.7.2. The Mouse Idiotype Systems

Although the first reports of idiotypic markers on mouse immunoglobulins lagged behind those for the human and rabbit by a number of years, the murine idiotype systems ultimately proved themselves the most powerful in elucidation of V-gene complexities. There were two major reasons for this. First, the availability of inbred mouse strains and the short generation time in this species allowed genetic studies not possible in the human or in the rabbit. Second, the transplantable myeloma or hybridoma cell lines producing single antibody molecules afforded a source of protein for structural and idiotypic studies and later a source of RNA for direct studies of antibody genes.

A number of the mouse idiotype systems have provided valuable information on idiotype inheritance; certain of these will be described in some detail here. For other systems a more rudimentary description will be given here and more detailed discussions of specific aspects will follow in later chapters (see Table 2.5).

The early experiments from the laboratories of Potter and of Cohn showed that the idiotype markers of murine myeloma proteins could provide valuable information. However, all studies did not use myeloma proteins. In addition to idiotype studies of murine plasmacytoma proteins, there was an alternative approach taken that was an extrapolation of the techniques used to study rabbit idiotypes. Antibodies were induced by normal immunization procedures, isolated by affinity chromatography, and used to induce anti-Id. This approach was taken by Nisonoff who used the phenylarsonate hapten, by Eichmann who used the streptococcal vaccines, by Mäkelä who used the hapten 4-hydroxy-3-nitrophenyl (NP) acetyl, and by Sachs who used staphyloccal nuclease (reviewed by Weigert and Potter, 1977).

Table 2.5. Mouse V_H Markers[a]

V_H marker	Assay	Reference antibody or myeloma protein	Reference strain
DEX	Idiotype	J558, MOPC104E	BALB/c
A5A	Idiotype, spectrotype	Induced anti-group A carbohydrate	A/J
A5A	Idiotype	Induced anti-group A carbohydrate	C57L
Ars	Idiotype	Induced anti-p-azophenyl arsonate	A/J
T15	Idiotype	T15	BALB/c
Nase	Idiotype	Induced antistaphylococcal nuclease	A/J-1 SJL-2
InuIdx	Idiotype	E109,A47,U61	BALB/c
U10-173	Idiotype	U10-MOPC173	BALB/c
NP	Fine specificity, idiotype, and spectrotype (N_1)	Induced anti-NP	C57BL/6
NBrP	Fine specificity	Induced anti-NBrP	C57BL/6-BALB/c[+]

[a] Adapted from Weigert and Potter (1977).

2.7.2.1. The Arsonate System

A 1972 paper by Nisonoff and his colleagues (Kuettner *et al.*, 1972) described initial experiments in the anti-arsonate (Ars) system. Antibodies against this hapten were induced in A/J and in BALB/c mice. The antibodies were affinity purified and rabbit anti-Id sera was prepared, appropriately absorbed, and shown to be specific for the anti-Ars antibodies. Controls on the specificity of the anti-Id sera included the demonstration that IgG from preimmune animals as well as antibodies directed against the carrier used to couple Ars for immunization were nonreactive.

The anti-Ars antibodies were radiolabeled and used in indirect (second antibody) precipitation reactions. Sera from Ars-immunized mice of the same and different strains were tested for their ability to inhibit the reaction between Ars antibodies and the anti-Id. It was found that the isologous sera from the majority of animals tested had inhibitory activity that would approach 75% of total if sufficient antibody were used. As shown in Fig. 2.14, the C57BL/6 anti-Ars sera had little effect on the reaction between A/J anti-Ars and the anti-Id, whereas nearly all samples of A/J sera showed significant inhibition.

Breeding studies on the A/J idiotype indicated that the idiotype, which was designated Ars, was linked to heavy chain C-region allotype of the e haplotype. It was later shown that a mouse strain that carried the A/J allotype on a BALB/c background had the Ars idiotype, whereas normal BALB/c mice did not. This congenic strain was the result of nine back-cross generations with selection at each generation for the C_H allotype. The fact that the idiotype remained in this strain indicates a close linkage between allotype and idiotype.

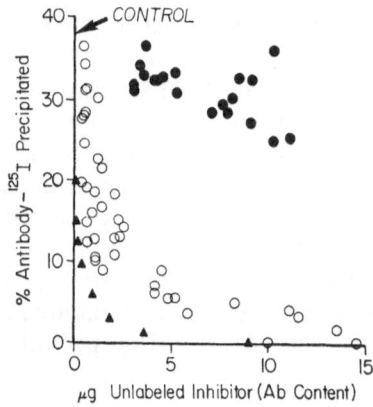

Figure 2.14. Inhibition of binding to its antiidiotypic antibodies of 0.02 μg of ^{125}I-labeled specifically purified anti-p-azophenylarsonate antibody from A/J mouse No. 413. Inhibitors are unlabeled antiazophenylarsonate antisera from individual mice. Data are plotted in terms of the weight of precipitable antibody in the serum. ▲, Autologous antiserum (from A/J mouse No. 413); ●, antisera from ten individual A/J mice, tested at varying concentrations; ○, antisera from 10 individual C57BL/6 mice. From Kuettner *et al.* (1972).

2.7.2.2. The A5A System

In a similar system, Eichmann (1972) studied the idiotype of an antibody directed against the group A streptococcal carbohydrate. The response to streptococcal immunization in A/J mice consistently included the idiotype designated A5A. The major difference between this study and that of the Ars idiotype was that the antibodies used to induce anti-Id were homogeneous, presumably the products of single clones. Guinea pigs were used to prepare heterologous anti-Id sera and isologous (A/J anti-A/J) antisera were also used.

It was observed that the idiotype of one of the antibodies studied, A5A, predominated in most A/J mice after immunization with streptococcal vaccine. Other mouse strains did not produce antibody with the A5A idiotype. Extensive breeding studies were carried out, and as with the Ars idiotype the A5A was linked to the heavy chain allotypes. However, an interesting exception to the linkage was observed, one that has had significant implications to the antibody problem and will be discussed further in Chapter 4. Later studies of the A5A idiotype showed that certain antisera had preference for heavy or light chains, and these preferences could be shown by the linkage data from breeding studies as well as by immunochemical procedures.

Aside from their value in studies on antibody diversity, the Ars and the A5A systems have given extremely good service in areas concerning regulation of idiotype expression. Data on suppression or induction of idiotypes and on the nature of the elusive T-cell component that bears an idiotype specificity have been obtained using these valuable systems.

2.7.2.3. The NP System

The antibodies that belong to the cross-reactive NP group studied by Imanishi and Mäkelä (1974) are peculiar in that they were first grouped on the basis of a fine binding specificity rather than on idiotypic specificity. When C57BL/6 mice are immunized with the hapten NP on a protein carrier, the resulting antibodies have higher affinity for certain analogues of NP than for NP itself. The property of an antibody to have a higher affinity for an antigen other than its immunogen had been defined as heteroclicity (Mäkelä, 1965). In contrast to the C57BL/6 mice, when BALB/c mice were immunized with the hapten NP similarly conjugated to a protein carrier, it was found that the antibodies raised in response were predominantly nonheteroclitic. It was further shown that the isoelectric focusing spectrotype of the heteroclitic NP antibodies was characteristic and different from that of nonheteroclitic NP antibodies. It was also shown that congenic mouse strains bearing the C57BL allotype (1.b) produced the heteroclitic antibody linking their synthesis to the heavy chain gene complex.

Later examination of the heteroclitic and nonheteroclitic antibodies by an anti-Id, designated NP^b, showed a strong positive correlation between heteroclitic antibodies and the presence of the NP^b idiotype. It was further shown that none of the antibodies produced in BALB/c mice would react with the anti-NP^b reagent. In a thorough analysis of the NP^b idiotype, it was shown that there were four or five spectrotypes present in the C57BL/6 response indicating some degree of heterogeneity within this idiotype. As will be seen in later chapters, examination of the factors underlying this heterogeneity have provided important new insights into the problem of inherited idiotypy.

2.7.2.4. The T15 Idiotype

A number of BALB/c myeloma proteins directed against phosphorylcholine (PC) were studied by Lieberman et al., (1974) using anti-Id reagents prepared in A/He mice. It was shown that two of these proteins, TEPC15 and HOPC8, were idiotypically identical to one another but different from other anti-PC binding plasmacytoma products.

A surprising feature of the T15 idiotype was its presence in the sera of normal, nonimmunized BALB/c mice. The concentrations of the idiotype in normal sera was estimated at 8 to 64 μg/ml, and reactivity could be removed by absorption with Sepharose-PC or the pneumococcal strain R36A. The T15 idiotype was not present in the sera of germ-free mice but on conventionalization T15 appeared, sometimes within five days.

The linkage of T15 to the BALB/c C_H allotype complex has been demonstrated conclusively. Recombinant inbred mouse strains, various congenic lines, and conventional breeding experiments were used to prove this linkage.

2.7.2.5. Antidextran Idiotypes

Studies of the antibodies directed against the alpha (1-3) linkage of dextran (DEX) were begun by using a myeloma protein, J558, that had specificity for this linkage (Blomberg et al., 1972). Antibodies from BALB/c mice cross-reacted with this idiotype but those from C57BL/6 mice did not. Genetic analysis indicated that the DEX idiotype was inherited and linked to the BALB/c C_H allotype complex.

In studies of mouse idiotypes, linkage to the C_H region allotypes was usually demonstrated and in most cases little was known about the light chain involvement in the idiotype. The DEX system is an exception in that the light chain has been the subject of intense study. The lambda light chain of the mouse, which composes only 1% to 2% of the total light chain in normal serum, is exclusively associated with anti-DEX antibodies. Primary structural data for the V regions of the anti-DEX lambda chains have provided an exciting data set for the theorist to consider and will be the subject of detailed analysis in later chapters.

In addition to the idiotype systems mentioned above, others based on induced antibodies directed against antigens, such as staphylococcal nuclease, or on myeloma proteins that bind specific antigens, such as galactans or inulins, were useful in the quest for information concerning the antibody V-region genes. In addition to the idiotypes, markers for fine specificity and isoelectric focusing spectrotypes of antibodies and isolated chains would be used to map V regions.

The unanimous conclusion from the studies on idiotypes in the mouse was that idiotypes are inherited and that their expression is linked to the C_H allotype genes. These idiotypic data suggest that V regions marked by the idiotype are encoded by single genes inherited in a simple Mendelian fashion. Before this conclusion is accepted, the contradictory findings should be reviewed. First and most relevant is the finding that not all antibodies appear to express inherited idiotypes. In nearly every study leading to the list of inherited idiotypes shown in Table 2.5, there were numerous examples of idiotypes that did not recur. A striking example of this is found in the Ars system. When the major idiotype marker is suppressed in neonates by injection of anti-Id serum, subsequent immunization with Ars induces levels of anti-Ars antibody comparable to those observed in normal nonsuppressed control animals. However *no* common idiotypes are found for the anti-Ars population elicited in the suppressed mice. Therefore, inherited idiotypes may represent an exception.

A second complexity of the idiotype systems is the occurrence of similar or cross-reactive antibodies that are not identical to the proband antibody. This raises the possibility that either mutation rates are very high for V-region genes or that single identical genes do not always encode the V region corresponding to a particular idiotype. The total data concerning genetic control of idiotypes leave us with the conclusion that demonstrations of inheritance of these V-region markers do not prove conclusively that antibody V regions are encoded as simple Mendelian alleles.

2.8. CONCLUSION

Serologists developed the foundations on which knowledge of the genetic basis of antibody diversity was built. Their studies yielded information concerning the arrangement of the immunoglobulin genes into a three-locus model with unlinked genes for the heavy chain and for the kappa and lambda light chains. This information made it possible to understand that the central question of diversity concerned the number and nature of V-region genes encoded within each of these complexes. Idiotype analyses indicated that V-region genes could be inherited, but the fact that idiotypes were not always inherited and that some idiotypes were cross-reactive rather than identical suggested that all V-region genes were not present in the germline. Further studies of antibodies using techniques other than serology would be required to construct a total picture of the antibody repertoire.

The next chapter will deal with studies by the protein chemists who determined primary structures for myeloma proteins and antibodies that complemented the serologic data. Great expectations accompanied the onset of these studies. It was thought by some that determination and comparison of amino acid sequences from just two different antibodies would provide answers to most questions concerning antibodies and their origins. It will be seen in the following chapter that although structural examination of antibodies further defined and fine tuned the problem of antibody diversity, the level of highest expectation was unfortunately not met.

REFERENCES AND BIBLIOGRAPHY

Blomberg, B., Geckeler, W. R., and Weigert, M., 1972, Genetics of the antibody response to dextran in mice, *Science* **177**:178.

Braun, D. G., and Jaton, J.-C., 1974, Homogeneous antibodies: Induction and value as a probe for the antibody problem, in: *Current Topics in Microbiology and Immunology*, Springer-Verlag, New York, p. 29.

Brient, B. W., and Nisonoff, A., 1970, Quantitative investigations of idiotypic antibodies. IV. Inhibition by specific haptens of the reaction of antihapten antibody with its anti-idiotypic antibody, *J. Exp. Med.* **132**:951.

Capra, J. D., and Kehoe, J. M., 1975, Hypervariable regions, idiotypy and the antibody combining site, *Adv. Immunol.* **20**:1.

Carson, D., and Weigert, M., 1973, Immunochemical analysis of the crossreacting idiotypes of mouse myeloma proteins with anti-dextran activity and normal anti-dextran antibody, *Proc. Natl. Acad. Sci. USA* **70**:235.

Claflin, J. L., and Davie, J. M., 1974, Clonal nature of the immune response to phosphorylcholine. IV. Idiotypic uniformity of binding site-associated antigenic determinants among mouse antiphosphorylcholine antibodies, *J. Exp. Med.* **140**:673.

Cohn, M., Notani, G., and Rice, S. A., 1969, Characterization of the antibody to the C-carbohydrate produced by a transplantable mouse plasmocytoma, *Immunochemistry*, **6**:111.

Dray, S., 1962, Effect of maternal isoantibodies on the quantitative expression of two allelic genes controlling the γ-globulin allotypic specificities, *Nature* **195**:677.

Dubiski, S., 1972, Genetics and regulation of immunoglobulin allotypes, *Med. Clin. North Am.* **56**:557.

Dubiski, S., Rapacz, J., and Dubiska, A., 1962, Heredity of rabbit gamma-globulin iso-antigens, *Acta Genet.* **12**:136.

Eichmann, K., 1972, Idiotypic identity of antibodies to streptococcal carbohydrate in inbred mice, *Eur. J. Immunol.* **2**:301.

Eichmann, K., 1975, Genetic control of antibody specificity in the mouse, *Immunogenetics* **2**:491.

Eichmann, K., and Kindt, T. J., 1971, The inheritance of individual antigenic specificities of rabbit antibodies to streptococcal carbohydrates, *J. Exp. Med.* **134**:532.

Feinstein, A., 1963, Character and allotypy of an immune globulin in rabbit colostrum, *Nature* **199**:1197.

Fleischman, J. B., Pain, R. H., and Porter, R. R., 1962, Reduction of the γ-globulins, *Arch. Biochem. Biophys. Suppl. I*, **99**:174.

Grey, H. M., Mannik, M., and Kunkel, H. G., 1965, Individual antigenic specificity of myeloma proteins: Characteristics and localization of subunits, *J. Exp. Med.* **121**:561.

Grubb, R., 1956, Agglutination of erythrocytes coated with "incomplete" anti-Rh by certain rheumatoid arthritic sera and some other sera, *Acta Pathol. Microbiol. Scand.* **39**:195.

Grubb, R., and Laurell, A. B., 1956, Hereditary serological human serum groups, *Acta Pathol. Microbiol. Scand.* **39**:390.

Gutman, G. A., 1977, Rat kappa chain allotypes. I. Distribution of RI-1 specificities among inbred strains and wild populations of *Rattus norvegicus*, *Immunogenetics*, **5**:597.

Haber, E., Margolies, M. N., and Cannon, L. E., 1976, Origins of antibody diversity: Insights gained from amino acid sequence studies of elicited antibodies, *Cold Spring Harbor Symp. Quant. Biol.* **41**:647.

Harboe, M., Osterland, C. K., Mannik, M., and Kunkel, H. G., 1962, Genetic characters of human γ-globulins in myeloma proteins, *J. Exp. Med.* **116**:719.

Herzenberg, L. A., McDevitt, H., and Herzenberg, L. A., 1968, Genetics of antibodies, *Annu. Rev. Genet.*, **2**,209.

Imanishi, T., and Mäkelä, O., 1974, Inheritance of antibody specificity. I. Anti-(4-hydroxy-3-nitrophenyl)-acetyl of mouse primary response, *J. Exp. Med.* **140**:1498.

Jerne, N. K., 1967, Summary: Waiting for the end, *Cold Spring Harbor Symp. Quant. Biol.* **32**:591.

Kelus, A. S., and Gell, P. G. H., 1967, Immunoglobulin allotypes of experimental animals, *Prog. Allergy*, **11**:141.

Kelus, A., and Moor-Jankowski, J. K., 1961, An iso-antigen (yBA) of mouse γ-globulin present in inbred strains, *Nature*, **191**:1405.

Kindt, T. J., 1975, Rabbit immunoglobulin allotypes: Structure, immunology, and genetics, *Adv. Immunol.* **21**:35.

Kindt, T. J., Thunberg, A. L., Mudgett, M., and Klapper, D. E., 1974, A study of V region genes using allotypic and idiotypic markers, in: *The Immune System* (A. Williamson, E. Sercarz, and C. F. Fox, eds.), Academic Press, New York, p. 69.

Krause, R. M., 1970, The search for antibodies with molecular uniformity, *Adv. Immunol.* **12**:1.

Kuettner, M. G., Wang, A., and Nisonoff, A., 1972, Quantitative investigations of idiotypic antibodies. VI. Idiotypic specificity as a potential genetic marker for the variable regions of mouse immunoglobulin polypeptide chains, *J. Exp. Med.* **135**:579.

Kunkel, H. G., 1965, Myeloma proteins and antibodies, *Harvey Lect.* **59**:219.

Kunkel, H. G., 1970, Individual antigenic specificity, cross specificity and diversity of human antibodies, *Fed. Proc.* **29**:55.

Kunkel, H. G., Mannik, M., and Williams, R. C., 1963, Individual antigenic specificity of isolated antibodies, *Science*, **140**:1218.

Lieberman, R., 1978, Genetics of IgCH (allotype) locus in the mouse, *Springer Semin. Immunopathol.* **1**:7.

Lieberman, R., 1979, Origin and characteristics of allotypic congenic strains, in: *Inbred and Genetically Defined Strains of Laboratory Animals*, Part 1, FASEB Handbook III (P. L. Altman and D. D. Katz, eds.), FASEB, Bethesda, p. 111.

Lieberman, R., and Potter, M., 1969, Crossing over between genes in the immunoglobulin heavy chain linkage group of the mouse, *J. Exp. Med.*, **130**:519.

Lieberman, R., Potter, M., Mushinski, E. B., Humphrey, J. R. W., and Rudikoff, S., 1974, Genetics of a new IgVH (T15 idiotype) marker in the mouse regulating natural antibody to phosphorylcholine, *J. Exp. Med.* **139**:983.

Mage, R., 1967, Quantitative studies on the regulation of expression of genes for immunoglobulin allotypes in heterozygous rabbits, *Cold Spring Harbor Symp. Quant. Biol.* **32**:203.

Mage, R. G., Lieberman, R., Potter, M., and Terry, W. D., 1973, Immunoglobulin allotypes, in: *The Antigens* (M. Sela, ed.), Academic Press, New York, p. 300.

Mäkelä, O., 1965, Single lymph node cells producing heteroclitic bacteriophage antibody, *J. Immunol.* **95**:378.

Natvig, J. G., and Kunkel, H. G., 1973, Human immunoglobulins: Classes, subclasses, genetic variants, and idiotypes, *Adv. Immunol.* **16**:1.

Oudin, J., 1956a, Réaction de précipitation spécifique entre des sérums d'animaux de même espèce, *C. R. Acad. Sci.* **242**:2489.

Oudin, J., 1956b, L'"allotypie" de certaines antigènes protéidiques du sérum, *C. R. Acad. Sci.* **242**:2606.

Oudin, J., 1966, Genetic regulation of immunoglobulin synthesis, *J. Cell. Physiol.* **67**:77.

Oudin, J., and Cazenave, P. A., 1971, Similar idiotypic specifications in immunoglobulin fractions with different antibody functions or even without detectable antibody function, *Proc. Natl. Acad. Sci. USA* **68**:2616.

Oudin, J., and Michel, M., 1963, A new allotype form of rabbit serum γ-globulins, apparently associated with antibody function and specificity, *C. R. Acad. Sci.* **257**:805.

Oudin, J., and Michel, M., 1969, Idiotypy of rabbit antibodies. II. Comparision of idiotypy of various kinds of antibodies formed in the same rabbits against *Salmonella typhi*, *J. Exp. Med.* **130**:619.

Pawlak, L. L., Mushinski, E. B., Nisonoff, A., and Potter, M., 1973, Evidence for the linkage of the IgCH locus to a gene controlling the idiotypic specificity of anti-p-azophenyl-arsonate antibodies in strain A mice, *J. Exp. Med.* **137**:22.

Pernis, B., 1967, Relationships between the heterogenicity of immunoglobulins and the differentiation of plasma cells, *Cold Spring Harbor Symp. Quant. Biol.* **32**:333.

Pernis, B., Chappino, G., Kelus, A., and Gell, P. G. H., 1965, Cellular localization of immunoglobulins with different allotypic specificities in rabbit lymphoid tissues, *J. Exp. Med.* **122**:853.

Potter, M., and Lieberman, R., 1970, Common individual antigenic determinants in five of eight BALB/c IgA myeloma proteins that bind phosphorylcholine, *J. Exp. Med.* **132**:737.

Ropartz, C., Lenoir, J., and Rivat, J., 1961, A new inheritable property of human sera: The Inv factor, *Nature* **189**:586.

Slater, R. J., Ward, S. M., and Kunkel, H. G., 1955, Immunological relationships among the myeloma proteins, *J. Exp. Med.* **101**:85.

Sogn, J. A. Coligan, J. E., and Kindt, T. J., 1977, The use of idiotypes as markers for antibody variable regions in the rabbit, *Fed. Proc.* **36**:214.

Stemke, G. W., 1964, Allotypic specificities of A- and B-chains of rabbit gamma globulin, *Science* **145**:403.

Todd, C. W., 1963, Allotypy in rabbit 19S protein, *Biochem. Biophys. Res. Comm.* **11**:170.

Todd, C. W., 1972, Genetic control of H chain biosynthesis in the rabbit, *Fed. Proc.* **31**:188.

Wang, A. C., Wilson, K., Hopper, J. E., Fudenberg, H. H., and Nisonoff, A., 1970, Evidence for control of synthesis of the variable regions of heavy chains of immunoglobulins G and M by the same gene, *Proc. Natl. Acad. Sci. USA* **66**:337.

Weigert, M., and Potter, M., 1977, Antibody varible-region genetics: Summary and abstracts of the homogeneous immunoglobulin workshop VII, *Immunogenetics* **4**:401.

Weiler, E., 1965, Differential activity of allelic γ-globulin genes in antibody-producing cells, *Proc. Natl. Acad. Sci. USA* **54**:1765.

Wells, J. V., Fudenberg, H. H., and Givol, D., 1973, Localization of idiotype antigenic determinants in the F_v region of murine myeloma protein MOPC 315, *Proc. Natl. Acad. Sci. USA* **70**:1585.

Williams, R., Kunkel, H. G., and Capra, J. D., 1968, Antigenic specificities related to the cold agglutinin activity in γM macroglobulins, *Science* **161**:379.

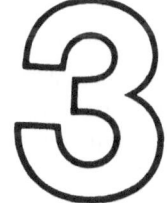

THE BIOCHEMIST'S APPROACH TO THE PROBLEM

Mystery, or unknowing, is energy. As soon as a mystery is explained, it ceases to be a source of energy.

—JOHN FOWLES *(The Aristos)*

Mixtures of antibodies were sufficient for serologic studies since extremely specific antisera could detect micrograms of an idiotype present in milligrams of an immunoglobulin mixture. The ground rules for the biochemical analysis of antibodies, however, are completely different. These studies require large amounts of antibodies that are not only directed against a single specificity, but that represent a single protein moiety.

3.1. BIOCHEMICAL STUDIES ON HETEROGENEOUS ANTIBODIES

The initial achievements in the elucidation of the chemical structure of immunoglobulins came painfully slowly because of the disconcerting degree of heterogeneity among the immunoglobulins. Defined originally as the slowest-moving electrophoretic group of serum proteins, gamma globulins had the unique properties of antibody activity and marked heterogeneity. The term gamma globulin was given more biologic and physiologic meaning than restriction to an electrophoretic group by Fahey, who in 1961 applied the term to all serum proteins "known to be found in plasmacytes and lymphoid cells." Further physiochemical and immunochemical procedures amplified the notion of diversity within this protein group. The molecular size range was immense. Most gamma globulins had molecular weights of 150,000, but ultracentrifugation studies demonstrated that about 10% of gamma globulins had molecular weights in the neighborhood of one million and were termed gamma macroglobulins or 19 S globulins. Appreciation of two major groups of globulins led to some of the first insights into the biologic complexity of the antibody response. For example, some antigens gave rise almost exclusively to macroglobulin antibodies and others largely to gamma G antibodies. The variety of antibody elicited further depended on the route and duration of immunization.

Despite the barricade presented by this unwieldly heterogeneity, immunoglobulins shared sufficient structural features that independently Porter and Edelman as well as others were able to unravel their basic structure. In a classic paper in 1950 that was a predecessor to his more definitive study in 1959, Porter cleaved rabbit antibodies into two fragments termed Fab for fragment antigen binding, and Fc for fragment

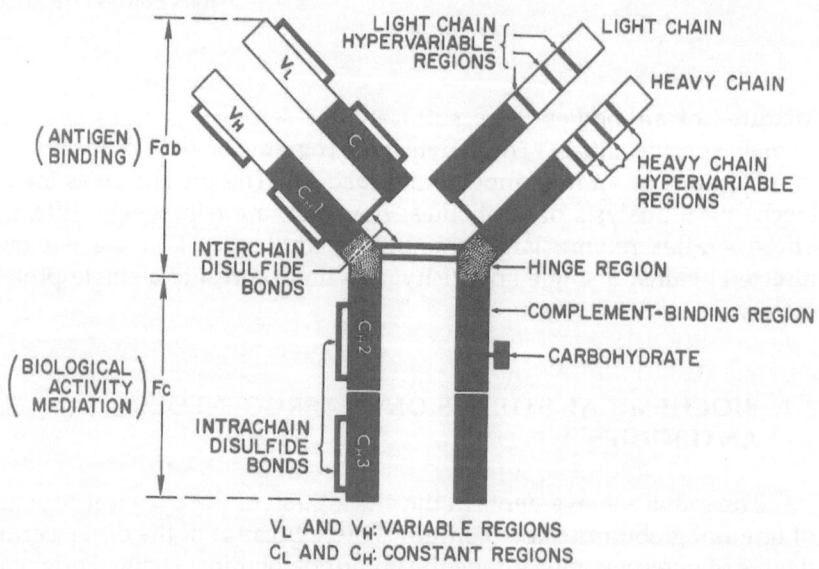

Figure 3.1. A modern version of the four-chain model for the IgG molecule.

crystallizable. Concurrently, studies were carried out on the susceptibility of gamma globulins to chemical reduction resulting in the notion
that gamma globulin molecules are composed of "discrete subunits or
polypeptide chains linked by disulfide bonds" as enunciated by Edelman
and Poulik in 1961. After demonstrating the dissociation of gamma globulins on reduction into polypeptides of differing molecular weight Porter
formulated the formal four-chain model of the immunoglobulin consisting of two identical heavy chains and two identical light chains in-
terlinked by disulfide bonds and noncovalent interactions. Although
there are some variations on this basic structure, the original model has
weathered remarkably well. An updated version of the four chain structure is shown in Fig. 3.1 and will serve as a focal point for much of this
chapter.

3.2. BIOCHEMICAL STUDIES ON HOMOGENEOUS ANTIBODIES

A more precise understanding of structure–function relationships
of the antibody molecule required circumvention of the heterogeneity
problem and a search for homogeneous immunoglobulins ensued. Nature was obliging in its capacity to expand a single immunoglobulin
species through the neoplastic process of myelomatosis. This neoplasm
has been observed in a number of species, but its products have been
most thoroughly explored in man and mouse. It was largely through
the persistent efforts of Kunkel (1965) that the human myeloma protein
came to center stage in studies of the human immune system and similarly through Potter (1967) that the BALB/c myeloma protein emerged
as the cornerstone of the murine immune system.

3.2.1. Human Myeloma

The early biochemical analysis of immunoglobulins of a homogeous
nature came largely through structural analyses of human multiple myeloma proteins. These were obtainable in relatively large amounts (10
to 50 mg/ml) from the blood of patients afflicted with this disorder (see
Fig. 3.2) and it was relatively easy to obtain enough homogeneous material for primary structural analysis. These proteins proved valuable in
defining the classes and subclasses and serving as prototypes for allotypic studies. Those with antibody activity such as the cold agglutinins

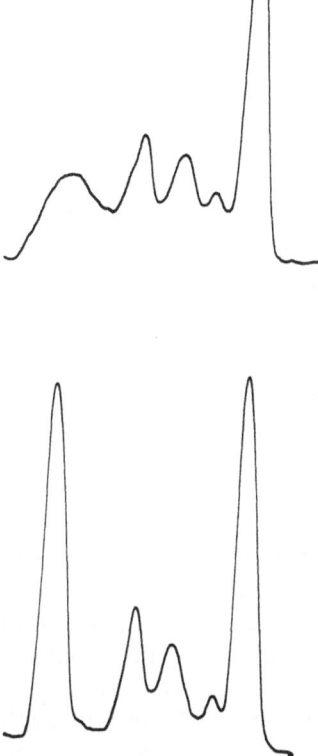

Figure 3.2. Paper electrophoresis of normal human serum (top) and a myeloma serum (bottom). The large peak on the right is albumin. Note the massive "spike" in the gamma region of the bottom profile. Both human and mouse myeloma sera have this characteristic component.

and antigamma globulins were crucial in deducing the principle of cross idiotypic specificity (see Chapter 2). With few exceptions, however, these proteins did not have defined antibody activity and, as such, whereas they provided important biochemical insights, they were generally uninformative in issues of antibody specificity. A second serious drawback of studies of human myeloma proteins is the outbred nature of the human population. Thus, structural variation could be attributable to allelic differences that had accumulated over evolutionary time. Thus, it was difficult to relate structural differences [particularly in the variable (V) region] of human immunoglobulins to issues of antibody diversity. Despite these difficulties human myeloma proteins were crucial in deducing a number of concepts.

3.2.2. Mouse Myeloma

In 1967, Potter reported the crucial discovery that myeloma can be induced through intraperitoneal injections of mineral oil in the BALB/c inbred mouse. The impact of that discovery cannot be overstated.

Although mouse myelomas were easily induced in the BALB/c strain, other strains did not respond to the injection of mineral oil. However, by clever breeding experiments, Potter was able to separate susceptibility to myeloma induction from heavy chain allotype and produced a number of heavy chain congenic mice on a BALB/c background. By raising myelomas in these mice, homogenous immunoglobulins from several other heavy chain allotypes soon became available for analysis. The primary structures of these molecules will be discussed later.

Although there is a perennial controversy concerning whether or not these paraprotein immunoglobulins truly represent normal antibody molecules, genetic, chemical, and physical criteria indicated that they did. Most influential, however, in the elevation of myeloma proteins to relevance, were observations of their binding capacity when tested against a variety of ligands. Many human myeloma proteins had demonstrated binding activities against gamma globulins, red cells, streptococcal products, and lipoproteins. Although the myeloma proteins in the BALB/c mouse could not be systematically induced to particular antigens, it became evident in the early 1970s that a number had antibody activity against certain polysaccharides. These may have arisen because the animals are colonized with gut flora with polysaccharide antigens on their surfaces. Many of these myeloma proteins spawned the idiotypic systems that have been so useful in analyses of the antibody repertoire, but for the present purpose they opened the avenue for detailed chemical analysis of antibodies by amino acid sequencing. Since immunoglobulins all had the same basic polypeptide chain structure, it was reasoned that heterogeneity must lie at the level of primary structure.

3.2.3. Other Homogeneous Antibodies

In 1965, Krause found that certain rabbits immunized with streptococcal vaccine produced antibodies with restricted heterogeneity in concentrations of 30 to 50 mg/ml of serum. This discovery made available homogeneous antibodies of defined specificity that proved crucial in the elucidation of antibody variation in yet another species. Even more important, the homogeneous rabbit antibodies allowed an unraveling of the mysteries of the structural basis of rabbit allotypy. This represented the first system in which homogeneous antibodies could be systematically raised to defined antigens. Several workers extended the antigenic repertoire of rabbit antibodies from streptococcal group A and C carbohydrates to the pneumococcal carbohydrates, and later to such diverse antigens as those on *Micrococcus lysodeikticus* and to various aromatic compounds. Figure 3.3 illustrates that the capacity of rabbits to develop homogeneous antibodies is a heritable characteristic.

Cebra's group pioneered studies on the induced antibody response of inbred guinea pigs and the amino acid sequences of the two subclasses IgG1 and IgG2 from two different strains of guinea pig were elucidated. More importantly, antibodies were raised against several different haptens such as arsonate so that structure-specificity correlations could be made for the first time. These relatively homogeneous antibodies, in addition, provided some of the first molecules to be affinity labeled in order to deduce the relationship between primary structure and the antibody-combining site.

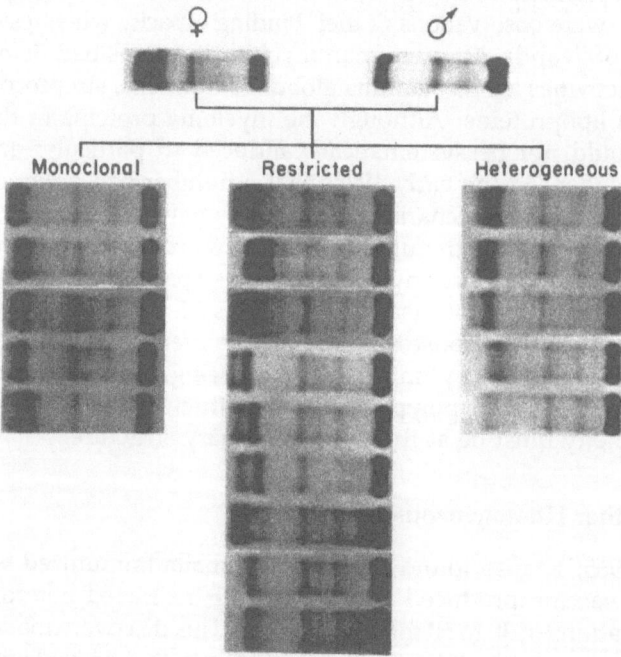

Figure 3.3. Microzone electrophoretic patterns of the second immunization antisera of one pair of rabbit breeders and their 19 offspring. All rabbits were immunized with group C streptococcal vaccine. This shows that rabbits who develop homogeneous antibodies on immunization tend to have offspring with similar homogeneous responses. (From Krause, 1970.)

Multiple myeloma was described in dogs, cats, and many other species and served as an important vehicle for the study of the structural basis of immunoglobulin evolution.

3.2.4. Hybridomas

Somatic cell fusion is a spontaneously occurring phenomenon originally described experimentally with plant protoplasts in the 1930s. The controlled experimental applicability of cell fusion was first brought to the attention of the immunological community by Kohler and Milstein in 1975. By fusing spleen cells from a mouse previously immunized with sheep erythrocytes with a drug-sensitive myeloma cell line, they were able to obtain in culture a continuous cell line with the growth characteristics of the tumor parent and the capacity to secrete not only the tumor immunoglobulin molecule but also antisheep red blood cell antibody. With the development of nonsecreting myeloma variants and techniques for fusion with polyethylene glycol, this procedure for isolating monoclonal antibody-secreting cell lines has gained widespread popularity. Since such cells can be grown indefinitely in vitro or as ascites tumors in mice, they are an excellent source of material for structural analysis. For induced antibody systems, they allow complete biochemical analysis at a level not previously obtainable: the single cell.

Contemporary immunoglobulin structural studies have almost exclusively turned to the hybridoma antibody as a molecule of defined specificity that can be generated in any inbred mouse strain and immortalized. Recent techniques for switching heavy chain isotypes in hybridoma cell lines have allowed extremely elegant experiments to be done with immunoglobulins expressing identical V regions but different C regions.

3.3. STRUCTURAL FEATURES OF IMMUNOGLOBULIN ISOTYPES AND ALLOTYPES

Although it was found that the major diversity of antibodies occurred in the variable region, background information on the constant regions is essential in order to appreciate the arguments that will be presented. At the present time, precise biochemical information is available on the five immunoglobulin classes of man and mouse. In man, these structures were achieved largely through the efforts of Hilschman and Putnam who independently sequenced kappa and lambda chains from human Bence Jones proteins and most of the heavy chain classes, subclasses, and allotypic variants. In the mouse, although much of this information was available at the protein level from the work of Hood (kappa), Appella (lambda), Fougereau (IgG2a), Milstein (IgG1), Hood (IgM), and Eisen (IgA), recently all of the murine immunoglobulin isotypes have been sequenced at the DNA level. In addition, kappa chains have been completely sequenced in rabbit and rat, IgG molecules have been completely sequenced in guinea pig and rabbit, and IgM molecules in the dog.

3.3.1. The Human Immunoglobulin Classes

The first complete structure of an immunoglobulin molecule was reported by Edelman in 1969. The structure not only verified many notions concerning immunoglobulin structure but, in addition, out of it emerged the domain concept that has permeated the field ever since. Edelman noted (as had Hill before) that certain regions of the molecule seemed to be homologous with other regions. With the entire structure available, he was able to study homology relationships and noted that the Ig molecule seemed to be constructed from domains consisting of 110 amino acid residues. Edelman reasoned that they might be the units of evolution and argued that the domains evolved to subserve separate and distinct biologic functions. Thus V_H and V_L (see Fig. 3.1) evolved as antigen-specificity regions, whereas CH2 evolved (as it was later shown) to serve as the "receptor" for the first component of complement. It has since been learned that each domain has a similar three-dimensional structure and, as will be discussed in a later chapter, the domain boundaries were remarkably close to the intron–exon junctions in the DNA.

With the recent publication of the amino acid sequence of human immunoglobulin D, the last of the immunoglobulins in man has been completely sequenced. Figure 3.4 presents the amino acid sequence in single letter code of the two C-terminal domains of all five immunoglobulin classes and illustrates several crucial points. Since this figure has been taken from a paper by Putnam, the comparisons have been made to the delta chain, which was the last of the human immunoglobulins to be sequenced. The alignment is so arranged that the top two and the bottom two groups of rows represent, respectively, amino acid residues encoded by putative exons for the last two constant domains of each heavy chain class. Gaps have been introduced into the alignment to account for possible deletion/insertion events and to achieve optimal homology among the five chains. The invariant cystine (C) and tryptophan (W) residues in each domain have been used to place the

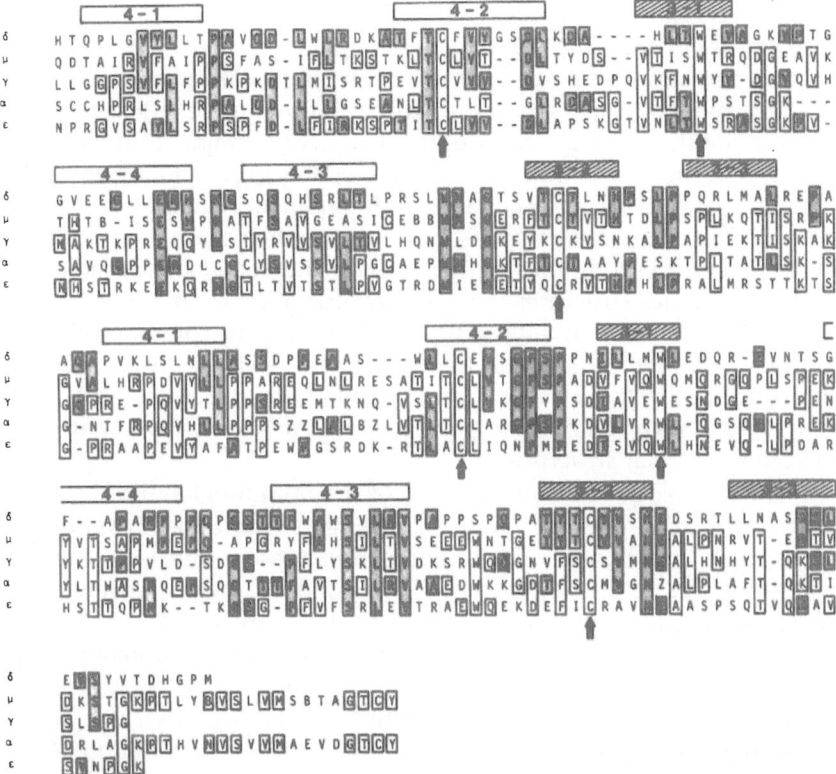

Figure 3.4. Comparison of the amino acid sequence of the Fc portions of all five immunoglobulin classes of man. Residues in the mu, gamma, alpha, or epsilon chains that share identity with the delta chain are outlined by a shaded box. Open boxes depict homologies that do not involve delta. See text for additional details. From Lin and Putnam (1981).

alignment in register, and these are indicated by the arrows. Residues in the mu, gamma, alpha, or epsilon chains that share their identity with the corresponding residues in the delta chain are outlined by a shaded box; residues that show homology among sequences other than the delta chain are outlined by open boxes. The beta strands are numbered according to the three-dimensional model proposed by Edmundson and are indicated above each row, with the four-stranded beta sheet elements in open bars, and the three-stranded beta sheet elements in hatchbars. Figure 3.5 can be used for reference in this regard, and represents a modification of data presented by Edmundson as modified by Putnam to illustrate the delta chain Fc region.

Several key points can be made from Fig. 3.4. First note that there are 17 positions in this stretch in which all immunoglobulin molecules have an identical amino acid residue. Thus, for example, in the top row of Fig. 3.4, there is a proline, a threonine, a cystine, and a tryptophan residue found in all five sequences. This homology among *all* the immunoglobulin constant regions is strong evidence for their common evolutionary origin. Interestingly enough, when one looks at molecules that have similar structures, such as beta-two microglobulin, rat Thy-1, and even histocompatibility antigens, they have in common with immunoglobulin molecules these same invariant residues. This argues for the common evolutionary origin of all of these structures and/or the convergent evolution of these particular residues to sustain a particular three-dimensional structure.

The homology between any two of the immunoglobulin classes in man is approximately 30%. Indeed, within a species, that is as close to a structural definition of an immunoglobulin class as there is. The amino acid sequences of C_κ, C_λ, C_α, C_μ, C_δ, C_γ, and C_ε, no matter how compared, are approximately 30% identical. This is in contrast to the subclasses of immunoglobulin G or A in man, where the homology is approximately 95%.

Further inspection of the Fc sequences for the five classes of human immunoglobulins shown in Fig. 3.4 shows that the distribution of ho-

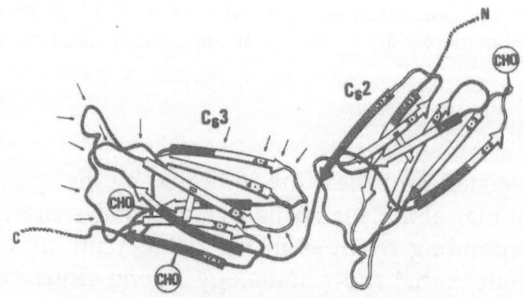

Figure 3.5. Spatial model of the IgD Fc region. The shading on the backbone indicates the extent of sequence homology between the five immunoglobulin classes. The open areas indicate areas of highest homology. Note the location of carbohydrate residues (CHO) largely on the surface. The large arrows indicate the direction of the polypeptide chain, and form the "beta-barrel" structure common to all immunoglobulin domains. Modified from Edmundson by Putnam. From Lin and Putnam, (1981).

mologous residues is not random, but fall into certain patterns that are revealed in the spatial model shown in Fig. 3.5. Residues that are highly conserved tend to be clustered within segments of beta-pleated sheets, especially around the two cystines that form the intrachain disulfide bond, and a tryptophan that is nearby in the three-dimensional structure.

3.3.2. The Carbohydrate Structures of Human Immunoglobulins

The classes of immunoglobulin differ considerably in the number and location of carbohydrate groups; however, oligosaccharide groups are often found in homologous positions, usually between domains or on the domain surface. Carbohydrate is usually found only on heavy chain C regions except for a few instances in which the tripeptide acceptor sequence Asn-X-Ser/Thr is found in the V region.

Figure 3.6 aligns the carbohydrate groups of seven human heavy chains. Homologous positions of carbohydrate attachment are represented by the solid boxes. Putnam described five sets of these homologous positions between the human immunoglobulin classes:

1. In the first constant domain of alpha 2, mu, and epsilon.
2. Before the hinge in alpha 2 A2m(2) and epsilon (in $C_\varepsilon 2$).
3. Within the hinge region (GalN moieties are found in alpha 1 and delta chains, GlcN in mu chains).
4. Forty residues into the first domain of Fc region in alpha 1, delta, mu, and epsilon, i.e., $C_\gamma 2$, $C_\delta 2$, $C_\mu 3$, $C_\varepsilon 3$. In gamma chains where the three-dimensional structure is known, this carbohydrate serves to separate the two $C_\gamma 2$ domains.
5. Fourteen residues from the carboxy-terminus of the extended "tail" in alpha and mu chains. This extension is found on the secreted form of these heavy chains and is replaced by a hydrophobic segment in the membrane-bound forms.

Carbohydrate attachment sites are often conserved between species in comparable classes of heavy chains. The single carbohydrate in human IgG1 is found in a homologous position in some gamma chains of mouse, rabbit, and guinea pig, suggesting that the carbohydrate may have structural and/or functional significance. Carbohydrate seems to play a role in the transport and secretion of glycosylated proteins. Inhibiting the glycosylation of polypeptide chains such as alpha or epsilon heavy chains has been shown to prevent secretion of IgA and IgE. This may also be true for the gamma chains, or carbohydrate may act as a scaffolding to hold domains in their proper functional positions and may protect the

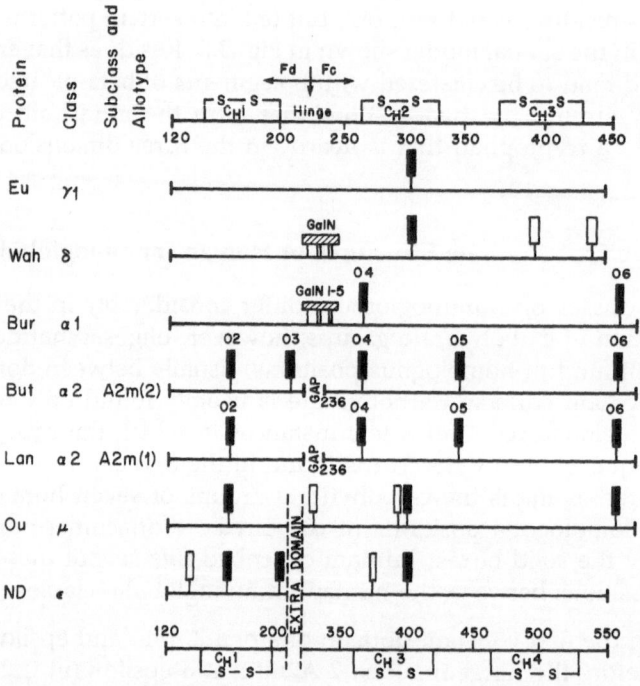

Figure 3.6. Location of the carbohydrate in human heavy chains. Glucosamine oligosaccharides are represented by vertical bars; shaded if in homologous positions in two or more chains, open if in unique positions. Horizontal striated bars show the positions of galactosamine oligosaccharides. The upper scale gives residue positions for the top five chains; the lower scale gives positions for mu and epsilon chains. Adapted from Lin and Putnam (1981).

molecule from degradation by protecting sites sensitive to proteolysis. Structure–function relationships may also be correlated with carbohydrates found in nonhomologous positions, since these may play a role in determining the unique functional properties of each class.

3.3.3. Comparisons of Immunoglobulins from Different Species

Figure 3.7 presents the C-region sequence of the kappa chain of four different species, rat, mouse, human, and rabbit. The sequences have been updated (in many instances by personal communication). Notice the tremendous homology from species to species documenting their common evolutionary origin. As expected, the closest homology is between the rat and mouse. Human and rabbits obviously derived

```
        110        120         130          140
Rat     R A N A A P T V S I F P P S T E Q L A T G G A S V V C L M N K F Y P R D I S V K
Mouse   R A D A A P T V S I F P P S S E Q L T S G G A S V V C F L N N F Y P K D I N V K
Human   R T V A A P S V F I F P P S D E Q L K S G T A S V V C L L N N F Y P R E A K V Q
Rabbit  G D P V A P T V L I F P P A A D Q V A T G T V T I V C V A N K Y F P R D V T V T
        150        160         170          180
Rat     W K I D G T E R R N G V L N S V T B Q D S K D S T Y S M S S T L S L T K A D Y Q
Mouse   W K I D G S E R Q N G V L N S D T Z W D S K D S T Y S M S S T L T L T K D E Y E
Human   W K V D N A L Q S G N S Q E S V T Z Q D S K D S T Y S L S S T L T L S K A D Y E
Rabbit  W E V D G T T Q T T G I E N S K T P Q D S A D C T Y N L S S T L T L T S T Q Y N
        190        200         210
Rat     S H N L Y T C Q V V H K T S S S P V V K N F N R N E C
Mouse   R H N S Y T C E A T H K T S T S P I V K S F N R N E C
Human   K H K L Y A C E V T H Q G L S S P V T K S F N R G E C
Rabbit  S H K E Y T C K V T H Q G T T S P V V Q S F N R G D C
```

Figure 3.7. The amino acid sequence of the kappa constant region from four species.

from separate phylogenetic orders, whereas rat and mouse belong to the same order. Typically, when immunoglobulins of the same class or light chain type from different species are compared, the homology is approximately 60%. An exception to this appears to be in the mu chain where comparison of the sequence between mouse, dog, and human IgM indicates homologies of greater than 90% (see Fig. 3.8). Thus, the

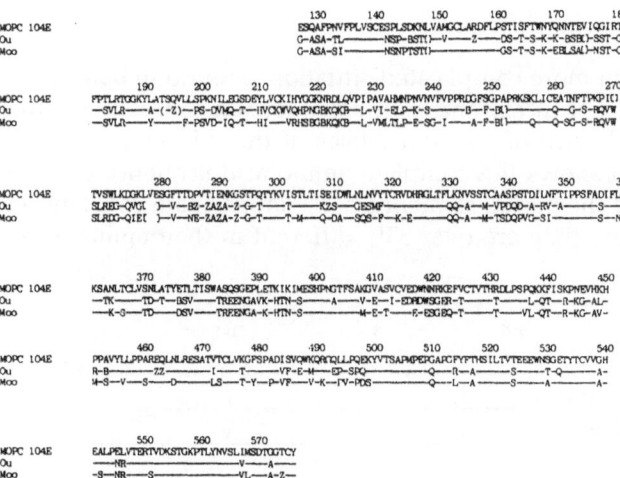

Figure 3.8. Amino acid sequence of mouse (104E), human (Ou), and canine (Moo) IgM heavy chain. A straight line indicates identity with the mouse sequence. This figure illustrates the extraordinary amino acid sequence homology of the IgM molecule between three species. Other classes are not so highly conserved. From McCumber *et al.* (1980).

structure of the mu chain has been more rigidly preserved in evolution than any of the other isotypes that have been sequenced to date.

3.3.4. Immunoglobulin Allotypes

3.3.4.1. Simple Allotypes

Perhaps the simplest example of allotypic variation in immunology is represented by the Inv or Km locus in man. There is but one kappa C region in man and it occurs in three known allelic forms termed Km 1, Km 1,2, and Km 3 as shown in Fig. 3.9. The entire sequence from position 108 to 214 of the C region of human kappa chains is identical in all humans, with the exception of positions 153 and 191, which vary as shown in Fig. 3.9. These amino acid variations have been definitively correlated with the allotype, and in three-dimensional models, positions 153 and 191 are adjacent and the epitope they define is on the surface.

There are a number of other examples of simple allotypes among the immunoglobulins, some of which have been alluded to already. Thus, the d and e allotypes of the rabbit gamma chain C region (Fig. 2.2) and most of the human Gm markers fall into this category of single amino acid substitutions.

3.3.4.2. Complex Allotypes

A much more complicated situation is found in both the rabbit and the rat. Except in extremely unusual circumstances, individual rabbits express only two of the four alleles of the b locus b4, b5, b6, and b9. Figure 3.10 shows the complete amino acid sequence of rabbit b4, b5, and b9 and the partial sequence of b6 kappa chain constant regions. As is illustrated, they are over 33% different in their amino acid sequence

	108	153	191	214
KM 1		V	L	OOO⁻
KM 1,2		A	L	OOO⁻
KM 3		A	V	OOO⁻

Figure 3.9. The human kappa chain and its three allelic forms. Only the variations are shown. Of all the human kappa constant regions sequenced, only these three variants have been described. In the three-dimensional structure, residues 153 and 191 come in close approximation and form a single epitope.

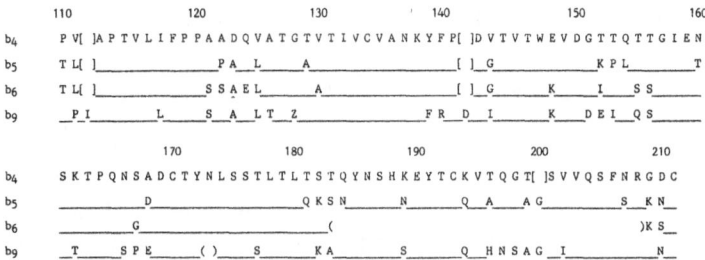

Figure 3.10. The complete amino acid sequence of the constant regions of rabbit kappa chains derived from rabbits with different C_K genetic markers. The structures are remarkable for their *differences* including insertions-deletions.

and require three sequence gaps for maximum homology. It is difficult, using conventional genetic arguments, to explain these dramatic differences in the products of presumably allelic genes.

A similar situation exists in rat C_κ system. Serologically, inbred rats express two distinct alleles. The amino acid sequence of the C regions of these two "alleles" is shown in Fig. 3.11. The variation, although not as great as in the rabbit, is nonetheless rather dramatic, and later studies (Chapter 7) will point out that it has been definitively shown that there is, in fact, a single C_κ gene in each rat.

The complex allotypes were important in pointing out unusual features of rabbit and rat immunogenetics and placed obstacles to certain theories of antibody diversity. The variations in these "constant" regions were as great as the variations in the variable region and many authors ascribed similar genetic mechanisms to the V regions as to the C regions.

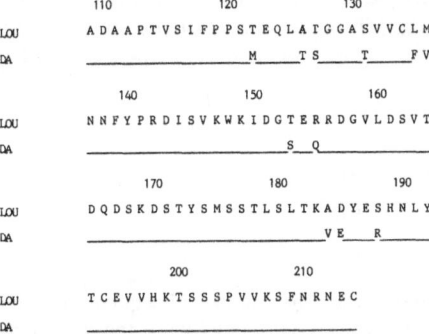

Figure 3.11. The complete amino acid sequence of the constant regions of rat kappa chains derived from rats with different C_K genetic markers (from G. Gutman, personal communication).

3.4. STRUCTURAL FEATURES OF V REGIONS

3.4.1. V-Region Subgroups

An appreciation of the detailed organization of immunoglobulin chains began with light chains and was obtained from sequencing efforts carried out in several laboratories, particularly those of Hilschmann and Craig, Putnam, Milstein, Hood, Niall and Edman, and Edelman. These studies in the late 1960s indicated that each kappa and lambda chain within a species could be divided into an amino terminal V region (positions 1 to 108), differing substantially among different proteins, and a carboxyterminal half or C region (positions 109 to 214), highly conserved among different proteins of the same isotype (see Fig. 3.1). Different light chains could be further classified into subgroups according to amino acid sequence of the V regions. The discovery of subgroups by Nial and Edman, Baglioni, Edelman and Gall, and Milstein was one of the most important advances of the late 1960s, and it had a direct bearing on the antibody problem.

As shown in Fig. 3.12, human immunoglobulin kappa chains can be easily divided into three subgroups based on the amino acid sequence of the amino terminal 108 residues. Only the first 25 residues are shown for illustrative purposes. The sequences shown have been chosen from the more than 100 human kappa chain V regions that have been sequenced to date. Virtually any representative of the three human V_κ subgroups could have been used for this purpose. Note that there are a number of positions (5,6,7,8,11,16,23,24) in which all three subgroups have the same amino acid. These are the so-called invariant positions, and in this illustration they represent about one third of the positions. The second structural feature of note is that there are several positions (1,3,4,10,12,14,15,17,18,20,21,22,25) in which two of the subgroups have one amino acid and the third subgroup has a second amino acid. This pattern occurs in 13 of the first 25 positions or roughly half, and suggests the existence of a common evolutionary ancestor for the three groups

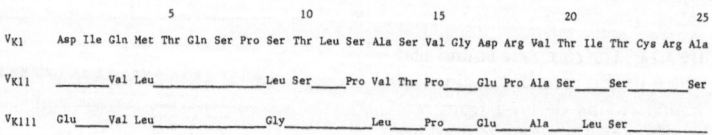

Figure 3.12. The amino acid sequence of the amino terminal 25 residues of three human kappa chains representative of the three major V_K subgroups. A line indicates identity with the topmost sequence.

that diverged subsequent to gene duplication. Note that there is no particular pattern in that neither of the two subgroups has more amino acids in common, suggesting that the three subgroups emerged relatively early in evolution. In only two positions of the N terminal 25 positions (9,13) are all three subgroups represented by different amino acids.

One of the most important consequences of the discovery of V-region subgroups in the kappa chain was evident at the 1967 Cold Spring Harbor Symposium when it became clear that more than one gene would be required to encode immunoglobulin V regions. The reasoning went as follows: As long as the variation observed among V_κ proteins appeared to be random, proponents of somatic mutation could argue that each amino acid substitution represented an independent somatic event. However, with the separation of human kappa chain V regions into three distinct subgroups, none of which could be easily generated by recombination with the other two, each subgroup had to be separately encoded. Thus, it was agreed that there had to be at least three human V_κ genes. There then came a semantic argument concerning exactly what constituted a subgroup, that is, how many substitutions would be required before designating a set of V regions as a separate V-region subgroup. The argument became more than semantic because the definition of the subgroup became one of the most hotly contested issues in the debate about the germline and somatic theories during the next decade. It was universally conceded that each subgroup required a separate germline gene; therefore, the "germliners" tended to use a very restrictive definition of a subgroup, whereas the "somaticists" used a looser definition.

Another important concept to be gleaned from Fig. 3.12 is that of "linked substitutions" that are at the core of the definition of a subgroup. For example, most proteins that have Gln-Met in positions 3 and 4 have serine at position 9, alanine at position 13, valine at position 19, and alanine at position 25. Thus, one can begin to predict the sequence of the entire V region based on a few positions.

The amino acid differences between members of different V-region subgroups cannot be precisely stated because of the imprecise definition of a subgroup. However, within the human system where three or four V_κ subgroups are fairly well defined, members of the same subgroup are identical at approximately 75% of their positions, whereas members of different subgroups are identical at only 50% of their amino acid positions. In the mouse, where there are many more subgroups, the subgroup distinction (particularly among the kappa subgroups) is less evident and there is less intra- and intersubgroup variation.

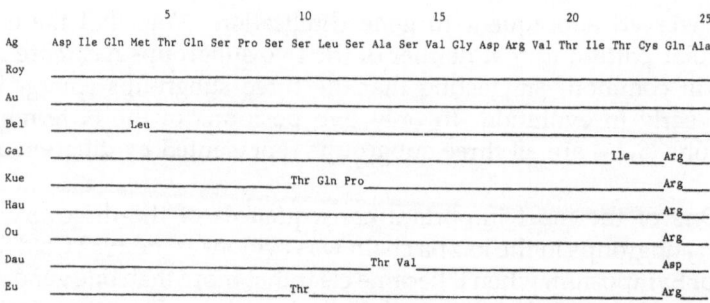

Figure 3.13. Amino terminal sequences of ten human V_K1 proteins. Residue positions identical with protein Ag are indicated by a straight line. Only variations are indicated.

Figure 3.13 illustrates the N-terminal 25 amino acid residues of ten different human proteins of the same subgroup ($V_\kappa 1$) in order to illustrate the variation that occurs within a V-region subgroup. The variations seen are largely random, although some exceptions will be discussed below. For the most part the substitutions tend to be conservative, both in terms of the genetic code and the hydrophilic–hydrophobic nature of the amino acid, as well as the size and bulkiness of the side chains involved. As the three-dimensional structure of the molecules became available, it was clear that the majority of these substitutions would have relatively little impact on the overall tertiary structure of an antibody molecule.

Similar sequence studies on human lambda chains have shown the presence of five V-region subgroups and three or four subgroups have been described for human heavy chains.

In the case of kappa chains, the three subgroups are isotypic rather than allotypic, since all three can be detected in the serum of any normal individual. Therefore, unless all subgroups are repeatedly reproduced in all individuals from one gene by somatic mutation and selection, they must be considered to be analogous to the classes of the C region. If this latter interpretation is accepted then for the human kappa, lambda, and heavy chains, there must be a minimum of three (kappa) to five (lambda) structural genes, each gene encoding one of the basic V-region subgroups.

In addition to differences specifying the three major subgroups within human kappa chains, there are also many positions in which either of two residues are equally likely to occur. For example, at position 24 of $V_\kappa 1$ (Fig. 3.13), glutamine is found in about half of the proteins and arginine in the other half. Milstein found no evidence of allelism associated with this position, both amino acids being present in all individuals tested. This and other similar analyses suggest further subdivision of the subgroups.

The subgroups of kappa, lambda, and heavy chains appear to be quite distinct, and furthermore, no kappa-type subgroup has been found in association with a lambda-type C region. Thus, it seems that each C-region gene or set of genes associates with a distinct pool of V-region genes.

Though V-region subgroup distinctions have often been subject to semantic controversy, differences of 40 of 108 V-region residues between light chains raised the possibility that the sequences were encoded by a single germline gene. In contrast, limited variation was found in the sequence of kappa C regions. This led to an early realization of the utility of amino acid sequencing in establishing a firm structural and genetic basis for the occurrence of serologic and genetic markers.

As described above, amino acid sequencing early revealed its power to provide insight into the nature of the antibody molecule; however, compilations of many sequences were required before fundamental questions about antigen binding and specificity could be addressed.

3.4.2. Framework and Hypervariable Regions

The sequence variability of the V region is not random but is organized on a surprisingly precise basis. Most notably, as first pointed out for light chains by Milstein and by Wu and Kabat (1970) and for heavy chains by Capra (1971), immunoglobulin V regions all contain hypervariable regions in which the sequence variation from protein to protein is especially marked. Figure 3.14 shows several human heavy chains of a single V-region subgroup (V_HIII). Four segments can be termed hypervariable. These include positions 31–37, 51–68, 84–91, and 101–110. Among these, the first, second and fourth hypervariable regions have been termed complementarity determining because x-ray defraction studies of immunoglobulins have shown that these segments do, indeed, line the antibody-combining site.

A parameter termed *variability* was introduced by Kabat (Wu and Kabat, 1970) and defined as follows:

$$\text{Variability} = \frac{\text{Number of different amino acids at a given position}}{\text{Frequency of the most common amino acid at that position}}$$

in which the denominator is the number of times the most common amino acid occurs divided by the number of proteins examined. For example, in Kabat's original study of position 7 of light chains, 63 pro-

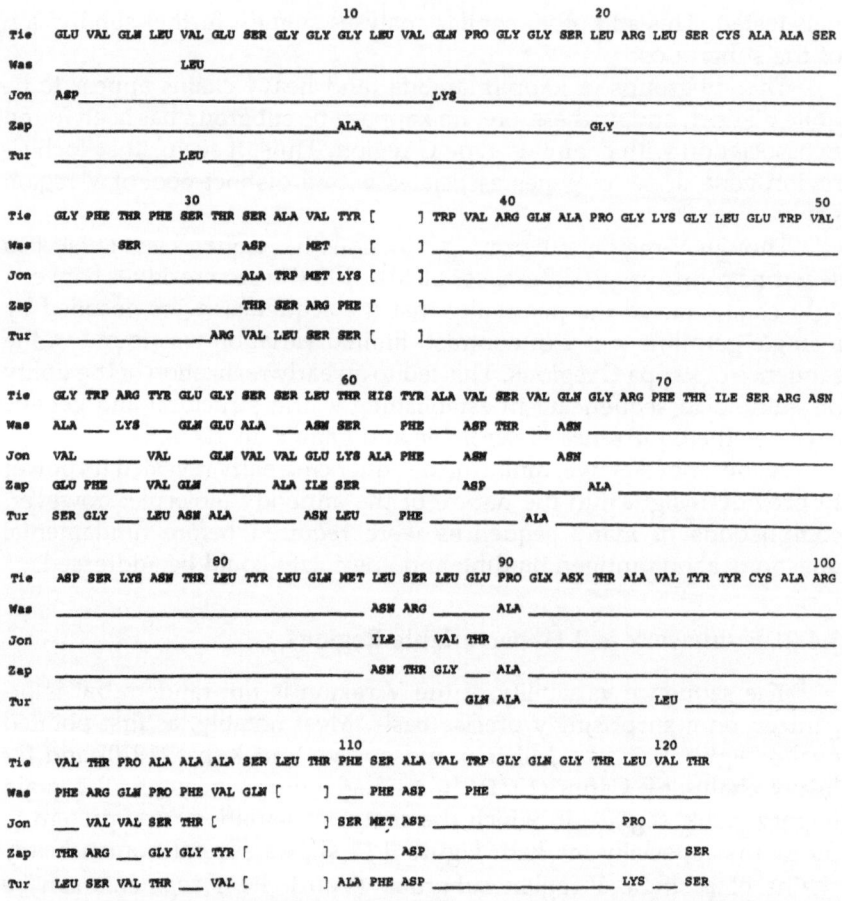

Figure 3.14. The amino acid sequence of five complete human $V_H III$ heavy chain V regions. All are compared with protein Tie, and only substitutions from the sequence are indicated. Deletions introduced to maximize homology to other V_H regions. From Capra and Kehoe (1975).

teins had been sequenced and serine occurred 41 times. Four different amino acids, proline, threonine, serine, and aspartic acid had been detected. The frequency of the most common amino acid was thus 41/63 = 0.65 and the variability was 4 divided by 0.65 = 6.15. In this equation, an invariant residue would have a variability of one, whereas the theoretical upper limit for 20 amino acids randomly occurring at any particular position would be 20 ÷ 1/20 or 400. The variability profile for the human heavy chain based on approximately four times as much data as is shown in Fig. 3.14, is shown in Fig. 3.15.

The function or significance of the heavy chain hypervariable region between positions 84 and 91 is not yet clear. It is conceivable that this segment reflects a V-region polymorphism that has yet to be elucidated. As mentioned earlier, any possible significance has been difficult to assess since until very recently the hypervariable regions in man have been defined using myeloma proteins, a system poorly suited to family studies aimed at tracing the genetic origin of a particular hypervariable region structure. Consequently, the reason for the existence of this hypervariable region remains unclear.

The position of the complementary-determining hypervariable regions in both the heavy and light chain is the same in a number of different species. This common location for hypervariable regions across a variety of animal species clearly indicates the selective advantage of this particular mechanism of generating antibody diversity in a wide variety of species existing in quite distinct environments.

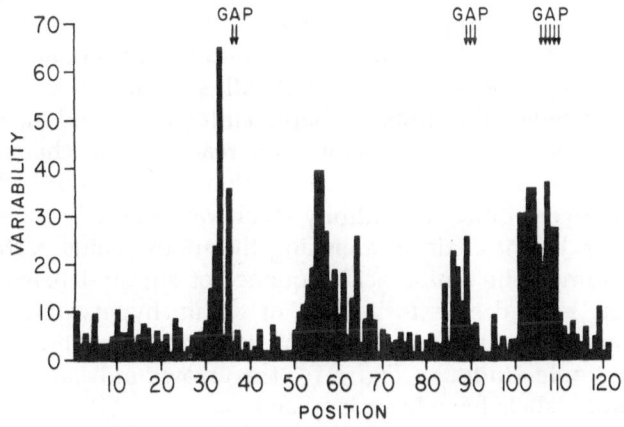

Figure 3.15. Variability of the human heavy chain V regions plotted according to the method of Wu and Kabat (1970). The arrows point to positions where deletions have been introduced in some sequences to attain maximum homology. The focus of variability around position 90 is not evident in murine heavy chains, although in rabbits it probably contributes to the heavy chain V region allotypes. It is not implicated in antigen binding. From Capra and Kehoe (1975).

Segments of the V region that are not included in the hypervariable regions (comprising approximately 80% to 85% of the total V region) have been termed the relatively invariant or *framework* regions. As shown by x-ray diffraction analysis, these segments provide a superstructure for positioning the complementarity-determining residues in an appropriate position to make contact with antigen. Especially within a given V-region subgroup, the variation between any two proteins in the framework segment is very modest (on the order of 5%). There is now no doubt that the relatively invariant segments of the V regions are responsible for the generally similar three-dimensional structure of the combining region of all antibodies. As with the hypervariable regions, the relatively invariant segments have very comparable dimensions in the immunoglobulins from the various higher animal species that have been studied to date, again, indicative of the general biologic unity reflected in this component of the humoral immune response.

3.4.3. The Antibody-Combining Site

Affinity-labeling studies of purified antibodies subsequently demonstrated that for the antibodies examined, the hypervariable regions are indeed those portions of the molecule likely containing the residues that made contact with antigen and, therefore, determine antigenic specificity. In this procedure, antibodies are first raised to a hapten-carrier complex. Then the hapten is modified, typically with a radioactive label. When the radioactive hapten is reacted with specific antibody, the specificity is provided by the antibody–hapten interaction, and the label then attaches (reacts) with amino acids with reactive side chains such as tyrosine (hydroxyl group) or lysine (epsilon amino group). When the experiments were done, the affinity label was generally found in *both* the heavy and light chain establishing that both chains participate in antigen binding. The amino acid sequence of affinity-labeled peptides revealed the labeled sites to be near or within hypervariable regions, although generally only a few hypervariable regions were ever implicated in a single study. In Fig. 3.16, the arrows indicate positions in which affinity labels have been localized.

Final support for the equation of hypervariable regions and the antigen-combining site emerged from x-ray crystallographic studies that established a cavity situated in the vicinity of the hypervariable regions. The three-dimensional structure of a Fab fragment provided a precise view of a combining site with hypervariable region sequences clustered spacially at one end of the molecule and fully exposed to solvent (Fig.

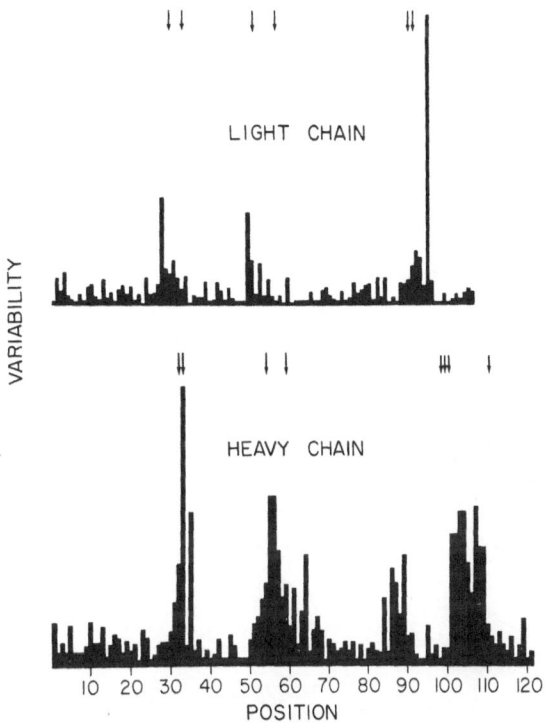

Figure 3.16. Variability at different positions for immunoglobulin heavy and light chains of all species. The positions in which affinity labels have been localized by various studies are indicated by arrows.

3.17). The structures of ligand–Fab complexes were solved in the mid 1970s for both human and mouse proteins (Fig. 3.18). This finalized the association of hypervariable regions and the antibody-combining site, a result anticipated by amino acid sequence analysis years before.

The mouse myeloma protein, MOPC 315, was originally described by Eisen as a DNP-binding protein. Its propagation and distribution throughout the world and the number of studies that have been done on this protein at the primary, secondary, and tertiary structural level have been instrumental in tying together the notions of idiotypy, hypervariable regions, and the antibody-combining site. Affinity-labeling studies of MOPC 315 were crucial in placing the hypervariable regions near the combining site, and this myeloma protein was the first in which an F_v (the heavy and light chain V regions noncovalently associated)

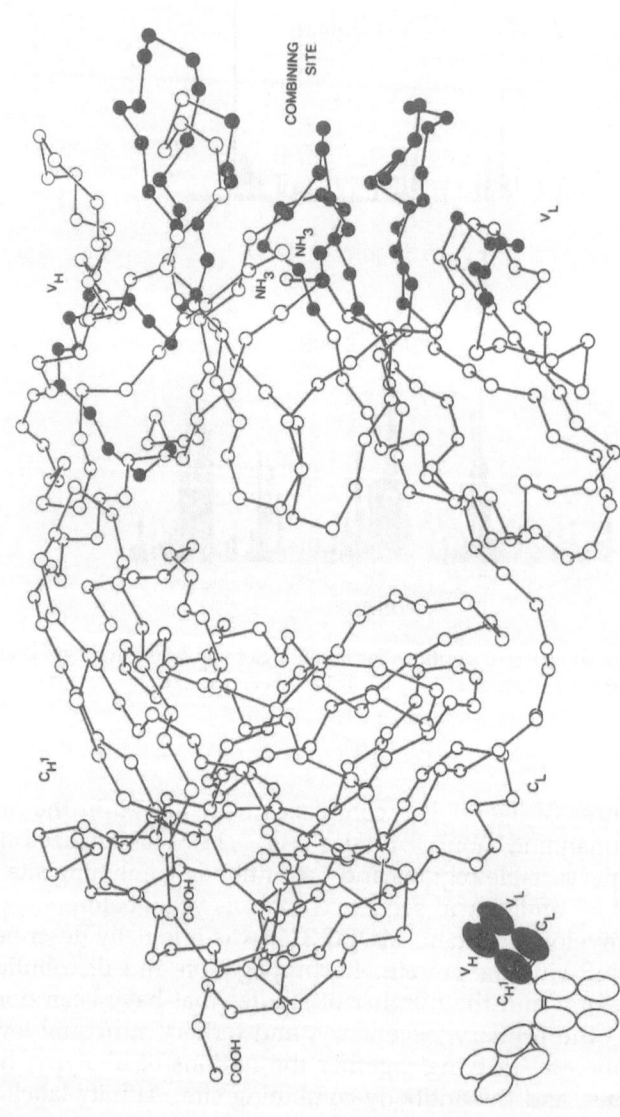

Figure 3.17. Carbon skeleton of a Fab fragment from a mouse myeloma protein designated McPC603 shows how the entire fragment is divided into closely packed C and V regions composed of paired domains from the heavy chain and light chain, and joined by extended segments called "switch regions." The combining site at the right-hand tip of the fragment is made up entirely of adjacent loops of hypervariable amino acids (shaded circles) contributed by both polypeptide chains. From Capra and Edmundson (1977).

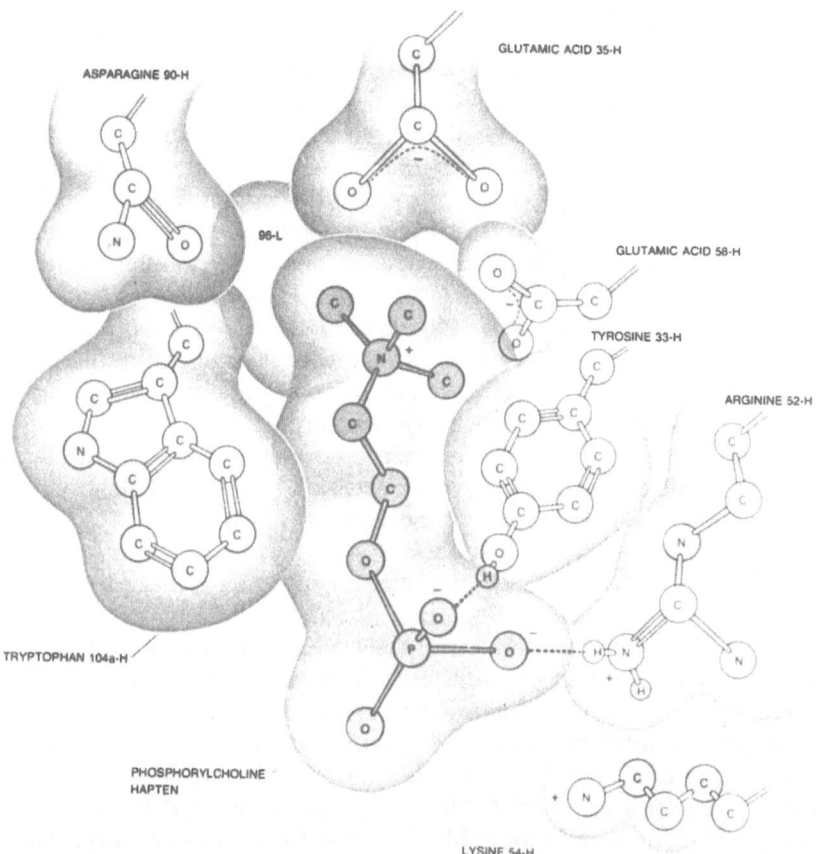

Figure 3.18. Model of the binding of the hapten phosphorylcholine to the binding site of McPC603 antibody illustrates how the shape of the site is precisely complementary to that of the hapten. In addition, amino acid side chains lining the cavity bind to hapten through weak, noncovalent interactions. Note from the designations that the combining site is composed of amino acids from all three hypervariable regions of the heavy chain but only one hypervariable region of the light chain. Three dimensional structures of several different molecules indicate a differing contribution of each of the six complementarity determining hypervariable regions to the combining site. Adapted from Davies *et al.* (1975) by Capra and Edmundson (1977).

fragment was produced that could still bind antigen. Later serologic analyses of this F_v fragment indicated that this fragment devoid of any C-region structure whatsoever bore the full complement of idiotypic determinants. These studies were the first to definitively show that the idiotype was associated with the V regions alone.

3.5. ARE THE C REGIONS REALLY CONSTANT?

One ancillary problem that should be addressed is the nature of the constancy in immunoglobulin C regions. When immunoglobulins are sequenced in two separate laboratories and minor variations are noted, the common assumption is that the minor variations are "technical" due to the enormous complexity of primary structural analysis. A few examples illustrate that the variability is, indeed, extremely minor within the C region. The complete amino acid sequence of a number of human kappa chains has been accomplished and with the exception of the positions that are known to be associated with allotypic (Km) markers, no sequence variability has been noted in over 50 proteins studied. This invariability had been revealed by extensive peptide map analysis over two decades ago. The slight variations noted between two human IgM molecules sequenced in two separate laboratories have recently been shown to be due to an allotypic variation as additional protein structures have been deduced with each of the variant structures.

In the mouse where such variation can not be due to an allelism, at least in the inbred strain, a large body of data confirms the notion that these molecules are indeed constant, although there are a few disturbing exceptions. The difference, for example, between the DNA sequence and the protein sequence of two different subclasses of IgG in different strains shows variation that remains unexplained. However, the degree of difference that may potentially exist within the C region is at the level of 1% (that is, one residue per hundred residues), whereas in the V region if no special selection processes is used (such as with idiotypic reagents), variation is likely to be at the 20% to 50% level. Thus, the extraordinary variability of the V region and the remarkable constancy of the C region seem clearly established.

3.6. STRUCTURAL ANALYSIS OF SELECTED V REGIONS

Results obtained by structural analysis of three separate systems will be examined in detail to illustrate certain principles of *subgroups*, *hypervariability*, and *idiotypy*. These are the BALB/c V_λ sequences, the BALB/c $V_\kappa 21$ sequences, and the A/J antiarsonate hybridoma light chains.

3.6.1. Mouse V_λ

Only 3% to 5% of all normal BALB/c mouse immunoglobulins contain lambda light chains. Weigert *et al.* (1970) collected approximately

18 such lambda chains and determined the amino acid sequence of the V regions of these molecules. Twelve were found to be identical. Six others differed from the twelve in from one to a maximum of three positions (see Fig. 3.19). In each instance, the variations fell within the hypervariable regions as defined by Kabat. These data were interpreted by Cohn and Weigert in the late 1960s to indicate that a single germline gene had given rise to six different somatic variants. Although two V_λ genes have been identified, both by amino acid sequence and DNA analysis, the prediction of Cohn and Weigert has proved to be remarkably precise. Over a decade ago, these structural data provided an important "test" for the germline and somatic theory polemic; the germline theory would demand that seven genes be found in the germline, whereas the somatic theory required but one. As additional mouse lambda sequences became available and "gene counting" by DNA analysis became more precise, the mouse V_λ system remained at the center of the controversy because the genes in lambda system were few enough to be actually counted. We shall return to this system in later chapters.

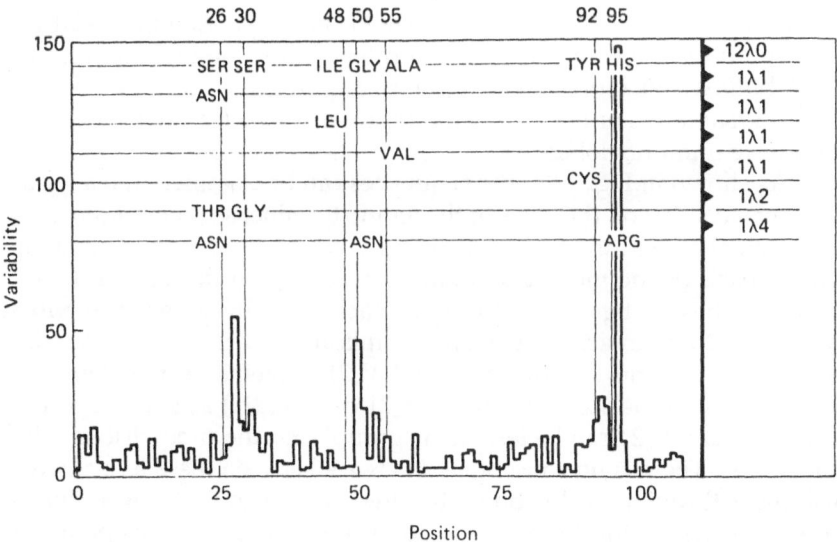

Figure 3.19. Location of amino acid substitutions in the variable region of mouse lambda chains superimposed on the variability plot for *all* light chains (see Fig. 3.18). Except where noted, all other positions were identical. To the right is noted the number of instances of each sequence and the number of changes required to generate that sequence from the top sequence. From Weigert *et al.* (1970).

3.6.2. Mouse V$_\kappa$21

The significance of the V$_\lambda$ structural analysis discussed above was controversial; many argued that the pattern of variation of V$_\lambda$ could not be extrapolated to V$_\kappa$. The argument was based on the fact that the mouse does not utilize its lambda chain locus as extensively as many other species (especially man). Weigert, who had done much of the early work in the lambda system began to approach the kappa system in much the same way. He, McKean, Potter, and others focused on a particular subgroup of mouse V$_\kappa$, termed V$_\kappa$21, which was defined by the framework structure of amino acid positions 1 to 23. The amino acid sequence of 14 mouse V$_\kappa$21 proteins was completed in the late 1970s; an update of these and several other unpublished sequences of V$_\kappa$21 proteins is shown in Fig. 3.20.

Early on, two distinct sets of V$_\kappa$21 kappa chains were identified serologically and were immediately appreciated to represent evolutionary divergent subgroups of V$_\kappa$21 chains. These serological reagents were useful in screening BALB/c myeloma tumors in order to identify further V$_\kappa$21 myelomas for sequence analysis. It was later shown that V$_\kappa$21 light chains composed a significant fraction of V$_\kappa$ chains, on the order of 10% in normal serum. Thus, V$_\kappa$21 light chains are expressed in a relatively high proportion of both myeloma proteins and normal serum immunoglobulins. This represents a significant approach to the argument that the V$_\lambda$ system was unusual in that it represented such a small percentage of mouse immunoglobulins.

As shown in Fig. 3.20, the sequences can be classified into a group, designated V$_\kappa$21, on the basis of the amino terminal sequence homology. They can also be further subdivided into seven or eight distinct subgroups on the basis of common sets of amino acids shared throughout their V regions. These subgroups differ from each other by as few as 6 and as many as 22 amino acids. A major complication of nomenclature arises at this point. One can designate all V$_\kappa$21 proteins as members of a subgroup, and the subdivisions of V$_\kappa$21 (i.e., V$_\kappa$21c) as sub-subgroups. Alternatively, V$_\kappa$21 can be termed a "group" and the subdivisions called subgroups. There is no conceptual difference between these terms, which will recur throughout this book, but the reader should be aware of the context in which the terms are used. The discussion at this point will not consider the diversity at the C-terminal end of the V$_\kappa$21 kappa chains because that portion of the chain is now known to be encoded by a set of genes distinct from the V-region genes. (Indeed, in Fig. 3.20, the C-terminal 12 amino acids have been "physically" separated. We shall return to this later.)

```
                                                         CDR1                     CDR2                                       CDR3
                                                                                                                                    1    1
                          1    1    2    2       3    3    4    4    5    5    6    6    7    7    8    8    9    9          9    0    0
Subgroup  L-chain  1...5....0....5....0....5..abcd..0....5....0....5....0....5....0....5....0....5....0....5....0....5     6...0....5...

VK21E     7175*    DIVLTQSPASLAVSLGQRATISCRASKSVSTSGYSYMHWYQQKPGQPPKLLIYLASNLESGVPARFSGSGSGTDFTLNIHPVEEEDAATYYCQHSRELP     LTFGAGTKLELK
          6684*    ---------------------------------------------------------------------  ---  ---------------------------     R---G-----I-
          7940*    ----------------------------AF--------------------------------------------------------------V--------     P---G-----I-
          2960*    ---------------------------N----I---GCL--------------------Y----------------------------       B--     Y---G-----I-
          B61      --------------------------  C------------------------------------------------------------
          T109     ------------------------------T---------------------

VK21?     2154*    ----A-------T--------------Q----------------------KY-----------------------------------D-A------W-I-     -----------
          A20      ------------D-----------------TS-T---I---------------AY---------------------------------------Q-N

VK21F     2485*    -------------------------------------------------------------S------------------Q---------I----  ---     ----------
          4039*    -------------------------------------------------------------S------------------Q---------I----

VK21D     7183*    ------------------------K--Q--DYD-D---N----------------A--------I-------------------------------Q-N-B-     -----------
          7043*    ------------------------K--Q--DYD-D---N----------------A--------I-------------------------------Q-B-D-     F---S-----I-
          6308*    ------------------------K--Q--DYD-D---N----------------T--------I-------------------------------Z-N-B-     W---G-----I-
          7210*    ------------------------K--Q-LDYD-D---N----------------A--------I------------------------  ------HQ- -B-     W---G-----I-
          7769*    ------------------------K--Q--DYD-D---N------------V--FA--------I-------------------------------Q-N-B-     W---G-----I-
          C101     ------------------------K--Q--DYT-E---N-----N---S------A--------I-------------------------------Q-N-B-     Y---G-----I-
          8701     ------------------------K--Q--DYD-D---N----------------A--------I-----------------------------      D-     ---S-----I-

VK21B     4050 ,*  N--------------------------E--DSY-N-F-------------------------------------R-----T-D---AD--------QNN-D-     -----------
          M63**    N--------------------------E--DSY-N-F-------------------------------------R-----T-D---AD--------QNN-D-     W---G-----I-
          A22      N--------------------------E--DSY-N-F-------------------------------------R-----T-D---AD--------QNN-D-     Y---G-----I-
          9245*    N--------------------------E--DSY-N-F-------------------------------------R-----T-D---AD--------QNN- -     Y---G-----I-
          11113    N--------------------------E--DSY-N-----------------     ------T-B---AB-----      -     W---G-----I-
          10400    N--------------------------Z--BSY-B-F-------------------------------------R--                             -I-
          11949    N-------------------M- ---EG-DSY-N-F-Y------------------------------------R-----T-D---AD------ -Z   D-     W---G-----I-
          7063*    N----------------------- -- Q--DGY-NTF-  -       ---     ---------------R-----T-                              ---G-----I-

VK21C     3741*    ---------------------------E--DSY-N-F-------------R--------I---------R-----T-N---AD-V-------Q-N-D-     Y---G-----I-
          T111     ---------------------------E--DSY-N-F-------------R--------I---------R-----T-N---AD-V-------Q-N-D-     Y---G-----I-
          A17      ---------------------------E--DSY-N-F-------------R--------I---------R-----T-N---AD-V-------Q-N-D-     W---G-----I-
          2242     ---------------------------E--DSY-N-F-------------R--------I---------R-----T-B---AB-V-------Z-  B-     W---G-----I-
          10916    ---------------------------E--DSY-N-F-------------R--------I---------R-----T-B---AB-V---        D-     F---S-----I-
          M321     ------------------------------D-Y-N-F-------------R--------I---------R-----T-N---AD-V-------Q-N-D-     F---S-----I-
          T124**   ---------------------------E--DWY-N-F-------------R--------I---------R-----T-B---AB-V-------Z-B-A-     ---S-----I-
          8982     ---------------------------E--DSS-N-F-----------      --------I---     ---T  --ABBV-------ZGB-D-     ----A--E----
          8153     ------------T--------------E--DSY-K--I-------S--S-------R--------I---------R-----T-N---AD-V-------QGN-D-     W---G-----I-

VK21A     2880*    ---------------------------E--DNY-I-F-N-F-------------A---QG-------------------S-----M--D-T-M-F--Q-K-V-     W---G-----I-
          1229*    ---------------------------E--DNY-I-F-N-F-------------A---QG-------------------S-----M--D-T-M-F--Q-K-V-     W---G-----I-
          B32      ---------------------------E--DNY-I-F-N-F-------------A---QG-------------------S-----M--D-T-M-F--Q-K-V-     Y---G-----I-
          7132*    ---------------------------E--DNY-I-F-N-F-------------A---QG-------------------S-----M--D-T-M-F--Q-K-V-     PY---G-----I-
          M70E     ---------------------------Q--DN--I-F-N-F-------------A---QG-------------------S-----M--D-T-M-F--Q-K-V-     W---G-----I-
          2413*    ---------------------------E--VNY-V-L---F-------------G---RG-------------------S-I---M--D-S-M-F-HQTK-V-     W---C-D---E
          4999*    ---------------------------E-IDNY-I-F-N
          3386     ---------------------------E--DNY-I-F-N-F-------------V---QG-------------------S--------D-T-M-F--Q-K-V-     Y---G-----I-

VK21?     8778     ---------------------------Z-ZEYY-T-L-Q---------------A---V--------------------S--------D-I-M-F--Q--KV-     W---G----ZI-
          7461     ---------------------------E--EYF-T-L-Q---------------V---V--------------------S--------D-I-L-F--Q--       ---G-----I-
```

Figure 3.20. The amino acid sequence of mouse V_K21 proteins. Many of these sequences are unpublished data of M. Weigert.

The sequences within subgroups share common amino acids throughout their V regions and these shared residues are different for different subgroups. It is unlikely that sequences in different subgroups could have been randomly generated in somatic cells from a common germline structural gene. The value of the mouse system over the human system for these comparisons is clearly evident. The variations seen in the human kappa chains could always be ascribed to allelic differences that had accumulated over evolutionary time and the single amino acid variations that are seen could similarly be viewed as genetic polymorphism. However, in the inbred BALB/c and NZB strains used for these $V_\kappa 21$ analyses, allelism cannot be invoked. As such, these $V_\kappa 21$ data brought the germline and somatic theories of diversity into sharp focus.

Figure 3.20 also serves to further illustrate the concept of "linked substitutions" that allow the further subdivision of the $V_\kappa 21$ into sub-subgroups. With the advent of the serologic definition of the sub-subgroups, it became evident to most that each of the sub-subgroups likely represented a different germline gene. However, despite the subdivisions of $V_\kappa 21$, it was extremely difficult to further subdivide these proteins beyond seven or eight sub-subgroups and yet additional proteins were observed with variations that often differed from the "germline" or "repeat" sequence. Taken together, these data provided strong evidence that somatic mutation occurred in immunoglobulin V regions. We shall return in Chapter 8 to a consideration of the $V_\kappa 21$ subgroup with DNA probes to "count the genes."

The observations of the workers in this area that the C-terminal portions of the molecule did not coincide with the sub-subgroup assignments of the N-terminal portions of the molecule were further fodder for the notion that two genes control the synthesis of an immunoglobulin V region. This had been suggested in the earliest discussions of subgroup variations in the human $V_\kappa III$ system by Milstein and by Capra in discussions of the human V_H subgroups. Both of these authors, along with the several workers who contributed to the $V_\kappa 21$ literature, appreciated that the lack of correlation between the N-terminal structure of the immunoglobulin chain and the C-terminal structure of the variable region suggested that separate genetic elements encoded the two portions of the chain. This concept will be further discussed in Chapter 6.

3.6.3. The Mouse V Ars Kappa Chains

Data concerning the mouse V_λ and $V_\kappa 21$ chains are crucial in understanding the issues concerning antibody diversity and, indeed, are important in understanding the structural characteristics of immunoglobulin variable regions. The deficiency of both these systems is that, at least in the early work, neither represent induced antibodies with defined specificities. The immune response to the simple hapten, *p*-azophenylarsonate, in the A/J mouse and the development of lymphocyte hybridomas circumvent this problem.

The induced antibody response to the hapten *p*-azophenylarsonate in the A/J mouse has provided a model system for the detailed examination of a heritable cross-reactive idiotype and its fine structural and serologic analysis. Five monoclonal antibodies, four cross-reactive idiotype positive, and one cross-reactive idiotype negative were selected by Siegelman and Capra (1981) for complete amino acid sequence analysis. These sequences are shown in Fig. 3.21.

These sequences illustrate a number of important points. First, when antibodies are selected on the basis of their binding to a specific hapten, and further selected for their possession of a cross-reactive idiotype, their amino acid sequences are highly conserved. Structural analyses of the heavy chains of these same antibodies indicate they are also very similar. Not only are the framework structures extremely similar, but the hypervariable regions (particularly the first and second) are virtually indistinguishable. These structural constraints are likely required for hapten binding as well as idiotypic reactivity. The focus of variability in the third hypervariable region is a point of particular interest in this series of molecules. The two amino acids at position 92 and 93 vary in almost all the molecules that have been sequenced. This is distinct from positions 96, the "V/J" junctional position (this will be discussed in detail in Chapter 7), and the reason for the variability is not at all clear.

These light chains thus demonstrate that in an inbred strain, variable

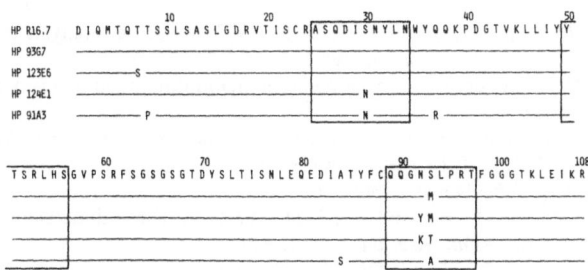

Figure 3.21. Antiarsonate hybridoma light chains. A comparison of amino acid sequences of the light chains derived from CRI+ (top four) and CRI− (bottom sequence) antibodies with that of the light chain of the CRI+ positive light chain, R16.7. A straight line indicates identical residues. Hypervariable regions are boxed. From Siegelman and Capra (1981).

regions derived from antibodies directed against a simple hapten and selected for idiotypic similarity are exceedingly similar in their primary structure. The data are consistent with the hypothesis that the light chains of these arsonate-binding hybridoma antibodies originate from a single germline V gene. The observed heterogeneity is more likely due to somatic mechanisms than to a selection of different although similar germline genes. The precise resolution of this issue would have to await direct analysis of the DNA itself.

3.7. PRECIS

The three systems discussed in detail were chosen to illustrate separate aspects of immunoglobulin V region diversity. All focused on the idea that immunoglobulin variable regions, although exceedingly similar, generally are separate and distinct one from the other. The origin of this primary *structural* diversity is the issue that is being directly addressed in this volume.

In the first chapter of this book, we defined the repertoire and discussed the fact that it required ten million binding specificities to deal with the myriad of antigens that constantly bombard the organism. In the second chapter we argued that the ten million different specificities could be viewed as ten million idiotypes. In this chapter we suggest that there must be ten million different primary structures of immunoglobulins. Since we have linked specificity, idiotype, and structure into a single molecular variable, we now turn to how these structures arise.

REFERENCES AND BIBLIOGRAPHY

Adetugbo, K., Milstein, C., and Secher, D. S., 1977, Molecular analysis of spontaneous somatic mutants, *Nature (London)* **265**:299.

Capra, J. D., 1971, A hypervariable region in human immunoglobulin heavy chains, *Nature (London)* **230**:62.

Capra, J. D., and Edmundson, A. B., 1977, The antibody combining site, *Sci. Am.* **236**:50.

Capra, J. D., and Kehoe, J. M., 1975, Hypervariable regions, idiotypy and the antibody combining site, *Adv. Immunol.* **30**: 1975.

Davies, Dr. R., Padlan, E. H., and Segal, D. M., 1975, Three dimensional structure of immunoglobulins, *Annu. Rev. Biochem.* **44**:639.

Edelman, G. M., and Poulik, M. D., 1961, Studies on structural units of the gamma-globulins, *J. Exp. Med.* **113**:861.

Fahey, J. L., 1961, Heterogeneity of gamma-globulins, *Adv. Immunol.* **2**:41.

Fougereau, M., Bourgois, A., De Preval, C., Rocca-Serra, J., and Schiff, C., 1976, *Ann. Immunol.* **127c**:607.

Francis, S. H., Leslie, R. G. Q., Hood, L., Eisen, H. N., 1974, Amino acid sequences of the variable region of the heavy (alpha) chain of a mouse myeloma protein with anti-hapten activity, *Proc. Natl. Acad. Sci. U.S.A.* **71**:1123.

Franek, F., 1969, The character of variable sequences in immunoglobulin and its evolutionary origin, in: *Symposium on Developmental Aspects of Antibody Formation and Structure* (J. Sterzl and I. Riha, eds.), Prague, p. 311.

Kohler, G., and Milstein, C., 1975, Continuous cultures of fused cells secreting antibody of predefined specificity, *Nature (London)* **256**:495.

Krause, R. M., 1970, The search for antibodies with molecular uniformity, *Adv. Immunol.* **12**:1.

Kunkel, H. G., 1965, Myeloma proteins and antibodies, Harvey Lect. **59**:219.

Lin, L., and Putnam, F. W., 1981, Primary structure of the Fc region of human immunoglobulin D, *Proc. Natl. Acad. Sci. U.S.A.* **78**:504.

McCumber, L. J., Wasserman, R., and Capra, J. D., 1980, Primary structural conservation in the evolution of IgM, *Biologic Basis of Immunodeficiency* (E. W. Gelfand and H.-M. Dosch, eds.), Raven Press, New York, pp. 169–176.

Siegelman, M., and Capra, J. D., 1981, Complete amino acid sequence of light chain variable regions derived from five monoclonal anti-p-azophenylarsonate antibodies differing with respect to a cross-reactive idiotype, *Proc. Natl. Acad. Sci. U.S.A.* **78**:7679.

Wasserman, R. L., and Capra, J. D., 1978, Amino acid sequence of the Fc region of a canine immunoglobulin M, *Science* **200**:1159.

Weigert, M. G., Cesari, I. M., Yonkovich, S. J., and Cohn, M., 1970, Variability in the lambda light chain sequences of mouse antibody, *Nature* **228**:1045.

Wu, T. T., and Kabat, E. A., 1970, An analysis of the sequences of the variable regions of Bence-Jones proteins and myeloma light chains and their implications for antibody complementarity, *J. Exp. Med.* **132**:211.

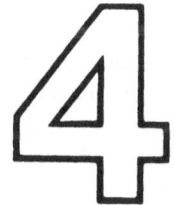

UNIQUE FEATURES OF THE ANTIBODY PROBLEM

Confusion is just a local view of things working out in general.
—JOHN UPDIKE *(Rabbit Redux)*

4.1. INTRODUCTION

Information obtained in the serologic and structural studies described in the previous chapters revealed several striking features of antibodies and the genes that encode them. First of all, it became obvious that there was no known precedent for the immune system. No other biologic process requires the synthesis, on demand, of numerous large molecules with diverse binding properties. There have been attempts to equate olfaction or the general function of the nervous system to the immune system but these are not appropriate comparisons because these systems are not known to use large numbers of structurally distinct proteins in their functionings. Other multigene families such as those encoding ribosomal RNA or histones are required to carry out fixed functions rather than maintain the ability to generate diversity. Although there are a number of similarities between immunoglobulins and proteins encoded at the major histocompatibility complex, the analogy does not include a similar type of diversity.

Antibodies are not only unique among biologic systems in their property of maintaining maximum diversity, they also demonstrate well-documented patterns of genetic behavior not observed for other proteins. Serologic and structural data indicate the existence in the same polypeptide chains of regions of extraordinary diversity along with regions with highly conserved primary structure. The following sections will discuss the structural variability of antibodies as compared with other protein families and will document additional features of antibodies and their genes that set this family well apart from the others.

4.2. STRUCTURAL VARIABILITY OF ANTIBODIES

A major theme of this volume is the diversity of binding functions required for the antibody system. This diversity first revealed by the multitude of antigens recognized by the immune system was later confirmed by serologic studies of the antibodies, especially those using idiotypic markers. Subsequent examination of the protein structures of antibodies indicated that this diversity was reflected in different variable (V) region structures. It must be emphasized that diversity among immunoglobulins is integral to their function, not an accumulation of differences that can be tolerated without loss of activity. This point is illustrated by an example taken from the compilation of immunoglobulin sequences by Kabat and his co-workers (1979).

The protein cytochrome c exercises a critical function in energy metabolism, serving in the electron transport system. Primary structural analyses of cytochromes from numerous species have been carried out. In addition, structure–function experiments have localized the active site of the molecule. If one plots the variability of cytochromes from numerous species on a Wu-Kabat plot (Fig. 4.1), it is seen that variations occur randomly throughout the molecule except in one region: the region of the active site. When similar plots are made for the V regions of immunoglobulin chains, the reverse is seen (see also Figs. 3.16 and 3.17, Chapter 3). In marked contrast to cytochromes, the antibody chains show reasonable conservation of structure everywhere *except* in the regions involved in antigen binding; that is, those areas that may be considered as the active site.

4.2.1. Immunoglobulins and Major Histocompatibility Complex Proteins

The major histocompatibility complex (MHC) like the immunoglobulin gene loci encodes families of proteins involved in immune function.

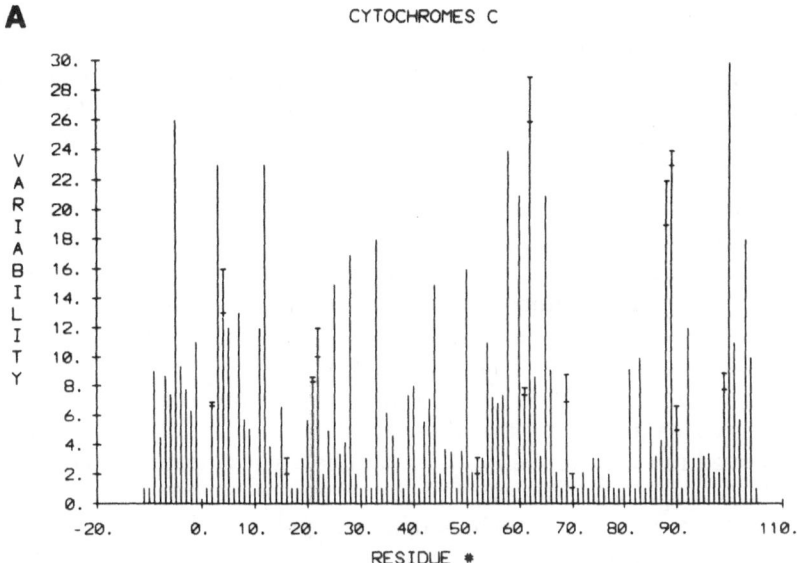

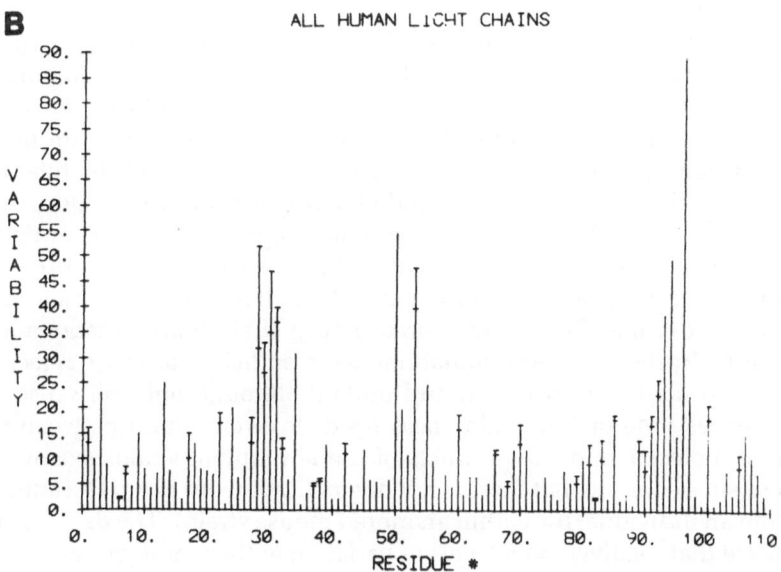

Figure 4.1. (A) Variability of cytochromes *c* from various species. The active site of the molecule is located around residues 70–80, the area of least variability. (B) Variability of human light chains, unselected for subgroup. The sites implicated in antigen-binding (residues 28–34, 50–58, and 90–98) show maximum variability. From Kabat, Wu, and Bilofsky (1979).

The gene products of both of these families consist of two-chain structures, and similar to the immunoglobulin heavy and light chains the component chains of the major transplantation antigens (class I antigens) are encoded at unlinked loci. The basic structural units of these two families are similar in that each has a larger chain that is a glycoprotein, a smaller chain that is not, and in each molecule both chains contain disulfide-linked domains. When either molecule is digested with proteolytic enzymes such as papain they are cleaved at restricted segments that are thought to be located between globular protein domains. Recent primary structural studies of human and murine major transplantation antigens indicate that one of the domains of the molecule has significant amino acid sequence homology to immunoglobulins. Although this homology is not high (about 30%), it has been pointed out by Strominger and his colleagues (1980) that there are a number of amino acid residues conserved in every protein of both families. These features, along with the large sequence differences observed between allelic forms of transplantation antigens and the high degree of polymorphism seen for MHC antigens in general, suggest that these proteins are closely related. It is reasonable to assume that the two gene families have derived from the same ancestoral gene.

In spite of this impressive list of similarities between MHC antigens and immunoglobulin molecules, there remains an extremely important difference between them. Structural studies of MHC antigens have not revealed diversity *among* the same molecules from individuals (or members of inbred populations), whereas sequence analysis of the total immunoglobulin fraction from an individual will show tremendous heterogeneity in the V regions. Unlike immunoglobulins, MHC antigens show no evidence of hypervariability. This consistency of structure was underscored by studies of Nathenson *et al.* (1981) on H-2K^b molecules isolated from members of an inbred mouse strain with mutations in a single H-2 product. These mutations were sufficient to cause rejection of skin grafts between parent and mutant although only very discrete differences (one or two amino acid residues) were found between the parent molecule and the products of the ten mutant strains examined. These studies argue that there is not diversification of a given H-2 antigen within an individual (or within an inbred mouse strain). The data further indicate that relatively low levels of variation in these antigens are easily recognized by the immune system. Therefore, in spite of the catalogue of similarities between MHC antigens and immunoglobulins, the immunoglobulins remain apart as a family of molecules maintaining an extraordinary primary structural diversity in their V regions.

4.2.2. Immunoglobulins and Hemoglobin

Primary structural data are available for a large number of hemoglobin chains, particularly for molecules from patients with clinical symptoms related to the function of hemoglobin. In contrast to immunoglobulins, a difference in a single amino acid in either chain of hemo-

Table 4.1. Clinical Manifestations Associated with Some Abnormal Hemoglobins[a]

Disorder	Abnormal Hb	Structural change		Comments
Hemolytic anemia	S	beta 6	glu--val	Forms molecular aggregates when deoxygenated, producing sickle cell anemia in homozygotes
	C	beta 6	glu--lys	Low solubility lessens plasticity of red cells, causing hemolytic anemia in homozygotes
	Torino	alpha 43	phe--val	
	Bibba	alpha 136	leu--pro	
	Savannah	beta 24	gly--val	
	Genova	beta 28	leu--pro	Unstable hemoglobin causes
	Hammersmith	beta 42	phe--ser	congenital nonspherocytic
	Bristol	beta 67	val--asp	hemolytic anemia in
	Christchurch	beta 71	phe--ser	heterozygotes; precipitated
	Sheph. Bush	beta 74	gly--asp	hemoglobin tends to form
	Santa Ana	beta 88	leu--pro	inclusion bodies within
	Sabine	beta 91	leu--pro	red cells
	Koln	beta 98	val--met	
	Casper	beta 106	leu--pro	
	Wien	beta 130	tyr--asp	
Cyanosis	M Boston	alpha 58	his--tyr	
	M Iwate	alpha 87	his--tyr	Methemoglobin causes cyanosis
	M Saskatoon	beta 63	his--tyr	in heterozygotes; some
	M Milwaukee	beta 67	val--glu	also have evidence of
	M Hyde Park	beta 92	his--tyr	hemolytic anemia
Polycythemia	J Capetown	alpha 92	arg--gln	
	Olympia	beta 20	val--met	Increased oxygen affinity
	Malmo	beta 97	his--gln	of hemoglobin hinders
	Kempsey	beta 99	asp--asn	release of oxygen to tissues,
	Hiroshima	beta 143	his--asp	causing compensatory polycythemia
	Ranier	beta 145	tyr--cys	in heterozygotes
	Bethesda	beta 145	tyr--his	
Anemia	Seattle	beta 76	ala--glu	Decreased oxygen affinity of
	Yoshizuka	beta 108	asn--asp	hemoglobin enhances release of oxygen to tissues and inhibits production of erythropoietin

[a] Adapted from Conley and Chanache (1973).

globin may give rise to significant functional aberrations. The best-known example is the sickle cell variant that involves a single amino acid interchange at position 6 in the hemoglobin beta chain. Many other similar mutant hemoglobin differences have been observed. As Table 4.1 indicates, these single amino acid differences that may occur in many different positions on either chain give rise to gross abnormalities. In this molecule even the slightest variability may alter the function of the molecule.

Although certain critical residues are necessary to their proper function, antibodies display an unprecedented level of variation in the region of the antigen-binding site. It may be stated as a general rule that the majority of proteins tolerate limited variability and still perform their intended role; antibodies, in marked contrast, require variability to perform their primary function of antigen binding.

4.3. TWO GENES–ONE POLYPEPTIDE CHAIN

The data accumulated from serologic and structural studies did not tell us how many antibodies could be synthesized by an individual nor did they reveal how many genes were involved in the generation of antibodies. However, the data did indicate that certain mechanisms operated to simplify the genetic burden acquired by the requirement for diversity. It will be seen that the antibody system has evolved certain economies to maintain and utilize genetic information. These features of the immune system placed questions concerning the number and nature of immunoglobulin genes in a new and different focus.

In the early 1960s, extensive information was obtained in support of the notion that the genes encoding the individual polypeptide chains of antibodies were not contiguous in the genome. Before documenting the studies that led to this heretical notion, it may be useful to briefly review the one gene–one polypeptide hypothesis in order to appreciate the background against which the observations for antibodies were made.

The concept of a single gene for a single enzymic function was first stated in Archibald Garrod's treatise on "Inborn Errors of Metabolism." Using the excretion of homogentisic acid in alkaptonuria as his example, Garrod postulated that the affected individual lacked the ability to carry out a single reaction in the oxidation of phenylalanine and tyrosine. He postulated that the genetically transmitted disease had its basis in a defect in a single gene encoding a single enzyme.

Garrod's work was extended in the 1940s in a brilliant study by Beadle and Tatum (1941). Using the bread mold *Neurospora crassa*, these investigators studied mutations in metabolic pathways and were able to pinpoint genetic lesions and show that these lesions altered single polypeptides. As a result of these studies, biochemical genetics would hold as dogma the dictum: one gene–one polypeptide chain.

Having shown the necessity for and the existence of many diverse protein structures for antibodies, one might ask whether the one gene–one polypeptide hypothesis applied to the genes encoding these proteins. The answer was a cautious yes, but there was a problem with its application—a problem of duplication. Antibodies have a bifunctional role and their functional duality is reflected in the structural division of both heavy and light chains into V and constant (C) regions. The C regions carry out various effector functions subsequent to the occurrence of antigen binding that is localized in the V region. Therefore, the most basic genetic model requires several sets of antibody genes, in each set every member would carry a replicate of the same C-region genes paired with a different V-region gene.

This minimal model must further take into consideration that many (although not all) binding sites would have to be duplicated for each C region. The overlap of binding site requirements for IgE and IgG may not be extensive, for example, but the overlap between IgM and IgG may be almost total. An additional serious problem with this model is the need to maintain, with little or no mutation, multiple copies of each of the C-region genes. Recall that C regions comprise greater than 75% of the mass of each heavy chain and 50% of each light chain. Therefore, the amount of DNA devoted to these replicates would be staggering. It is furthermore conceivable that serious problems with immune function could be latent in such a genetic arrangement.

Having considered these problems concerning a one gene–one immunoglobulin chain model, let us examine the data relevant to the question, from which there emerged a more attractive alternative.

4.3.1. The Todd Phenomenon

In 1963, Todd demonstrated that the rabbit heavy chain allotypes (group a allotypes) were present on both IgG and IgM. He used the technique of gel filtration on Sephadex to separate the two immunoglobulin classes and tested the pools for reactivity with anti-allotype sera (see Fig. 4.2). The finding that the a (heavy chain) markers as well as the b (light chain) markers were common to two classes was recognized to be an unusual and significant finding. Interpretation of the result, however, was not simple because there was an experimental uncertainty. The uncertainty did not center about whether three genes (a allotype, b allotype, and mu or gamma region) were involved in synthesis of these molecules, but whether *three different chains* were present in the molecule. The two-chain model for immunoglobulin had not yet been established and therefore there was no basis for drawing the now obvious conclusion that two of the three genes encoded *one* of the two chains.

Within the same year, Feinstein (1963), demonstrated that IgA also carries the group a allotypes. In Feinstein's study, immunoelectrophoresis was used to show reactivity of distinct molecules with the heavy chain anti-allotype. These reports were the first in a series of findings that suggested that antibodies violate the one gene–one polypeptide chain dogma. Supporting the serologic data of Todd and of Feinstein on sharing of group a allotypes in IgM, IgA, and IgG were the compositional studies of Koshland *et al.* (1969) demonstrating amino acid differences within immunoglobulin classes that correlated with the al-

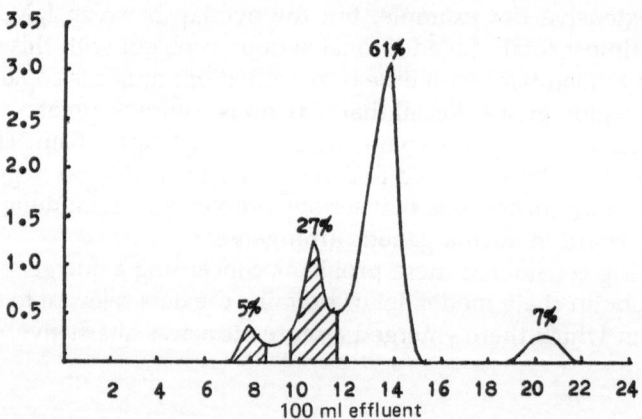

Figure 4.2. Gel filtration on Sephadex of serum from an a1/b4 rabbit. Shaded areas indicate fractions that gave positive tests for both allotypic specificities. Percentages at the top of each peak represent the percent of the total optical density units (OD × volume) found in each peak. The fraction at the center of the first peak gave a positive test for a1 at a dilution of 1/4 and for b4 at a dilution of 1/8. It was negative for anti-Fc specificity. The fraction at the center of the second peak gave a positive test for a1, b4, and for gamma chain antigens. From Todd (1963).

lotypes and to functional differences of the chains. It was further shown by Kindt and Todd (1969) that rabbit IgE also expressed the a allotypes.

4.3.2. Structural Differentiation of V and C Regions

In addition to the results obtained for rabbit allotypes, there was evidence of another type that hinted of an unusual relationship between portions of the immunoglobulin chains. Peptide-mapping studies of light chains from human or mouse myeloma proteins by Baglioni *et al.* (1967) and others revealed that one set of peptides comprising approximately half of the total were present for all chains studied. Each enzymatically digested chain also contained, however, a second set of peptides that distinguished it from all others studied. The peptide-mapping studies were soon followed by amino acid sequence determinations by Hilschmann and Craig (1965) and by Putnam *et al.* (1967) showing that the amino terminal portion was variable and that the carboxy-terminal portion was constant in the immunoglobulin light chains.

4.3.3. Statement of the Two-Gene Hypothesis

The demonstrations that immunoglobulin light chains had a C and a V region set the stage for the postulation of Dreyer and Bennett (1965) that there were two genes involved in their synthesis. They first examined the question of whether there was an extra (third) chain present in the immunoglobulin molecule by looking for nonpeptide linkages that might have joined two separate molecules into C and V regions. Finding no such evidence, the authors suggested that the presence in the same polypeptide chain of C and V parts was "paradoxical."

There was the evidence from studies of the human Inv (now Km) allotypes that C regions were inherited as simple Mendelian alleles; with the exception of the minor genetically determined variations, the amino acid sequences of C regions from light chains of the same type were identical. However, the same protein that displayed these properties also contained a set of peptides that differed in every sample that had been tested (see Fig. 4.3). The genetic implications of these results is very well stated in a direct quotation from the 1965 paper of Dreyer and Bennett:

> An attempt to explain the genetic mechanism required to synthesize these proteins in a normal way leads to a genetic paradox. The paradox results from the observation that one end of the light chain behaves as if it were made by the genetic code contained in any one of more than 1000 genes,

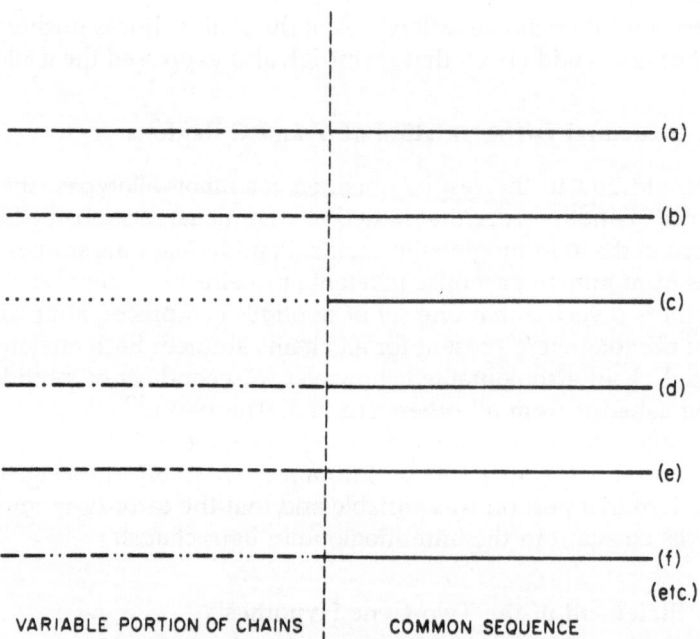

Figure 4.3. Graphical illustration of the general type of amino acid sequence variation found in light chains of both mouse and man. From Dreyer and Bennett (1965).

while the other end of the L chains can be shown to be the product of a single gene. That this latter portion is under the control of a single locus is evidenced by the fact that it can undergo mutation (allotypes), Mendelian segregation, and that it is rigidly constant in amino acid sequence whenever produced. These facts rule out the possibility that each of the complete polypeptide chains is synthesized under the genetic control of a separate and independent gene contained in the germ line. It appears therefore that immunologically competent cells have evolved a pattern of somatic genetic behavior which is radically different from anything normally found in modern molecular genetics.

Several explanations for this paradoxical behavior were considered by these authors including hypermutability of the variable portion during differentiation. This possibility was rejected because of the heritable nature of the capacity to respond to certain antigens. The authors favored the possibility that the many V-region genes were present in the germline and that they combined with the single C-region gene in the process of differentiation.

It would be a number of years before it was conclusively demonstrated that *two* genes encoded a single immunoglobulin chain, and the suggestion that two genes were responsible for one antibody chain would be considered only a hypothesis during this period. The possibility that the one gene–one polypeptide chain dogma had an exception was generally ignored by geneticists and biochemists for many years. For the immunologist, this hypothesis would stimulate many experiments and these experiments would confirm and extend this remarkably prescient hypothesis.

In the 1967 Cold Spring Harbor Symposium, there were numerous references to the two-gene hypothesis; many reported studies supported the notion and the general tone in this meeting was one of acceptance. Certainly all reported structural data appeared to confirm the two-gene hypothesis. In a round table discussion on theories of antibody variability that was chaired by Crick, it was assumed a priori that the C region was the product of a single gene. The discussion in this session dealt almost entirely with the problem of V region diversity.

Not only was there support for the general notion of the two-gene hypothesis, but interesting and novel experimental approaches intended to further extend and explore this hypothesis were reported. Experiments reported by Fleischman (1967) and by Lennox et al. (1967) explored the possible levels at which the interaction could occur: at the level of DNA, mRNA, or at a posttranslational stage. In the words of Lennox:

> These facts (concerning the possibility that immunoglobulin chains are under the control of two genes) then encourage experiments that look for such control of light and heavy chains. Since, in any case, heavy and light chains are each single polypeptide chains apparently without nonpeptide links there would have to be a fusion of separate peptides to make a single polypeptide chain, prior fusion of two messenger RNAs or fusion of two genes. The last would seem most likely and the first is easiest to look for. It is possible to test whether a light chain or heavy chain is synthesized as a single unit by examining the rate of synthesis of different portions of the chain during time intervals which are short compared to the synthesis time of the whole chain.

Lennox used the light and heavy chains of mouse myeloma proteins as a model system. He separated the heavy chain Fc and Fd fragments after splitting them with papain. He also studied peptides from light chains of myeloma proteins for which the amino acid sequence was already determined. This study and that of Fleischman, who used the rabbit heavy chain as his model system, involved what is commonly known as a pulse-chase experiment (Fig. 4.4). The mouse myeloma cells or the rabbit lymph node suspension were radiolabeled in culture, the experiment stopped after varying amounts of time had elapsed, the chain isolated, and fragments prepared and analyzed for their relative specific activity. In both experiments, it was shown that immunoglobulins are

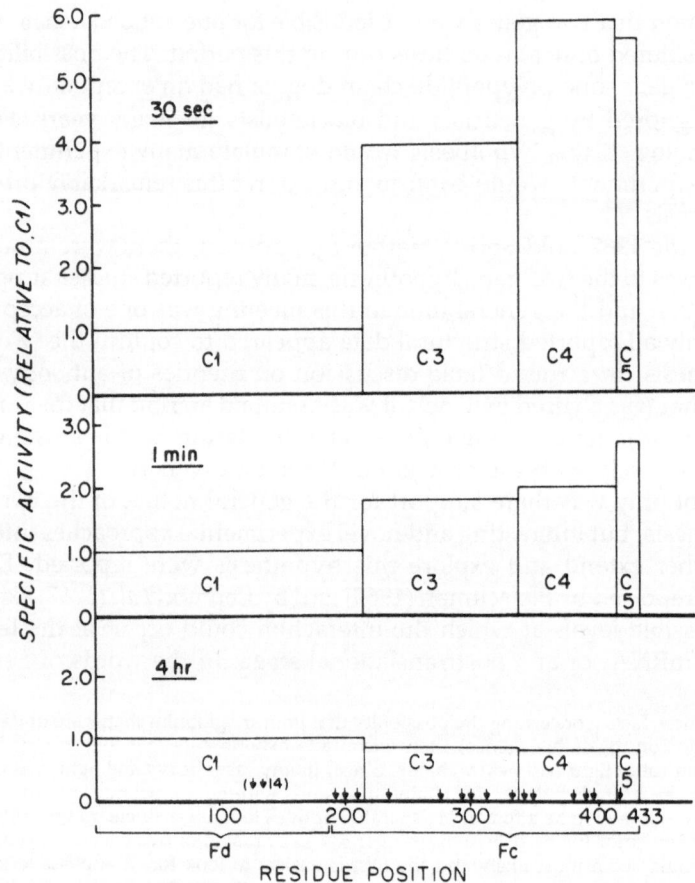

Figure 4.4. Relative specific activities of the CNBr fragments of heavy chain radiolabeled with leucine in a pulse-chase experiment. The size and order of the fragments and the numbering of residues are tentative. Arrows indicate the known positions of leucine residues. From Fleischman (1967).

synthesized as single units growing from the amino to the carboxyl terminus. These data ruled out any posttranslational joining of peptide units to form the C and V portions of the immunoglobulin chain. The data however, did not distinguish whether the joining took place at the DNA or at the RNA level. In his discussion, Lennox argued that joining should occur at the DNA level because it would then not be necessary for fusion to take place at each division of the cell committed to make heavy and light chains.

4.3.4. Cis or Trans Synthesis

The discovery of allotype markers for the C portion of the rabbit heavy chain by Mandy and Todd (1968) and by Dubiski (1969) along with the V_H allotypes made possible a new type of experiment to test the two-gene hypothesis. Two new different C_H allotype systems, the group d (d11, d12) and e (e14, e15) allotypes, were reported for the rabbit within a short period of time. The group d allotypes were localized to position 225 in the hinge region, and the structural correlates of the allotypes were methionine for d11 and threonine for d12. The group e allotypes were in the C_H2 domain; e14 was defined by a threonine residue at position 309, whereas e15 had alanine in this position. Therefore, the rabbit heavy chain had a combination of V_H (group a allotypes) and C_H genetic markers that could be used to observe the interactions of the putative V and C genes that were postulated to encode this chain.

Information concerning the genetics of the group d allotypes indicated that they were closely linked to the group a allotypes. It was also known that most of the a allotypes (1, 2, 3) could occur in linkage with either d11 or d12. The occurrence of most of the possible combinations in rabbit populations indicated that cross-overs between V and C genes had previously occurred. With this background information, the following experiments were carried out.

A rabbit doe homozygous for the a3-d11 allotypes was mated to a buck with the a1-d12 combination. A mating to give the reciprocal types was also carried out (see Fig. 4.5 for pedigrees). Immunoglobulin G was isolated from the sera of the doubly heterozygous offspring and the d11 molecules were separated from d12 molecules by gel filtration after cleavage of the methionine residues with CNBr. This separation was possible because d11 IgG has an additional methionine and yields a smaller fragment. The separated molecules were then typed for the group a markers by a quantitative method (Fig. 4.6). If the two pools of d11 and d12 molecules had each contained both a1 and a3 molecules, or had the d11 pool contained all or mostly all a1, and the d12 contained a3, this would have shown conclusively that the two genes inherited from the different parents interacted to form the heavy chains in the heterozygote. This was not the result observed. The d11 pool contained the maternal a3 allotype, whereas the d12 consisted almost entirely of a1 from the buck. The heterozygote from the opposite mating types (a1, d11; a3, d12) gave results confirming these. An identical finding was observed for the allotype combination a and e. Therefore, the majority of heavy chains retained the inherited association of V- and C-region allotypes.

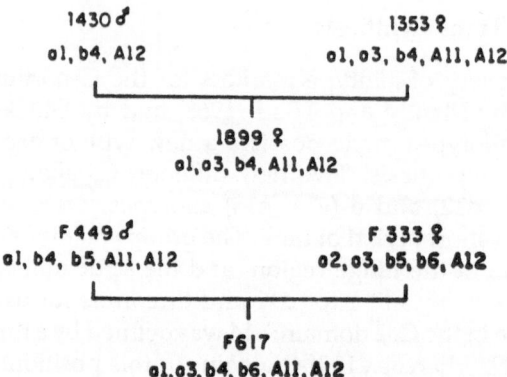

Figure 4.5. Pedigrees for rabbits 1899 and F617. Because of the linkage observed in the inheritance of the group a and the d11 (A11) and d12 (A12) allotypes, it could be concluded that rabbit 1899 had inherited a1 and A12 from the father and a3 and A11 from the mother. Contrariwise, rabbit F617 inherited a1 and A11 from the mother and a3 and A12 from the father.

The C- and V-allotype experiment did not demonstrate interaction of maternal and paternal genes in the somatic cell. It did, however, provide an informative answer. These data placed a constraint on the mode of interaction between immunoglobulin genes: they reacted in a *cis* as opposed to a *trans* fashion. That means that V- and C-region genes on the same chromosome interact with one another rather than with the homologous genes on the other chromosome.

Studies on rabbit V- and C-region allotypes addressed an additional aspect of V- and C-region genes. When the data concerning *cis* synthesis were first obtained, the methods for typing group a allotypes were such that a pool containing 95% of one allotype was not readily distinguished from one containing 100% of the allotype. Therefore, the question of whether the 5% or less of *trans* synthesis products were artifacts or alternatively represented a minor population was left open. Using more sensitive solid-phase techniques, it was later shown that the *trans* IgG products do exist in serum at a level of about 1%. When IgA samples were tested by Knight *et al.* (1974) for combinations of alpha chain allotypes with group a allotypes from the antithetical chromosome, a somewhat higher frequency of *trans* products was observed.

When immunoglobulin-producing cells from doubly heterozygous rabbits were examined by fluorescent antibody techniques for cells carrying combinations of group a and d or group a and e markers from

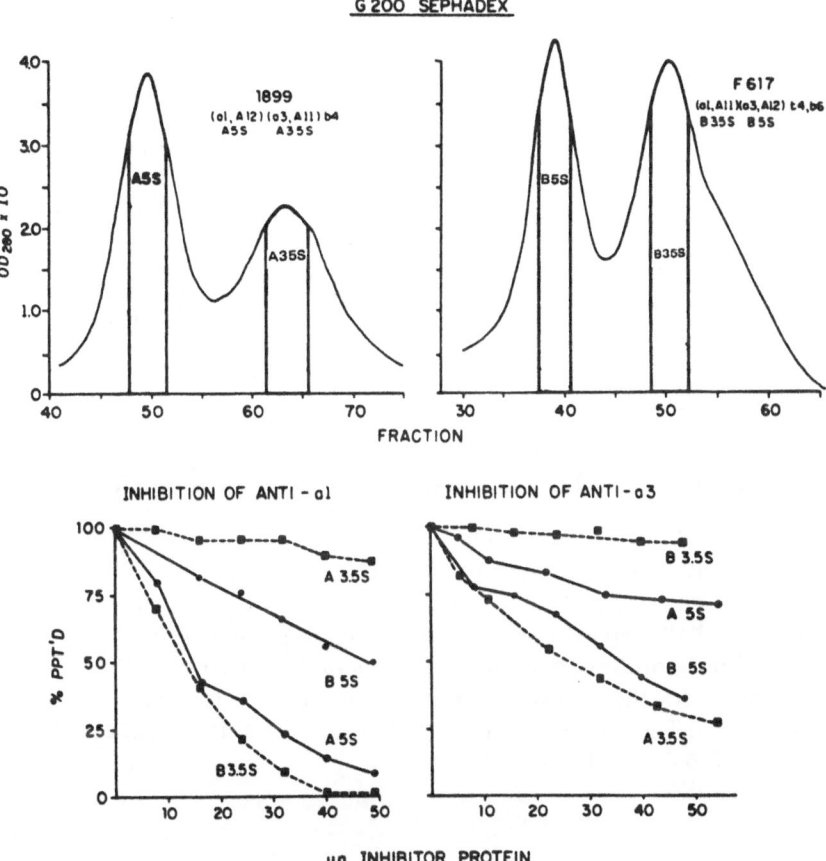

Figure 4.6. Upper panels: gel filtration of limited CNBr digests of IgG from rabbits 1899 and F617 (see Fig. 4.5). The fractions indicated by bars were pooled and concentrated. The major peak to which these allotypic combinations contribute is indicated below the parenthesized specificities. The 5S peaks contain molecules positive for the 12 allotype and the 3.5S peaks the 11 positive. Lower left: inhibition of the precipitation of 35 μg of [125]I a1, b4, d12 IgG with 0.1 ml of anti-a1 by the column pools. The percent precipitated is relative to the number of ^{125}I counts precipitated in the absence of inhibitor. Lower right: inhibition of a3 IgG precipitation under the same conditions. From Kindt *et al.* (1970).

different linkage groups, the 1% level of *trans* synthesis was again recorded. It is not certain what mechanism gives rise to these products; they may be the products of *trans* synthesis or they may result from mitotic (not to be confused with recombination in germ cells during meiosis) cross-over events of the V- and C-region genes.

Table 4.2. Recombination between V_H and C_H Markers[a]

	V_H	C_H	Recombinants found	Frequency in percentage and 95% confidence interval
Rabbit	a	d	2/460	0.43 (0.05–1.58)
	a	e	1/366	0.27 (0.01–1.53)
	a	de	3/1011	0.30 (0.06–0.87)
Mouse	Dex	Ig-1a	8/1949	0.41 (0.20–0.84)
	Dex	Ig-1b	5/843	0.59 (0.19–1.36)
	Inuldx	Ig-1a	2/82	2.44 (0.30–8.53)
	A5A+	Ig-1e	2/82	2.44 (0.30–8.53)
	S117+	Ig-1a	3/78	3.84 (0.80–10.83)

[a] Adapted from Weigert and Potter (1977).

4.3.5. Genetic Recombination between V- and C-Region Allotypes

Shortly after the description of the *cis* interaction, a cross-over was observed between the group e and the group a allotypes in the laboratory of Mage *et al.* (1971). Two other V-C cross-overs have since been reported, one between group d and group a allotypes and another between e and a. These findings not only strengthened the two-gene theory, but also allowed for the first time estimates of distances between V- and C-region genes. The frequency of cross-over in these studies was estimated at around 0.5% (see Table 4.2).

4.3.6. Biclonal Myeloma Proteins

As mentioned in Chapter 2, the finding by Oudin and Michel (1969) of identical idiotypes on IgG and IgM antibodies supported the two-gene hypothesis. It was found that IgG and IgM antibodies directed against the bacterium *Salmonella typhi* had identical idiotypic markers. This demonstration was made more remarkable by the fact that these idiotypes were not found in the sera of related rabbits that had been immunized with the same bacterium. This finding extended the results concerning common V-region allotypes on heavy chains of different classes to include V regions that were functionally identical and that expressed the same highly individualistic marker. It was therefore suggested that IgG and IgM antibodies had identical V regions. Confirmation and extension of this result came from studies of human idiotypes that provided a convincing demonstration that identical V regions could be found in association with different C regions.

The laboratories of Kunkel (1970) and of Fudenberg (Wang *et al.*, 1969) first showed that in certain patients with multiple myeloma, the serum contains two discrete monoclonal components; that is, two distinct immunoglobulin molecules that often are of different classes. In one instance, an IgG2 and an IgM molecule were isolated from a patient's serum, and it was shown that although the C regions displayed the expected class-related differences, *the V regions of the heavy chains of these proteins were identical.* When the IgG2 and IgM monoclonal proteins were compared using anti-Id, no differences were observed. These data were extended by studies on additional polyclonal myeloma proteins (Fig. 4.7) and the results added a new dimension to the two-gene studies by showing conclusively that polypeptides could have in common identical V regions and be totally distinct in their C regions.

The results concerning identical V regions in antibodies of different classes prompt a mention of "switching," that is, the change during maturation of an antibody-producing cell from production of an antibody of one class to an antibody with identical binding site but of a different class. The two-gene hypothesis adds an attractive aspect to models of maturation of the immune response. The problem of how the response shifts from predominantly IgM to IgG without loss of specificity is nicely answered by switching C-region genes while maintaining the same V-region genes in the selected cells.

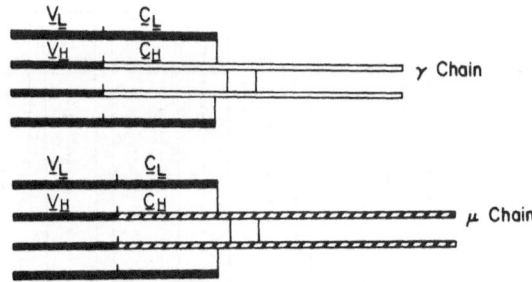

Figure 4.7. Shared amino sequences (shaded areas) in the heavy and light chains of the monotypic IgG and IgM of patient Til, and, hypothetically, in normal IgG and IgM antibodies produced by a single clone of cells. It is assumed that genes controlling V_L, C_L and V_H segments are the same for the two classes of molecule. From Hopper and Nisonoff (1971).

4.3.7. Cross-overs between Idiotypes and C Regions

It would be possible to continue the discussion of data directly supportive of the two-gene hypothesis for many additional pages. However, it may be best to conclude with one final example that typifies an area of research most directly relevant to the issue of antibody diversity. The area involves idiotype inheritance in inbred strains of mice.

As mentioned in Chapter 2, the discovery in inbred mice of cross-reactive idiotypes and of their polymorphic expression provided a new approach for the genetic analysis of immunoglobulins. One of the more valuable idiotypes was the A5A marker for the antibody to group A streptococcal carbohydrate that was secreted by lymphocytes from the A/J strain mice. It had been shown in studies by Eichmann and Berek (1973) that the A5A idiotype was linked to the IgG-1e allele of the A/J heavy chain C-region genes. It was further shown in these studies that the BALB/c strain that expressed the immunoglobulin heavy chain C-region allotype 1a did not make the idiotype A5A.

In a series of experiments designed to test the linkage of the A5A idiotype to the 1.e haplotype, back-cross experiments were carried out in which (A/J × BALB/c)F₁ mice were bred back to BALB/c mice (Fig. 4.8). In this back-cross, half of the progeny would be expected to have the allotype a/e and the other half, the allotype a/a. Only those mice containing the e allotype genes would be expected to express the A5A idiotype if the A5A gene were closely linked to the heavy chain C-region

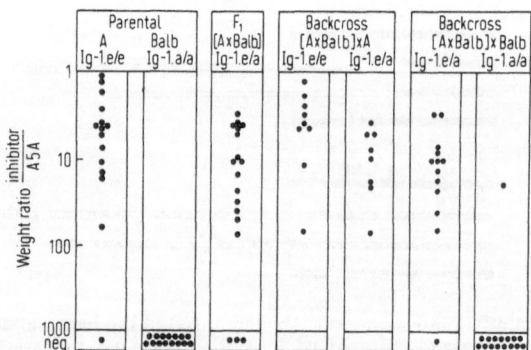

Figure 4.8. The expression of the A5A idiotype in antibodies to streptococcal A carbohydrate (A-CHO) from A/J mice, BALB/c mice, F₁ hybrids, and back-cross mice. Each dot represents the result on a single mouse. The ordinate gives the ratio of the weight of an inhibitor to that of antibody A5A causing equal inhibition. Eichmann and Berek (1973).

allotype. Eichmann observed, however, that in one of 16 back-cross mice that were typed homozygous for the Ig-1a allele, there was expression of the A5A idiotype (Fig. 4.9). The mouse (BB ♂ 7), showing the putative recombinant haplotype, was a male and therefore was subsequently bred to a number of mice in order to demonstrate that a cross-over had occurred in the germ cells.

As mentioned in Chapter 2, there was another well-studied idiotype, Ars, which was a marker for anti-*p*-azophenylarsonate antibodies in A/J mouse. Because Ars (like A5A) was not found in BALB/c it was of interest to know if the recombinant produced antibodies positive for this idiotype. It was possible using the recombinant A5A mouse with the BALB/c allotype to determine whether A5A and Ars mapped in the same position relative to the immunoglobulin heavy chain C-region allotype. Because the recombinant mice responded like BALB/c rather than like A/J to immunization with arsonate (i.e., negative for Ars idiotype), it was concluded that the recombinant haplotype did not include the Ars gene. This experiment and a number of similar results (see Table 4.2) confirmed the fact that C- and V-region genes could be separated by cross-over as shown by the earlier results obtained with the rabbit C- and V-region allotypes. These mouse idiotype data further revealed that cross-over events could separate genes encoding different idiotypes; this strongly suggested that there are multiple V-region genes.

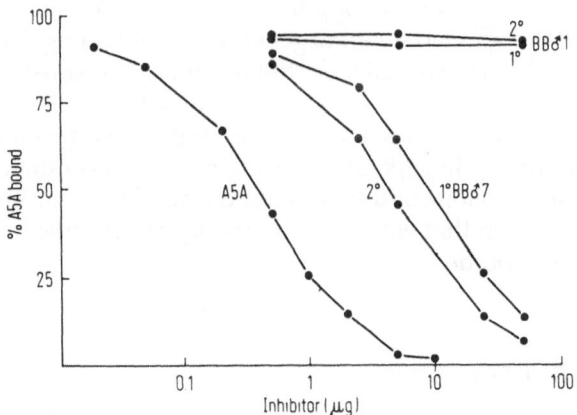

Figure 4.9. Inhibition curves of the antibodies from BB♂7 after the first (1°) and second (2°) immunization series. The inhibition curves of antibody A5A and of the antibodies from another Ig-1a/a homozygous back-cross mouse (BB♂1) are included for comparison. The ordinate gives the percent of 20 ng radiolabeled antibody A5A bound, the abscissa gives the amount of cold inhibitor per test tube. From Eichmann and Berek (1973).

4.3.8. Theoretical Impact of the Two-Gene Hypothesis

A wealth of data supporting the revolutionary concept that two genes participated in the synthesis of a single polypeptide chain had been accumulated. These data that permeated the literature after 1965 comprised a body of consistent information obtained by several different techniques. However, for some reason, this revolutionary idea did not extend beyond the immunology community and the two-gene hypothesis was largely ignored by biochemists and geneticists until formal proof was obtained by recombinant DNA techniques. The hypothesis had, however, a profound impact on theories of antibody diversity.

It should be emphasized that the two-gene hypothesis neither confirms nor precludes either germline or somatic mutation theories. Nearly all data supporting the two-gene hypothesis can be interpreted as supportive of either multiple germline gene theories or of those calling for few V-region genes with somatic mutation generating the necessary diversity. The fact that there are two genes that interact to synthesize a single immunoglobulin chain says little about the number of V-region genes that are encoded in the genome. The two-gene hypothesis does, however, make either theory more plausible. On one hand, it is easier to deal with the genetic burden imposed by many V-region genes in the germline if it is not necessary to replicate the constant region genes for each V region contained in the genome. By the same token, if there are small numbers of V-region genes, say 3 or 4, it is easier to consider mutation and subsequent joining to a constant region gene than it is to consider mutation in two separate genes, each containing C and V region information. This is especially pertinent when one considers the data from allotype and idiotype studies indicating that different classes of heavy chain may have the same V region. It is very difficult to postulate mutations occurring in separate genes that would eventually lead to an identity in the V regions of the products encoded by these genes. Therefore, it may be seen that either type of theory can profitably incorporate the two-gene hypothesis.

4.4. ALLELIC EXCLUSION

A diploid cell from a heterozygous individual contains genetic information for two different allelic proteins, and if the cell synthesizes one it will synthesize both allelic products. Except in special cases, the two products will be synthesized in approximately equal amounts. By contrast, a germ cell that is derived by the process of meiosis and contains a haploid complement of chromosomes can express only those proteins encoded in their chromosomal complement. Examination of a population of sperm cells from a heterozygote would reveal that approximately half of the cells contain one allele and the remainder contain the other. Therefore, it may be stated as a general rule that aside from germ cells and the special case introduced by the X chromosome, all somatic cells express the products of both homologous autosomal gene loci. That is, all cells *except* those producing immunoglobulins.

4.4.1. The Lyon Hypothesis

Prior to studies on immunoglobulin biosynthesis, the most well-studied deviation from normal autosomal allelic expression involved the X chromosome in females. It was known that female, but not male, mice exhibited dappled or mottled coat colors and that human females with the XO karyotype, that is, with only half the normal complement of X chromosomes, were normal in most respects. On the basis of this and other information, Lyon in 1961 formulated a hypothesis concerning X-linked genes. This hypothesis states that in early embryogenesis, one of the two X chromosomes becomes genetically inactive and forms the Barr body that is observed in cells from a female. The Lyon hypothesis further states that random chance dictates which X chromosome in any single cell (whether the one from the father or the one from the mother) is inactivated. Furthermore, once the X chromosome inactivation has occurred in a given cell, the same X chromosome will remain inactive in all descendants of that cell (Fig. 4.10). This inactivation process occurs in all cells of the female with the exception of the germ cells, which do not participate in X chromosome inactivation.

The Lyon hypothesis predicts that the cells of the female should display mosaicism for any X-linked variable trait. This was verified by Beutler in 1962 for glucose-6-phosphate dehydrogenase deficiency. It was found that heterozygous females have two distinct populations of cells, those with normal enzyme activity and those with diminished enzyme activity.

4.4.2. Selective Expression of Immunoglobulin Alleles

As discussed in Chapter 2, immunoglobulins are inherited as autosomal codominant alleles. This means that the products of both the maternally inherited and the paternally inherited genes are expressed in the organism. It is also known that the immunoglobulin molecule was a symmetrical four-chain structure containing two identical heavy

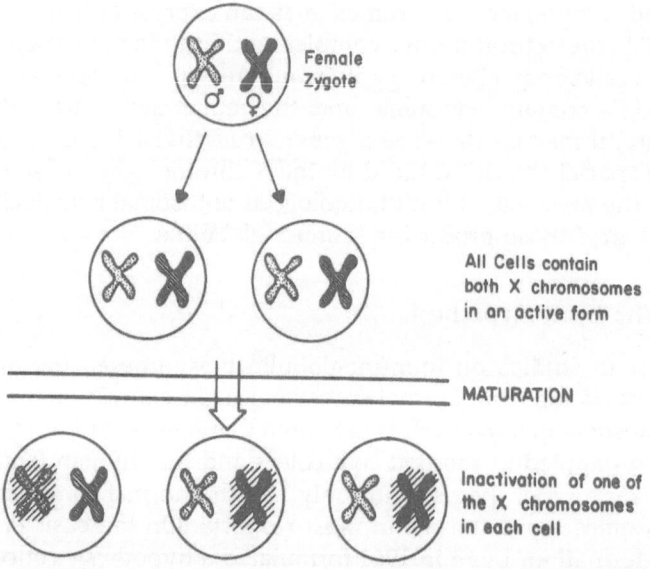

Figure 4.10. The Lyon hypothesis states that one of the two X chromosomes in female cells is randomly inactivated at some point early in embryogenesis. All daughter cells will retain the same inactive and active chromosomes.

and two identical light chains. Therefore, in each four-chain molecule from a heterozygous individual, only *single* allotypic specificities for the light chain and for the heavy chain were found. This exclusion was thought to require a special mechanism in the intracellular assembly of the polypeptide chains because if both allelic specificities were present in a single cell, mixed molecules would be formed. In early studies of human myeloma proteins, it was observed that only one of the possible alleles was expressed in any given homogeneous immunoglobulin. If myeloma cells were truly products of a single clone, then that clone had to be producing only a single allelic product from the heavy and light chain genes. This raised the possibility that immunoglobulin-synthesizing cells violated the principle of allelic expression, a possibility that was independently tested by the experiments of Pernis *et al.* (1965) and of Weiler (1965).

Pernis used the technique of fluorescent antibody staining of lymphoid cells to determine that a single cell produced only a single allelic product. Antisera directed against the rabbit allotypes of the group a (heavy chain) and group b (light chain) indicated that the products of allelic genes were always present in different cells. Pernis' study further showed that the products of nonallelic genes, for example, those of the heavy and light chain, randomly associated in the cells producing the immunoglobulins. Therefore, a given cell could express the light chain allotype from the buck in combination with the heavy chain allotype of the doe but *never* expressed more than one allelic product (Fig. 4.11).

In the same year that Pernis described the phenomenon of allelic exclusion of rabbit allotypes using immunofluorescence, Weiler (1965) reported a similar finding for mice. In his study, Weiler used Jerne's newly developed technique of plaque formation (Jerne and Norden, 1963). In this technique, spleen cells taken from mice immunized against sheep red blood cells are mixed in soft agar with sheep red blood cells. The antibody secreted by the spleen cells can lyse the red blood cells in their vicinity, thus forming a clear plaque of lysis. In order for lysis to occur, complement must be present and furthermore, if the antibody is not of the IgM type, a second (facilitating) antibody must be used in order to affect complement-mediated lysis of red blood cells. In Weiler's study the spleens were taken from mice that were heterozygous for the heavy chain C-region allotypes a and b, and the facilitating reagent used

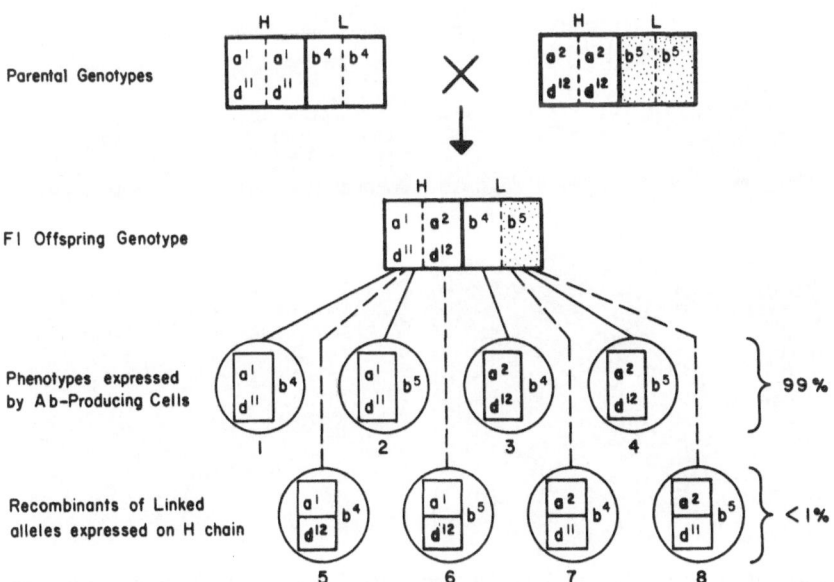

Figure 4.11. Antibody-producing cells display phenotypes indicative of allelic exclusion. In the example shown the complexity of the mosaic trait is increased by the possibility of cells with recombinant (a–d) IgG heavy chains.

was either anti-a or anti-b. A given spleen cell produced antibody of either one allotype or the other; no cell produced antibody of both allotypes (Fig. 4.12). Weiler concluded:

> Phenotypic mosaicism exists in female mammals with respect to genes on the X chromosome. It can be understood as a dosage regulation effect, since males have only one X chromosome but females have two. On the other hand, such a phenomenon has not been demonstrated previously for autosomal genes. In fact, there are examples where both parental alleles are known to be expressed in each cell, such as transplantation and blood group antigens, or polypeptide chains of hemoglobin. The differential activity of genes specifying gamma globulin, as reported in the present work, so far constitutes an exception among autosomal loci. This finding may be related to the fact that in plasma cell tumors only one of two parental allotypes is expressed.

There was speculation regarding the mechanism of allelic exclusion for immunoglobulin genes. Ohno *et al.* (1966) proposed that the non-

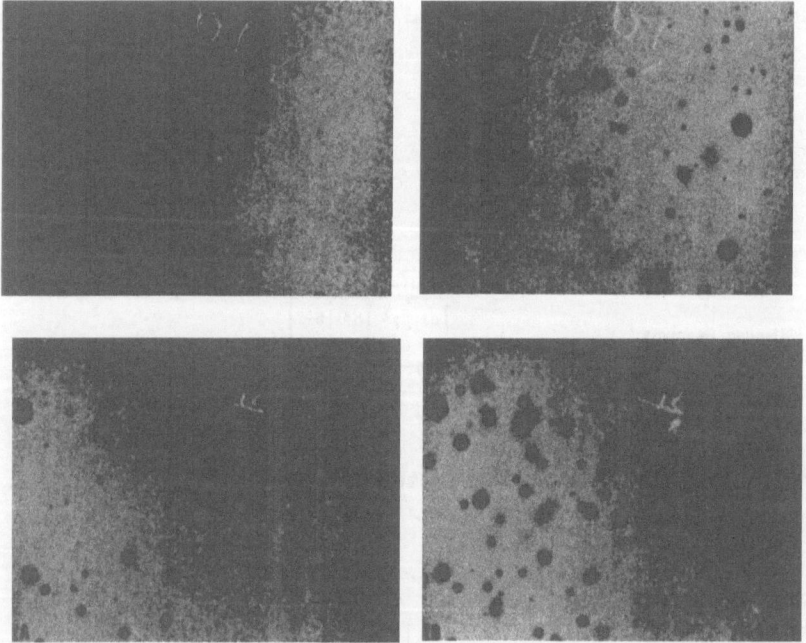

Figure 4.12. First- and second-round facilitation with heterozygous a/b murine spleen cells in Jerne plaque assays. (1A) Normal serum in the first round; (1B) allotype antiserum Ab in the second round of the same preparation. (2A) Allotype antiserum Aa in the first round; (2B) additional facilitation by Ab in the second round. Dark field illumination from one side. About 1/3 of the preparations are shown. Magnification 3.6×. From Weiler (1965).

active chromosome was not present in the antibody-producing cell, and that this exclusion involved somatic segregation of chromosomes carrying the genes for immunoglobulins. Recent data obtained by Wabl and Tenkhoff (1982) using markers for the chromosomes carrying these genes have shown that both chromosomes are present in the cells showing allelic exclusion. Mechanistic models of allelic exclusion will be discussed in Chapter 7, but the total process remains undefined. Therefore, it was quite clear by 1965 that immunoglobulins were exceptional in yet another respect. Of all proteins known to be encoded on autosomes, the immunoglobulins alone stood out as an exception to the general rules for the synthesis of allelic proteins. This finding of allelic exclusion fit nicely with the known facts about immunoglobulins and similar to the two-gene hypothesis was quickly incorporated into the mainstream of immunologic thought.

4.5. THE THREE LOCI FOR IMMUNOGLOBULINS

Throughout all discussions of the two gene–one polypeptide chain hypothesis and the phenomenon of allelic exclusion for immunoglobulin genes, the examples used have concentrated on the actions of single loci. However, as pointed out in a graphic manner by Fig. 4.13, the

Locus	V Region	C Region
H Chains	V_{HI} ———	——— μ
	V_{HII} ———	——— δ
	V_{HIII} ———	——— γ_1
	V_{HIV} ———	——— γ_2
		——— γ_3
		——— γ_4
		——— ϵ
		——— α
Kappa Chains	V_{KI} ———	——— C_K
	V_{KII} ———	
	V_{KIII} ———	
Lambda Chains	$V_{\lambda I}$ ———	——— $C_{\lambda I}$
	$V_{\lambda II}$ ———	——— $C_{\lambda II}$
	$V_{\lambda III}$ ———	——— $C_{\lambda III}$
	$V_{\lambda IV}$ ———	——— $C_{\lambda IV}$
	$V_{\lambda V}$ ———	

Figure 4.13. Diagrammatic representation of human immunoglobulin structural genes. Each group includes a set of linked genes. Each bar represents at least one gene; the numbers of genes in each group are minimum numbers based on subgroup sequence. One V-region gene and one C-region gene interact in the synthesis of each immunoglobulin chain. The order of genes is arbitrary and this representation depicts only a haploid complement of genes.

active chromosome was not present in the antibody-producing cell, and that this exclusion involved somatic segregation of chromosomes carrying the genes for immunoglobulins. Recent data obtained by Wabl and Tenkhoff (1982) using markers for the chromosomes carrying these genes have shown that both chromosomes are present in the cells showing allelic exclusion. Mechanistic models of allelic exclusion will be discussed in Chapter 7, but the total process remains undefined. Therefore, it was quite clear by 1965 that immunoglobulins were exceptional in yet another respect. Of all proteins known to be encoded on autosomes, the immunoglobulins alone stood out as an exception to the general rules for the synthesis of allelic proteins. This finding of allelic exclusion fit nicely with the known facts about immunoglobulins and similar to the two-gene hypothesis was quickly incorporated into the mainstream of immunologic thought.

4.5. THE THREE LOCI FOR IMMUNOGLOBULINS

Throughout all discussions of the two gene–one polypeptide chain hypothesis and the phenomenon of allelic exclusion for immunoglobulin genes, the examples used have concentrated on the actions of single loci. However, as pointed out in a graphic manner by Fig. 4.13, the

Locus	V Region	C Region
H Chains	V_{HI}	μ
	V_{HII}	δ
	V_{HIII}	γ_1
	V_{HIV}	γ_2
		γ_3
		γ_4
		ϵ
		α
Kappa Chains	V_{KI}	C_K
	V_{KII}	
	V_{KIII}	
Lambda Chains	$V_{\lambda I}$	$C_{\lambda I}$
	$V_{\lambda II}$	$C_{\lambda II}$
	$V_{\lambda III}$	$C_{\lambda III}$
	$V_{\lambda IV}$	$C_{\lambda IV}$
	$V_{\lambda V}$	

Figure 4.13. Diagrammatic representation of human immunoglobulin structural genes. Each group includes a set of linked genes. Each bar represents at least one gene; the numbers of genes in each group are minimum numbers based on subgroup sequence. One V-region gene and one C-region gene interact in the synthesis of each immunoglobulin chain. The order of genes is arbitrary and this representation depicts only a haploid complement of genes.

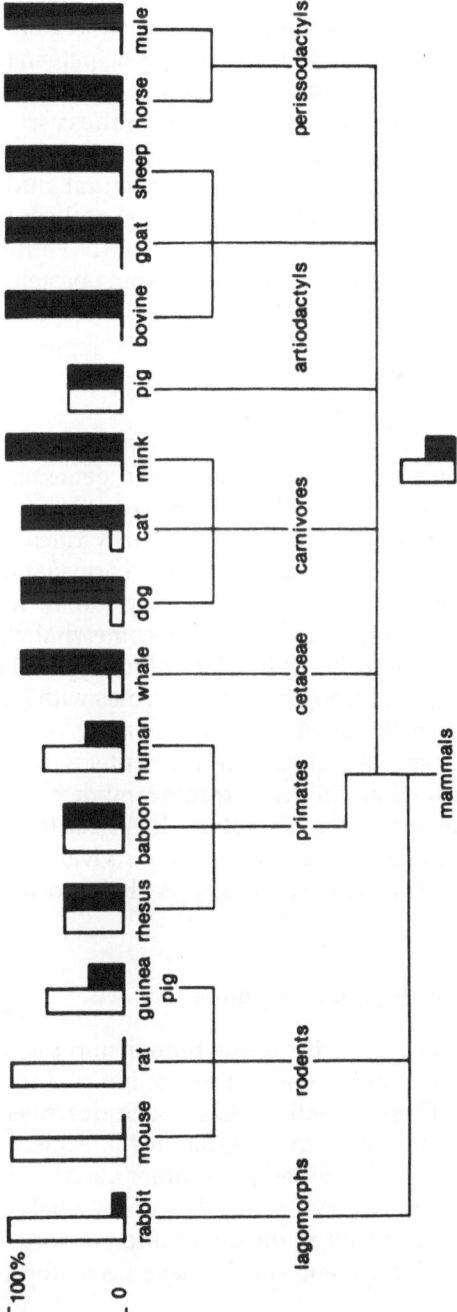

Figure 4.14. Frequency distribution of lambda and kappa light chains in sera of different mammals. From Hood *et al.* (1970).

the V-region gene sets associated with each light chain type contain overlapping information for binding sites. If the V regions of one light chain type were deficient in that they did not participate in the formation of useful and protective antibodies, then these would not be selected and the variance in ratio would be explained. In the case of the mouse, the response to the polysaccharide dextran gives rise to antibodies that express only the lambda chains. Extensive structural studies indicated that the lambda chains of the mouse varied only slightly in their V region structure. This restricted variation in the V region was verified by studies of lambda chains from a number of mouse myeloma proteins. Therefore, it may be assumed from these restrictions in variations that only certain antibody-binding functions can be served by the V regions of the mouse lambda chains and this is the reason that it is represented in very low amounts in the normal IgG population.

In spite of the low representation of lambda chains in mouse immunoglobulin, the number of C-region lambda genes is greater than kappa. The same is true in man where there are at least six lambda C-region genes and only one C_κ gene. This disparity rules out the possibility that C-region gene numbers influence the kappa/lambda ratios. In the rabbit, the amount of lambda chain is very low in normal immunoglobulin samples, but the amount may vary somewhat with the kappa chain allotype. A rabbit with the light chain phenotype b4/b4 may have approximately 4% of its immunoglobulin molecules with lambda chains; on the other hand, a b9/b9 animal may have as much as 20% of its light chains as the lambda type. As discussed in Chapter 2, nearly the entire complement of immunoglobulin may express lambda chains in the case of an allotype suppressed rabbit. Therefore, it is clear that lambda light chains contain sufficient information for the survival of an individual rabbit. What is not evident is why the kappa chain normally predominates.

4.5.2. Expression of V-Region Subgroups

The V regions of heavy chains of the human and the mouse can be classified into subgroups on the basis of the amino acid sequence of the framework residues. These variations have been described in detail in Chapter 3. Because subgroups are isotypic in the same sense as light chain types, their selection provides yet another variable in the process of gene selection for antibody synthesis. The distribution of subgroups among different species as well as the distribution of subgroups among the heavy chain classes of a single species have been studied by several investigators.

The V_HIII subgroup is readily identified by amino acid sequence analysis because it is not blocked at the amino terminus as are the heavy chains of subgroups I and II. This property was exploited by Capra *et al.* (1973) in a survey of the amount of V_HIII subgroup present in pooled heavy chains that were isolated from a number of mammalian species. It was found that the percentage of V_HIII varied from no detectable level to nearly 100% of the heavy chain in the samples tested (Fig. 4.15). More surprising than this wide range was the fact that the species tested fell into three discrete categories having 100%, 20%, or 0%, respectively, of this subgroup in their heavy chains. These groupings neatly coincided with phylogenetic origins of the various species.

Within a species, the subgroup distribution differs for heavy chains of the different classes. It has been shown from studies of normal pools of immunoglobulins and myeloma proteins that large disproportions occur in the distribution of subgroups among the various classes. For example, Capra showed that in humans the V_HIII subgroup is greatly overrepresented in IgA, whereas IgG has a much lower level of V_HIII than would be expected on the basis of immunoglobulin class distribution.

The obvious selection of the V-region framework by the various species may relate to the options available to members of that species. For example, if 90% of the V-region genes are encoded as genes with the V_HIII structure, the antibodies must reflect this proportion. It is difficult to explain selection of V-region subgroups by the different heavy chain classes. This may relate to the types of antigens most frequently encountered by the different heavy chain classes, or alternatively it may have to do with switching mechanisms that make certain combinations of V- and C-region genes more difficult to attain than others.

4.5.3. Allelic Selection of Immunoglobulin Genes

The antibody-producing cell in a heterozygote must not only choose between kappa and lambda light chains and among heavy chain subgroups, it must further select one of the two alternative alleles from each locus. In the interest of survival of an outbred species, it would seem that the selection would be made on a more or less random basis and that the ratio of immunoglobulins expressing a given allele would approximate 50/50. Experimental data have shown that this is not always the case, however, and certain alleles are selected over others in a number of immune responses. For example, in the human the responses to Rh antigens of red blood cells and to bacterial flagellin have been shown to select one Gm type almost exclusively over another.

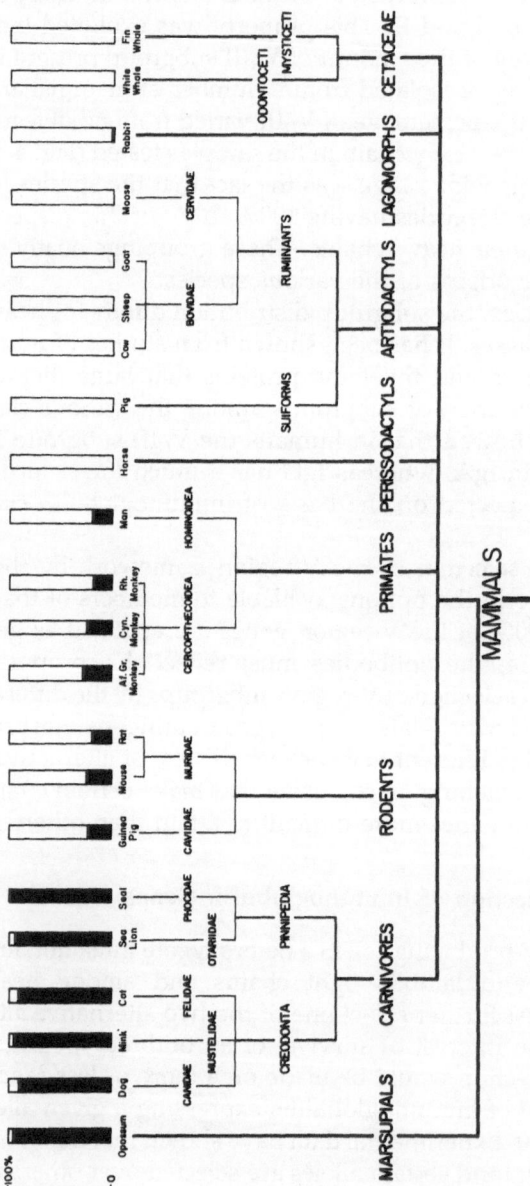

Figure 4.15. Phylogenetic distribution of the V_HIII subgroup of immunoglobulin heavy chains among mammals. The percent of unblocked V_HIII subgroup is depicted in black. From Capra *et al.* (1973).

In the rabbit response to certain antigens, allotype selection has been noted. Haurowitz and co-workers (Foshay *et al.*, 1976) showed that the response to *p*-azophenylarsonate preferentially selected one group a allotype over another. Similarly, Catty *et al.* (1969) showed that anti-pneumococcal antibodies had a strong selective preference for one group b allotype over another.

An extended family of rabbits derived from a b4/b4 doe and a b9/b9 buck were used for detailed studies of the allotypes in the response to streptococcal antigens, indicating that in heterozygous (F_1 or F_2) rabbits with the light chain allotype b4/b9, the b4 allele was overwhelmingly selected. It was further shown that in the F_2 generation those rabbits with the allotype b9/b9 produced as much antistreptococcal antibody as did those with the b4/b4 or b4/b9 type. The response was not linked to the b allotype. It had been shown earlier by Dubiski (1972) and by others that there was a "pecking" order or allotype preference in certain heterozygous animals. That is, one allotype would be represented more frequently on immunoglobulin molecules than would its alleles. This finding was extended to show that antibody-producing cells showed similar allotype ratios; this finding precluded allotype-related defects in rate of synthesis as the explanation for the pecking order.

Studies of the V regions associated with different kappa light chains in the rabbit by primary structural analysis have shown that different sets of V regions exist and these may be inherited in linkage to the C-region allotypes. It is not known, however, what factors govern the selection of one set over another in the majority of instances in a heterozygous animal. Attempts to explain these selections on the basis of antibody affinity or other factors have not been convincing.

4.6. CONCLUSION

There is much evidence to show that the antibody system is unique in many ways. The antibody V regions display a pattern of structural variability not mimicked in any other protein system. The expression of immunoglobulin genes reveals further surprising features. A number of experimental findings suggest that immunoglobulin genes violate the one gene–one polypeptide chain dogma. Additionally, the inheritance of immunoglobulin allotypes indicates that although immunoglobulins are encoded by autosomal codominant alleles, a single antibody-producing cell expresses only one allele. Further peculiarities relate to the relative levels of expression of immunoglobulin isotypes and allotypes and have no easy explanation. In light of the exceptional behavior of the immunoglobulin system, it was not surprising that theorists would attempt to explain this collection of bizarre facts.

To this point the discussion of antibody diversity has been mainly descriptive and has included listing the basic elements of the problem, describing the immunoglobulin molecules, and determining what was learned about the nature of immunoglobulin genes in structural and serologic studies. An attempt will be made in the next two chapters to integrate the available data concerning the peculiar behavior of immunoglobulins and their genes and in a formal way outline the theories that were put forth to explain the genetic basis of antibody diversity. In the next chapter, the two most fundamental theories, the germline theory and the somatic mutation theory, will be discussed in light of their respective insights to the unique problems of antibody diversity.

REFERENCES AND BIBLIOGRAPHY

Baglioni, C., Cioli, D., Gorini, G., Ruffilli, A., and Alescio-Zonta, L., 1967, Studies on fragments of light chains of human immunoglobulins: Genetic and biochemical implications, *Cold Spring Harbor Symp. Quant. Biol.* **32**:147.

Beutler, E., Yeh, M., and Fairbanks, V. F., 1962, The normal human female as a mosaic of X chromosome activity: Studies using the gene for G-6-PD deficiency as a marker, *Proc. Natl. Acad. Sci. U.S.A.* **48**:9.

Beadle, G. W., and Tatum, E. L., 1941, Genetic control of biochemical reactions in neurospora, *Proc. Natl. Acad. Sci. U.S.A.* **27**:499.

Capra, J. D., Wasserman, R. L., and Kehoe, J. M., 1973, Phylogenetically associated residues with the V_HIII subgroup of several mammalian species: Evidence for a "Pauci-Gene" basis for antibody diversity, *J. Exp. Med.* **138**:410.

Catty, D., Humphrey, J. H., and Gell, P. G. H., 1969, The proportion of two b locus allotypic determinants in rabbit antisera raised against pneumococcal polysaccharide SSS-III antigen, *Immunology* **16**:409.

Conley, C. L., and Charache, S., 1973, Inherited hemoglobinopathies, in: *Medical Genetics* (V. A. McKusick and R. Claiborne, eds.), H. P. Publishing Company, Inc., p. 53.

Dreyer, W. N., and Bennett, J. C., 1965, The molecular basis of antibody formation: A paradox, *Proc. Natl. Acad. Sci. U.S.A.* **54**:864.

Dubiski, S., 1969, Immunochemistry and genetics of a "new" allotypic specificity A_e^{14} of rabbit γG immunoglobulins: Recombination in somatic cells, *J. Immunol.* **103**:120.

Dubiski, S., 1972, Genetics and regulation of immunoglobulin allotypes, *Med. Clin. North Am.* **56**:557.

Eichmann, K., and Berek, C., 1973, Mendelian segregation of a mouse antibody idiotype, *Eur. J. Immunol.* **3**:599.

Eichmann, K., and Kindt, T. J., 1971, The inheritance of individual antigenic specificities of rabbit antibodies to streptococcal carbohydrates, *J. Exp. Med.* **134**:532.

Feinstein, A., 1963, Character and allotypy of an immune globulin in rabbit colostrum, *Nature* **199**:1197.

Fleischman, J. B., 1967, Synthesis of the rabbit gamma G heavy chain, *Cold Spring Harbor Symp. Quant. Biol.* **32**:233.

Foshay, M. C., Zimmerman, S. E., Spencer, L. K., Haurowitz, F., and Knight, K., 1976, Perferential expression of anti-azobenzenearsonate antibodies of heterozygous at a³ rabbits in the a1 allotype, *J. Immunol.* **116**:1010.

Fu, S. M., Winchester, R. J., and Kunkel, H. G., 1975, Similar idiotypic specificity for the membrane IgD and IgM of human B lymphocytes, *J. Immunol.* **114**:250.

Garrod, A. E., 1923, *Inborn Errors of Metabolism*, 2nd Ed., Oxford University Press, London.

Harboe, M., Osterland, C. K., Mannik, M., and Kunkel, H. G., 1962, Genetic characters of human γ-globulins and myeloma proteins, *J. Exp. Med.* **116**:719.

Hilschmann, N., and Craig, L. C., 1965, Amino acid sequence studies with Bence-Jones proteins, *Proc. Natl. Acad. Sci. U.S.A.* **53**:1403.

Hood, L., Grant, J. A., and Sox, H. C., 1970, On the structure of normal light chains from mammals and birds: Evolutionary and genetic implications, in: *Developmental Aspects of Antibody Formation and Structure*, Vol. 1, (J. Sterzl and I. Riha eds.), Academia Publishing House of the Czechoslovak Acadamy of Science, Prague, p. 283.

Hopper, J. E., and Nisonoff, A., 1971, Individual antigenic specificity of immunoglobulins, *Adv. Immunol.* **13**:57.

Jerne, N. K., and Nordin, A. A., 1963, Plaque formation in agar by single antibody-producing cells, *Science* **140**:405.

Kabat, E., Wu, T. T., and Bilofsky, H., 1979, Sequence of immunoglobulin chains, U. S. Dept. Health, Education and Welfare, PHS, NIH, p. 121.

Kindt, T. J., Mandy, W. J., and Todd, C. W., 1970, Association of allotypic specificities of group a with allotypic specificities A11 and A12 in rabbit immunoglobulin, *Biochemistry* **9**:2028.

Kindt, T. J., and Todd, C. W., 1969, Heavy and light chain allotypic markers on rabbit homocytotropic antibody, *J. Exp. Med.* **130**:859.

Knight, K. L., Malek, T. R., and Hanly, W. C., 1974, Recombinant rabbit secretory immunoglobulin molecules: Alpha chains with maternal (paternal) variable-region allotypes and paternal (maternal) constant-region allotypes, *Proc. Natl. Acad. Sci. U.S.A.* **71**:1169.

Koshland, M. E., Davis, J. J., and Fujita, N. J., 1969, Evidence for multiple gene control of a single polypeptide chain: The heavy chain of rabbit immunoglobulin, *Proc. Natl. Acad. Sci. U.S.A.* **63**:1274.

Kuettner, M. G., Wang, A., and Nisonoff, A., 1972, Quantitative investigations of idiotypic antibodies. VI. Idiotypic specificity as a potential genetic marker for the variable regions of mouse immunoglobulin polypeptide chains, *J. Exp. Med.* **135**:579.

Kunkel, H. G., 1970, Experimental approaches to homogeneous antibody populations: Individual antigenic specificity, cross specificity and diversity of human antibodies, *Fed. Proc.* **29**:55.

Lennox, E. S., Knopf, P. M., Munro, A. J., and Parkhouse, R. M. E., 1967, A search for biosynthetic subunits of light and heavy chains of immunoglobulins, *Cold Spring Harbor Symp. Quant. Biol.* **32**:249.

Lyon, M. F., 1961, Gene action in the X-chromosome of the mouse *(mus musculus L.)*, *Nature (London)* **190**:372.

Mage, R. G., Young-Cooper, G. O., and Alexander, C., 1971, Genetic control of variable and constant regions of immunoglobulin heavy chains, *Nature (New Biol.)* **230**:63.

Mandy, W. J., and Todd, C. W., 1968, Allotypy of rabbit immunoglobulin: An agglutinating specificity, *Vox Sanguinis* **14**:264.

Nathenson, S. G., Uehara, H., Ewenstein, B. M., Kindt, T. J., and Coligan, J. E., 1981, Primary structural analysis of the transplantation antigens of the murine H-2 major histocompatibility complex, *Annu. Rev. Biochem.* **50**:1025.

Ohno, S., Weiler, C., Poole, J., Christian, L., and Stenius, C., 1966, Autosomal polymorphism due to Pericentric inversions in the deer mouse *(Peromyscus maniculatus)*
and some evidence of somatic segregation, *Chromosoma (Berlin)* **18:**177.

Oudin, J., and Michel, M., 1969, Idiotypy of rabbit antibodies. II. Comparison of idiotypy
of various kinds of antibodies formed in the same rabbits against *Salmonella typhi*, *J.
Exp. Med.* **130:**619.

Pernis, B., Chiappino, G., Kelus, A., and Gell, P. G. H., 1965, Cellular localization of
immunoglobulins with different allotypic specificities in rabbit lymphoid tissues, *J.
Exp. Med.* **122:**853.

Putnam, F. W., Titani, K., Wikler, M., and Shinoda, T., 1967, Structure and evolution of
kappa and lambda light chains, *Cold Spring Harbor Symp. Quant. Biol.* **32:**9.

Strominger, J. L., Orr, H. T., Parham, P., Ploegh, H. L., Mann, D. L., Bilofsky, H., Saroff,
H. A., Wu, T. T., and Kabat, E. A., 1980, An evaluation of the significance of amino
acid sequence homologies in human histocompatibility antigens (HLA-A and HLA-
B) with immunoglobulins and other proteins, using relatively short sequences, *Scand.
J. Immunol.* **11:**573.

Todd, C. W., 1963, Allotypy in rabbit 19S protein, *Biochem. Biophys. Res. Commun.* **11:**170.

Wabl, M. R., and Tenkhoff, M., 1982, Allelic exclusion of immunoglobulin expression is
not caused by somatic segregation, *Proc. Natl. Acad. Sci. U.S.A.* **79:**606–607.

Wang, A.-C., Wang, I. Y. F., McCormick, J. N., and Fudenberg, H. H., 1969, The identity
of light chains of monoclonal IgG and monoclonal IgM in one patient, *Immunochemistry*
6:451.

Wang, A. C., Wang, I. Y. F., and Fudenberg, H. H., 1977, Immunoglobulin structure and
genetics: Identity between variable regions of a μ and a γ2 chain, *J. Biol. Chem.* **252:**7192.

Weigert, M., and Potter, M., 1977, Antibody variable-region genetics: Summary and ab-
stract of the Homogeneous Immunoglobulin Workshop VII, *Immunogenetics* **4:**401.

Weiler, E., 1965, Differential activity of allelic γ-globulin genes in antibody-producing cells,
Proc. Natl. Acad. Sci. U.S.A. **54:**1765.

Wilkinson, J. M., 1969, Variation in the N-terminal sequence of heavy chains of immunoglobulin G from rabbits of different allotype, *Biochem. J.* **112:**173.

Wu, T. T., and Kabat, E. A., 1970, The analysis of the sequence of the variable regions
of Bence Jones proteins and myeloma light chains and their implications for antibody
complementarity, *J. Exp. Med.* **132:**211.

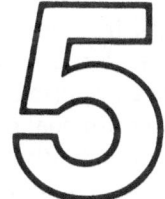

THE POLAR SOLUTIONS

There is one great difficulty with a good hypothesis. When it is completed and rounded, the corners smooth and the content cohesive and coherent, it is likely to become a thing in itself, a work of art. It is then like a finished sonnet or a painting completed. One hates to disturb it. Even if subsequent information should shoot a hole in it, one hates to tear it down because it once was beautiful and whole.

—JOHN STEINBECK *(Log from the Sea of Cortez)*

.1. INTRODUCTION

As detailed in previous chapters, the description of antibody diversity moved rapidly in the wake of sophisticated experiments designed to probe the extent of the repertoire. Data obtained by serologists, biochemists, and geneticists all revealed the complexity of immunoglobulin populations and indicated that the capability to produce a large number of antibody molecules was present in a single organism. Whether one arrived at this large number by counting antibody-binding sites, idiotypes, or amino acid sequences of heavy and light chain V regions, the data strongly supported the two-gene hypothesis and underscored the bifunctional nature of the antibody molecule. However, this body of serologic and structural data failed to answer an overriding question, one that dominated the area of immunoglobulin genetics during this time: What was the precise number and nature of V-region genes?

Although the experimentalists could readily agree on the major descriptive aspects of antibody diversity, the theorists seeking to explain it found no such easy agreement. Although there were several theories advanced to explain antibody diversity, the majority of immunologists fell into one of two camps, each dealing with the same experimental data but arriving at almost diametrically opposing conclusions. Because the opposing theorists were required to explain the same data, it was not unusual during this period to see two speakers in a symposium on antibody diversity using identical slides to reach opposing positions. As new data became available, each group modified their theory to explain these new facets of antibody diversity.

The two major theories that were advanced to explain antibody diversity differed in their estimates of how many V-region genes were present in the germline. There were, on the one hand, theorists contending that every antibody V region required a separate germline gene. On the other hand there were those arguing that the number of germline V genes was very low, perhaps as low as one, and that V-region diversity arose from mutations occurring in somatic cells. Theories calling for a large number of V-region genes in the germline were called *germline* theories. Theories calling for a small number of germline genes that would mutate to form the necessary binding sites were called *somatic mutation* theories. The question of whether few or many V-region genes are present in the germline became for many the major question in immunology.

Before going on to explain how each of these theories dealt with the accumulated body of experimental facts concerning antibody diversity, it may be useful to state the major tenets of each of the theories. For the purpose of this discussion the theories will be considered in their modern forms that take into account the two-gene hypothesis. Major objections to each of the theories of antibody diversity were removed by the postulate that V and C genes were separated in the genome as discussed in Chapter 4. For the germline theory this allowed a tremendous reduction in the number of DNA base pairs required for antibody synthesis. It would not be necessary for each of the multiple heavy chain classes or light chain types to have their own contiguous V regions. Furthermore, it removed the need for replicate copies of C genes and the accompanying possibility of mutations affecting biologic function. The somatic mutation theory was spared the difficulties inherent in having identical V regions in two different antibody classes arise by parallel mutational events. Therefore, it is difficult to say which theory was most greatly advanced by the two-gene hypothesis because each became more believable in the light of this "simplification" of the antibody genes. It should be emphasized that the two-gene hypothesis did not favor one theory over the other; on the contrary, it gave to each theory a new level of plausibility.

5.2. THE GERMLINE THEORY

Although it may be argued (see Chapter 1, Fig 1.3) that Ehrlich's side-chain theory is the first mention of such an hypothesis, the germline theory has no easily defined historical starting point. It is based on the classic genetic theme that for each protein there is a corresponding gene. In its purest form it requires no ad hoc assumptions and is supported by a large number of precedents. Application of the germline theory to immunoglobulins requires a rather large commitment of DNA to antibody synthesis but, as will be discussed immediately below, the proportion of the genome required is not unreasonable. In addition, the advent of the two-gene hypothesis relieved much of the pressure for such a large genomic investment in the function of antibody synthesis.

The germline or multigene hypothesis states that each organism has one gene in its germline for each unique (V region) antibody polypeptide chain that it can synthesize. Separate genes present as single copies encode each of the C regions of the heavy or light chains. During differentiation of the antibody-forming cell, a single V-region gene is joined to a C-region gene for the heavy chain. Similarly, a V-region gene is joined to the C-region gene for the light chain and the resulting differentiated cell produces one antibody molecule. The numerous genes encoding the V regions arise by the normal process of chemical evolution; that is, by gene duplication followed by mutation and selection.

Application of the germline theory to the problem of antibody diversity requires that approximately 10 million antibodies are encoded in the germline. It may be asked whether there is sufficient DNA for the synthesis of all of the antibodies required in the germline theory. This question was approached in an early paper by Hood and Talmage (1970) who used the following reasoning to show that there was no problem in having sufficient DNA for the required 10 million antibodies. They argued that if most combinations of heavy and light chains form unique antibody binding sites, then approximately 3000 genes are required for the variable portion of the light chain and 3000 genes for the variable portion of the heavy chain. Since the V region of the antibody is approximately 110 amino acid residues long, 330 base pairs would be required for each V gene. Accordingly, about 1 million base pairs would be devoted to V-region genes for the light chain and another million for V-region genes for the heavy chain. If the genome contains 10^9 base pairs, it would require approximately 0.2% of the total genomic material to encode the necessary antibody V regions. Although proponents of the germline theory may argue for larger or smaller numbers of V_H or

V_L genes, the postulated variations would not have a significant impact on this figure. Whether 0.2% is an unreasonable proportion of the genome to devote to a function that is as important as antibody synthesis is difficult to ascertain based on any available data. Certainly no one could argue that DNA available in the genome is not sufficient to encode the number of antibodies specified by the germline theory.

The germline theory was definitely alluring and its major attraction was its simplicity. Without invoking any novel genetic mechanisms (other than the two-gene hypothesis), the problem of antibody diversity could be concisely solved. The theory was very simple to understand and as a consequence was also quite simple to criticize in light of experimental data. There were certain data concerning antibody diversity that did not fit neatly into the simple pattern predicted by the germline hypothesis. It is these exceptional data that precluded universal acceptance of the germline theory and that were a major factor in leading to the lengthy and polarized controversy over the origin of antibody diversity.

5.3. THE SOMATIC MUTATION THEORY

In polar opposition to the germline theory was the somatic mutation theory. This theory calls for the presence of only a relatively few V genes in the germline as opposed to the presence of all V genes as in the germline theory. The somatic mutation theory had its roots in the instructive hypothesis (see Chapter 1) and in 1959, Lederberg advanced a more modern version calling for mutation of antibody genes as a means of generating diversity. In the somatic mutation theory developed by Milstein, Cohn, Weigert and others, the role of somatic events in shaping the antibody-binding site was not perceived in the drastic terms of the Breinl-Haurowitz theory (see Chapter 1, Section 1.3.2), but rather involved selection by antigen following somatic alterations of the protein structure. However, the bulk of the repertoire would still arise de novo in the host rather than be inherited. In more recent versions of the theory, terms such as point mutation, contact residue, and hypervariable region were used to develop a cogent hypothesis to explain the manner in which this universe of necessary binding sites was generated.

In the somatic mutation model, antibody diversity is generated by mutations in as few as one V-region gene. The basic set of antibodies that is encoded in the germline may have binding sites directed against the most common pathogens or alternatively, as stated in a variation of this concept advanced by Jerne (1971), may be directed against certain alloantigens. In any case, the majority of useful antibodies are produced by mutation of this small set of V-region genes and the newly generated antibodies are selected by antigen. The selection step occurs following each mutation.

In sharp contrast to the germline theory, which in its most basic form requires no ad hoc assumptions, the somatic mutation theory raises the immediate need for several clarifying explanations. These explanations, however, can be given without invoking unprecedented mechanisms. The first issue concerns whether the mutational frequency of the antibody V-region genes is sufficient to generate the necessary binding sites during ontogeny. The second issue concerns the mechanism of selection and how this fits into the general functioning of the immune system.

The issue of mutational frequency was handled by Cohn (1970) who used the following argument. Assume that the mutational frequency of antibody genes is the same as that measured for bacterial genes (about 10^{-7} per base pair per division). If approximately 100 base pairs are involved in encoding the residues that compose the antigen-binding site (hypervariable regions), there would be a frequency of 10^{-5} for base pairs encoding an antibody-binding site. At this rate, if one begins with 10^8 cells that divide between three and four times per day, there could be generated 2×10^4 antibodies within ten days. If the frequency of mutation were slightly higher for the antibody V region as might be expected for this system, say 10^{-3}, then 2×10^6 new antibodies would result within the same period of time. It should be pointed out that a mutational frequency lower than 10^{-5} would pose serious obstacles to this form of the somatic mutation theory. This calculation further assumes that each mutation in the hypervariable region sequences will give rise to a new antibody; therefore, silent mutations are not considered in the calculation.

The second issue to be raised concerns the selection of useful antibodies from the dynamic pool of antibody mutants that are constantly being formed. It is envisioned that only those cells that produced and displayed an antibody that was selected by antigen would divide and mature into antibody-secreting plasma cells and long-lived memory cells. Those other cells bearing the unselected binding sites would not divide and mature.

Thus under this broad outline, the somatic mutation theory was viewed by many as a feasible alternative to the germline theory. Although the germline theory was favored by many because of its apparent simplicity, it was difficult to choose either of the theories on any a priori basis. For example, considering the question of economy to the organism, the germline theory would require maintenance of considerably more DNA devoted to antibody synthesis than the somatic mutation theory. On the other hand, however, the somatic model required production of many cells that are not selected by antigen. Arguments can be made favoring either situation but it would require experimental data to resolve the question of which theory better explained the facts of antibody diversity. It was unusual to find experimental data that fit precisely and exclusively one or the other theory. In fact, the choice was not substantially simplified by consideration of all the data from protein sequence analysis and from serologic analyses of antibodies.

5.4. DATA FAVORING GERMLINE THEORIES

Although it was rarely possible to point to experimental data that precisely fit one or the other of the polar theories to the absolute exclusion of the other, there emerged data from certain systems that favored one of the theories. In general, however, it was difficult to predict how a certain type of experiment would ultimately be interpreted. For example, serologic studies of allotypes yielded data that favored somatic mutation models. On the other hand, serologic studies of inherited idiotypes that sprang directly from the allotype experiments were clearly easier to explain in terms of germline models. Similarly, the structural studies of antibody V regions yielded data in support of the germline theory in that there were a large number of subgroups; however, the identical studies yielded data concerning phylogenetically associated residues that strongly favored somatic theories. In the following sections, several examples in which one or the other theory had a distinct advantage in explaining the data will be considered.

5.4.1. V-Region Subgroups

Amino acid sequences of antibodies were scrutinized in great detail by theorists attempting to explain antibody diversity. If antibodies were primary gene products (and there was no reason to consider any other possibility), then the V-region genes were revealed by the V-region amino acid sequences. In this respect, sequence data were much easier to interpret than serologic data that required that the observed antigenic differences corresponded to differences in primary protein structure. Although the two-gene hypothesis that was postulated on structural data found universal acceptance within a very short time, the same data did not so easily reveal a universally acceptable answer to the question of how many V regions are encoded in the genome.

The findings related to V-region structure had multiple interpretations and each group of theorists found reasons why a new data fragment was supportive of their theory. Some experimental findings, however, posed real difficulty for one theory or the other and in these cases a typical strategy was denial of the validity of the data. In the case of data obtained using the serologically detected allotypes and idiotypes, interpretations could be disputed on the basis of the sometimes subjective data. In the case of the description of V-region subgroups that were based only on the objective criterion of protein sequence data, the validity of the primary data could scarcely be challenged. However, in this instance disputes may have centered about the sources of starting material used to obtain the data. For example, it may be asked whether randomly chosen BALB/c myeloma proteins represented a valid window through which to view the entire antibody repertoire. Therefore, although the amino acid sequence data were themselves quite straightforward, their interpretation was often highly controversial. Perhaps the most controversial question that developed in this area concerned the concept of V-region subgroups.

A thorough description of V-region subgroups was given in Chapter 3, and the present discussion will emphasize subgroup variation and the ramifications of subgroups to the two major theories of antibody diversity. Perhaps the key element to be considered here in the definition of the subgroup is the fact that the amino acid substitutions observed among the various subgroups were nonrandom. There were positions that were constant to all subgroups and then there were positions at which variations could be observed. The nonrandom nature of this variation was interpreted to indicate that each well-defined subgroup could represent the product of a germline gene. This interpretation then led to an experimental test of the polar theories: if you can count the subgroups, then you can count the minimum number of germline genes. Because there was no substantial disagreement on this point, the antibody diversity argument focused on the definition of a subgroup and it is about this definition that controversy raged for a number of years.

Because the germline theory called for multiple genes, a very restrictive definition of subgroups was favored. There could be as many subgroups as one wished, so there was pressure to disallow lumping of a great many sequences into one subgroup. The somatic mutation theory, on the other hand, was more consistent with a loose definition of subgroups because the presence of many variants within one single subgroup would imply that these all were derived by mutations from one single subgroup gene.

The role of genetic polymorphism in V region diversity was also an issue. The existence of allelic forms of the same subgroup was favored by somatic mutation proponents because it allowed multiple forms of the same gene to exist in the population without raising the number present in any one individual. When the human V_κ subgroups were initially described, it was postulated that much of the observed variation within a subgroup was of an allelic nature. This was an acceptable view because the myeloma proteins were derived from outbred human patients. However, arguments concerning the role of genetic polymorphism lost ground as increasing amounts of amino acid sequence data for kappa light chains from the inbred BALB/c mouse strain became available. Because this was an inbred strain, every animal was, in principle, homozygous at all loci and one BALB/c mouse was presumed identical to another. Therefore, the polymorphism arguments could not be applied to the data obtained from inbred mice. As will be seen in Section 5.5.3, the question of V-region genetic polymorphism persisted as a problem to be considered for both of the theories. In fact, there were two polymorphic systems, the rabbit heavy chain V-region allotypes and the mouse kappa light chain V-region allotypes that provided arguments against a pure germline theory.

Several points of the subgroup definition could be agreed on and these centered first about the nature of the data to be considered. Most reported V-region sequences were not complete but rather represented data from a single amino terminal sequence analysis of the light chain or heavy chain using an automated sequencer. Accordingly, it was conceded that examination of the amino terminal 23 residues of an immunoglobulin chain could validly predict its relationship to other chains. However, it was also thought that counting the number of subgroups based on the amino terminal residues would underestimate the total number by a factor of two.

Another important point in the definition of a subgroup is related to framework versus hypervariable residues. As discussed earlier, hypervariable regions were shown to form the antigen combining site. With few exceptions the three hypervariable regions of the heavy or the light chain contain all of the most variable positions. Therefore, these regions provide areas for localization of mutations in the somatic mutation theory. One would expect that variations among different chains within a single subgroup to be confined solely to these positions. In the somatic mutation theory, hypervariable substitutions were postulated to be the major driving force in the generation of diversity. Two chains that were identical in their framework sequence but different in the hypervariable regions would have to be considered as the prime example of antibody diversity generated by somatic mutation. Therefore, it was postulated that only framework substitutions were relevant to the delineation of different V-region subgroups; recall that the most well-defined hypervariable regions were found for chains within a single subgroup (Chapter 3). This not only made sense for the subgroup definition but also provided implicit support for somatic mutation theories. This fact provided the basis for analysis of data from the mouse lambda and mouse kappa systems that supported the somatic mutation theory. However, in spite of this support, studies on V-region subgroups would ultimately favor the germline, not the somatic mutation theory.

An inevitable consequence of counting C-region genes by counting V-region sequences was that the number of postulated germline genes always had to increase. As new sequences were completed, there was no easy way to include them all in the existing subgroups. New subgroups were then postulated, raising the number of germline genes. Furthermore, certain subgroups had to be divided into sub-subgroups in order to accommodate all of the related sequences. By 1975, the estimates for the number of V-region subgroups in the BALB/c kappa genes reached as high as 250. As the V-region gene number estimated from the amino acid sequence data increased, the germline hypothesis became more attractive. However, the numbers that were being obtained by counting in this fashion were still not high enough to account for the several thousand V-region genes that would be needed by this theory. On the other hand, the somatic mutation theories lost much of their appeal when estimates of gene numbers reached 50 or 100. Except for the special case of the mouse lambda light chain (Section 5.5.2), most V-region families in which some form of V-gene counting was possible reached numbers of this magnitude. Thus, the subgroup data favored the germline theory although many questions remained, especially concerning the precise number of V genes. The number of genes estimated by these studies was too high to be consistent with a somatic mutation model.

5.4.2. Evolutionary Divergence (Trees)

There was an additional aspect of the V-region subgroup data that was used mainly by Hood and Talmage (1970) to support germline theories. The amino acid sequence data for antibody V regions were analyzed by computer programs. These programs had been originally developed by Fitch and Margoliash (1967) to show phylogenetic relationships among protein homologues from different species. Figure 5.1 depicts a

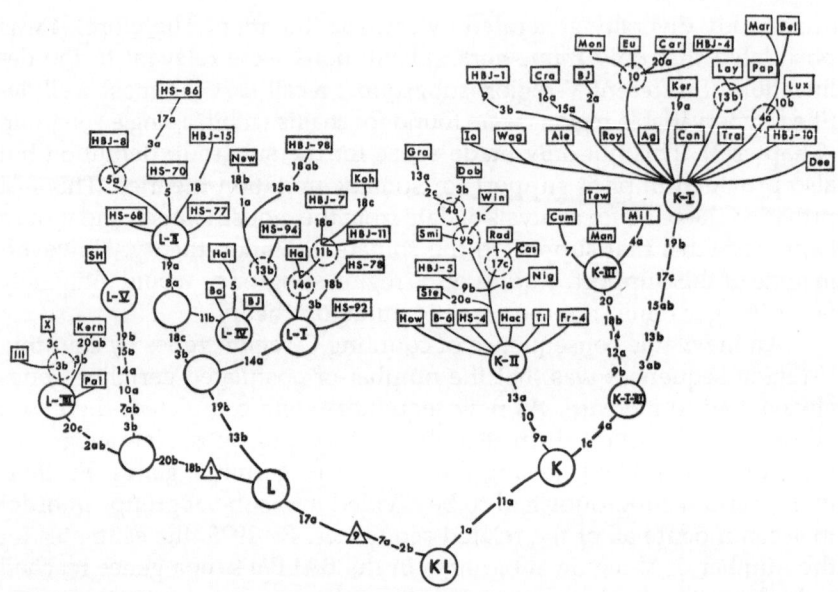

Figure 5.1. A "phylogenetic" tree constructed from the amino terminal 20 residues of 41 human kappa and 23 human lambda proteins by the method of Fitch and Margoliash (1967), which reduces the number of mutations to a minimum. The 64 proteins are indicated by closed rectangles. Deletions are indicated by triangles and mutations by numbers. The letters a, b, or c indicate which nucleotide is changed according to the genetic code. Closed circles indicate major subgroups. Dotted circles indicate subdivisions of the subgroups or highly improbable identical somatic mutations occurring in two different individuals. From Hood and Talmage (1970).

tree constructed from amino terminal sequence data of human kappa and lambda light chains. The position of the differences among the chains are noted on the branches. The number indicates the amino acid position beginning with number one as the amino terminal; the letters a, b, and c refer to substitutions of the nucleotides within the codons for the amino acids.

Several points may be made based on these representations of amino acid sequence data. First of all, the separation of kappa and lambda chains is easily seen in this analysis. Next, it should be noted that although subgroups can be recognized, there are large numbers of intrasubgroup variants within some of these subgroups. It may be argued in these cases (for example, see K-1 in Fig. 5.1) that intrasubgroup variation is as marked as intersubgroup variation. When this occurs, the distribution between subgroups blurs and there is pressure to define more subgroups to explain the variation. This tendency to increase subgroups according to our earlier definition means increasing the number of germline genes and, of course, favors the germline theory.

Thus, the amino acid sequence data could be further interpreted by this computer-aided analysis to project that more germline genes were required for the antibody repertoire. As arguments based on phylogenetically associated residues and V-region allotypes were developed in support of somatic mutation theories, the computer analyses were used to show that these situations as well could be explained by simple divergence of multi-gene families.

5.4.3. Inheritance of Idiotypes

Although data concerning immunoglobulin V-region subgroups obtained from N-terminal sequences played a role in shaping questions about V gene numbers, it was evident that complete variable region sequences were needed. After all, the real question concerned the antigen-binding sites of antibodies, and ultimately it was the germline complement of these that had to be enumerated. With the discovery of idiotypes and the subsequent realization that these were indeed markers for the V region of antibodies came the possibility that inheritance of antibody-binding sites could be followed by simple serologic tests. In the ultimate case, idiotype identity could infer total identity of the V-region sequence. The labor of determining complete V-region amino acid sequences, therefore, could be circumvented and the germline genes counted in a much simpler fashion. Obviously, there are certain flaws in this reasoning, a number of which were pointed out in Chapter 2. However, assuming that an anti-Id reagent detects either a V_H or V_L region and the recognized determinants are in the hypervariable region, then a reasonably clear test of the polar theories becomes possible using the idiotype systems.

If all antibody V regions are encoded in the germline, then observations of the same idiotype, at least in family members or members of the same inbred animal strain, should be a common occurrence. Conversely, the somatic mutation theory argues that random mutation of hypervariable residues would generate so many different solutions to the problem of binding a given antigen that finding two identical antibodies in different animals should be an infrequent occurrence and idiotype markers should be more or less unique to the animal in which they were originally produced.

The first descriptions of idiotype inheritance were interpreted as supportive of the germline theory as illustrated by the following quote by Eichmann and Kindt (1971):

> In such a rabbit family with limited idiotypic variability, antigenic stimulation frequently selects antibodies with similar or identical individual antigenic specificity, and this individual antigenic specificity can be preserved over several generations. This observation argues against the occurrence of somatic mutation as the major mechanism of idiotypic variability. Rather it appears that each idiotype is an inherited gene product. . . .

The inheritance of idiotypes was demonstrated for antibodies directed against a number of antigens in different mouse strains. As described in Chapter 2, the idiotypes in many cases were linked to heavy chain allotype genes of the mouse. In several cases, when more than one idiotype was followed in a single mouse strain, there was evidence to indicate that there was sufficient distance between the V genes to allow for cross-over. In one example (previously mentioned in Chapter 4), the A5A and Ars idiotypes were observed to segregate in a mouse that was identified as an exception to the linkage between the allotype gene Ig-1e and the idiotype of the antistreptococcal antibody A5A. The cross-over animal carried the BALB/c C-region allotype Ig-1a along with A5A, which was normally absent in BALB/c animals. When the recombinants were tested for the Ars idiotype, which is present in animals with the A/J haplotype but absent in BALB/c, it was not found. Therefore, the recombinant haplotype contained a V region associated with A/J idiotype A5A but not the V region encoding the Ars idiotype. These data were presumptive evidence that the variable region locus had sufficient length to allow cross-over between two distantly spaced V-region genes. Obviously, such data suggest that a large number of V-region genes are maintained in coupling and are most easily interpreted by germline models.

There were, however, certain aspects of idiotypic inheritance that could be interpreted in terms of somatic mutation theory. In one such study, Hart et al. (1973) used antibodies directed against the Ars idiotype to suppress expression of this idiotype in A/J mice. When the suppressed animals were immunized with a protein–arsonate conjugate, the animals responded with anti-Ars antibodies at levels similar to the nonsuppressed mice. However, none of the mice produced idiotype-positive antibodies. This is not suprising, but merely shows that the idiotype suppression was effective. However, when antibodies were taken from the suppressed animals, isolated, and used to prepare new anti-idiotype reagents, no cross-reactions were detected among the antibodies from different suppressed mice. This finding was interpreted by Nisonoff to indicate that there was a germline gene that encoded Ars but that its suppression led to the selection of mutants that were sufficiently distant from Ars that no idiotypic cross-reaction would occur. The fact that there were no cross-reactions among the antibodies in the suppressed animals indicated that many directions of mutation could be taken to solve the problem of binding arsonate.

The difficulty of interpreting inherited idiotypes as representative of germline genes and noninherited idiotypes as products of somatic mutation leads to a situation similar to that observed in studies of V-region subgroups. Every discovery of an inherited idiotype means a new germline gene and how many one finds probably depends on how long and hard one looks. Inevitably, the number of inherited idiotypes increased to the point where somatic mutation theories could not provide an adequate explanation.

5.5. DATA FAVORING SOMATIC MUTATION MODELS

Although the germline theory was the perennial favorite and was given increasing support by the structural data showing a multiplicity of subgroups and serologic data showing inheritance of an increasing number of idiotypes, there was never universal acceptance of this model. There were, in fact, several aspects of the structural data that did not easily fit the germline theory. In a similar fashion certain serologic studies, especially those concerned with V-region allotypes, were also better explained by paucigene theories.

The somatic mutation theory had its proponents and they had data to support their position. As will be seen in Sections 5.5.1–5.5.4, there are certain data that placed stumbling blocks in the smooth progression toward acceptance of a simple multigene theory. The explanations required for these difficulties in a germline model would be forthcoming, but each qualification of the theory detracted from its strongest point that was its simplicity.

5.5.1. Phylogenetically Associated Residues

Although the general trend of subgroup identification and the proliferation of subgroups with the new sequence information favor multigene theories, several findings from the amino acid sequence data were most compatible with the somatic mutation theory. One of these in particular was the identification of residues that were found at certain positions for all (or nearly all) V-region sequences derived from one species and that were different for proteins of other species. These were called species-specific or phylogenetically associated residues. The *distribution* of phylogenetically associated residues along immunoglobulin chains will be further developed in Chapter 6; here we will discuss their existence and interpretation.

In its simplest form, a multigene theory calls for a set of V-region genes that evolve and are selected throughout the evolutionary process just as any other protein. The observation of phylogenetically associated residues in given positions in each member of the inherited set required a special mechanism not specified by this theory. Obviously, it is highly unlikely that several positions in each gene of the set mutated to the identical residue by convergent evolution of a variable gene family. Phylogenetically associated residues were therefore far more acceptable to paucigene theories wherein the species had one or very few germline genes that carried the phylogenetically associated residues. Proponents of the germline theory advanced two possible explanations to reconcile the data concerning phylogenetically associated residues to the germline theory: these were gene expansion–contraction and coevolution or gene conversion models.

In a gene expansion–contraction model, the set of related genes on a given chromosome can be expanded or contracted by homologous but unequal cross-over events. These events must operate within certain defined limits that preclude significant expansion of the total complement of genomic DNA. Such cross-overs can be seen to lead to dominance of a given sequence in a species and the absence of that sequence in another species. This would occur by duplication of certain genes and the deletion of others following an unequal cross-over event.

A second possibility for maintenance of phylogenetically associated residues in a multigene set involves a variation on gene conversion theories (described in Chapter 8). In the pure form of this model, all genes in a given set would be rectified against a master gene leading to identity among all members of the set. This master–slave hypothesis does not fit the immunoglobulin genes because they are not all identical one to another. Accordingly, a modified version of the theory that allows conversion of only certain genes, say those within a subgroup, or alternatively, only a defined sequence within each gene, could explain the phylogenetically associated residues.

The necessity for such complex explanations, however, detracted seriously from the germline theory. As mentioned above, the beauty of the germline theory lay in its simplicity and the lack of necessity for *ad hoc* explanations.

5.5.2. Mouse Lambda Light Chains

Occasionally certain data were compatible with both theories but could be much better explained by one of them. A case in point is the pattern of diversity observed for the mouse lambda light chains. The structural information for these chains more easily fits somatic mutation theories. In fact, these data were extremely important in demonstrating that this was indeed a viable alternative to the germline theory.

Mainly through the efforts of Weigert *et al.* (1970), amino acid sequence data were obtained for the variable regions of 18 mouse lambda chains. In most cases complete variable-region sequences were determined for these proteins. The data indicated that 12 of the 18 chains were indistinguishable and that all the rest were unique, but that the variation observed among them fell within the hypervariable regions. The majority of the variants differed from the prototype (that is, the sequence that was observed 12 times) by a single amino acid substitution; two variants differed by one and another by three amino acid substitutions (the data are illustrated in Chapter 3, Fig. 3.20). The most straightforward explanation of these data is given by the somatic mutation theory wherein a single subgroup gene exists for V_λ. Variations of this subgroup are generated by somatic mutation and are selected by antigen in a stepwise fashion. The fact that all the lambda variants have the same framework sequence defines this as a single subgroup. Recall that only framework differences were important to the definition of a subgroup. Although the counter argument, that there are multiple V_λ genes in the germline that evolved with differences only in the hypervariable regions, is also feasible, this situation is much more easily explained by the somatic mutation theory.

Perhaps the most damning criticism of the lambda light chain data was that since only a few percent of mouse immunoglobulin molecules express lambda chains, this system was not an important element in the generation of antibody diversity. This criticism, however, was nicely answered by application of the principles illustrated by this system to subgroups of mouse kappa chains, most importantly those of the V_κ 21 subgroup (see Chapter 3, Fig. 3.21). Similar results were obtained by these analyses.

It is difficult to overstate the importance of the detailed analysis of the lambda system to models for somatic mutation. Although the data do not explain why there are so many subgroups in other systems, the data strengthened the argument that somatic mutation could operate on hypervariable regions of genes within a single subgroup. This clear demonstration was a major factor in keeping this theory alive in spite of heavy criticism based on increasing numbers of germline genes as postulated from the proliferation of V-region subgroups.

5.5.3. Rabbit Group a Allotypes

As discussed in Chapter 2, the discovery of a heavy chain V-region genetic polymorphism for rabbit antibodies had a profound impact on theories of antibody diversity and was interpreted by most authors as favoring the existence of relatively few germline genes. There were two major reasons for this: One was the difficulty of maintaining genetic purity in a multiple gene set and the second was the difficulty in explaining how the mutations (there were multiple mutations for these complex allotypes) giving rise to the different allotypes spread throughout an entire gene set. By contrast, the somatic mutation theory easily dealt with the allotypes as markers for the framework residues of one or very few germline genes.

The allotypes a1, a2, and a3 had been observed in a number of rabbit colonies in several countries to be inherited as Mendelian alleles. Although there were some reports to the contrary, the vast majority of immunoglobulin heavy chains from a domestic rabbit will express these allotypes and the types expressed by a given rabbit can be accurately predicted by the parental types. It has further been shown that the sequences giving rise to the allotype specificities are present in V-region peptides. The amino acid interchanges correlating with the allotypes are, with some minor variations, consistent. Application of these data to a multigene model makes it extremely difficult to understand why cross-overs have not mixed the a1, a2, and a3 sets of germline genes to the point where no genetic distinction could be found. As noted in Chapter 2, Fig. 2.3, a set of several thousand allelic V-region genes bearing a given allotype would be next to impossible to maintain. Because of this aspect of allelism, the rabbit V-region allotypes are even more difficult to reconcile with the germline theory than are the phylogenetically associated residues.

The second difficulty that rabbit allotypes pose for the germline theory is very similar to that which is outlined above for phylogenetically associated residues: How did these mutations spread over a set of several thousand germline genes that are themselves different in other respects? The answer to this question would have to be much the same as that postulated above for the phylogenetically associated residues and would involve the need for lengthy explanations and hypotheses to bring these data in line with the germline theory.

How did proponents of the germline theory deal with the question of rabbit allotypes? An answer to the first objection can be simply that cross-overs for the V_H region are suppressed. That is to say that the homologous genes that encode the rabbit V_H regions are prevented from cross-over during meiosis and therefore there is no possibility of cross-contaminating the pure sets of allotype-specific V-region genes. The second type of explanation that would answer both objections is that the sequences that specify the different allotypes diverged in evolution not as alleles, but as gene duplications just as did the V-region subgroups. Different rabbit chromosomes, however, could have undergone deletions and duplications so that they now contain allelic genes for different subgroups. In this way, linked genes may have become allelic genes in the evolutionary process. An alternative explanation called for inherited regulator genes that control the synthesis of the V_H allotypes. In this model each genome would contain information for more than one of the allotypes but only the one corresponding to the regulator would be expressed.

Therefore, although the rabbit allotypes posed a special problem for the proponents of the germline theory, they were willing to admit their existence and to propose a number of mechanisms for the evolution of a multigene set carrying for each member a similar genetic marker. In this respect a quote from a 1973 article by Hood is relevant:

> . . . . Perhaps the same is true for the allotype differences among rabbit V_H regions. If so perhaps the differences among the V_H genes of different allotypes may have arisen by the same mechanism that explains the evolution of clusters of genes in antibody families. The mechanism I favor in this regard is gene expansion and contraction. In a multigene model, however, this process would have to involve multiple crossing over events, which would inevitably scramble the differences as fast as they arose unless crossing over between the three types of chromosomes was in some way prevented. These populations of rabbit may have evolved three chromosomes independently as if they were separate species. (These populations may have been remixed too recently for detectable recombination to have occurred.) These features might be explained if the a1 and a3 sequences diverged not as alleles but as gene duplications just as with the variable region subgroups. Different rabbit chromosomes however might have undergone subsequent gene deletions and/or duplications so that they now contain genes for different subgroups. In this way, linked genes which diverged long before the rabbit became a species and thus have accumulated a large number of differences might have become alleles (or pseudoalleles) in contemporary rabbits. If the number of genes is very limited, only a few deletions and duplications could be required. Second, interchromosomal crossing over may have for some reason been prevented. (The proposed gene expansion–contraction could be due to *intra*chromosomal crossing over.) The assumption that intrachromosomal crossing over occurs frequently while interchromosomal crossing over is undetectable might be regarded as somewhat contrived. . . .

Therefore although the rabbit group a allotypes were a problem for proponents of the germline theory, the theorists were equal to the problem and could come up with explanations to cover every aspect of this system. However, as seen in the above quote, each explanation required further adjustments of the theory.

5.5.4. A V-Region Allotype for the Mouse Kappa Chain

There was another V-region allotype described by Edelman and Gottlieb (1970) who found a cysteine-containing tryptic peptide in peptide maps of light chains from AKR mice. This peptide, which was detected by derivatization of the cysteine residue with a radioactive label, was absent in similar maps made from light chains derived from IgG of the DBA/2, CE/J, and most other strains tested. It was shown that this peptide was derived from the variable region of kappa chains and that it included the cys residue at position 23, which is in the framework region. Breeding studies indicated that F_1 mice produced by a cross of AKR to DBA/2 mice expressed the marker at levels of approximately one

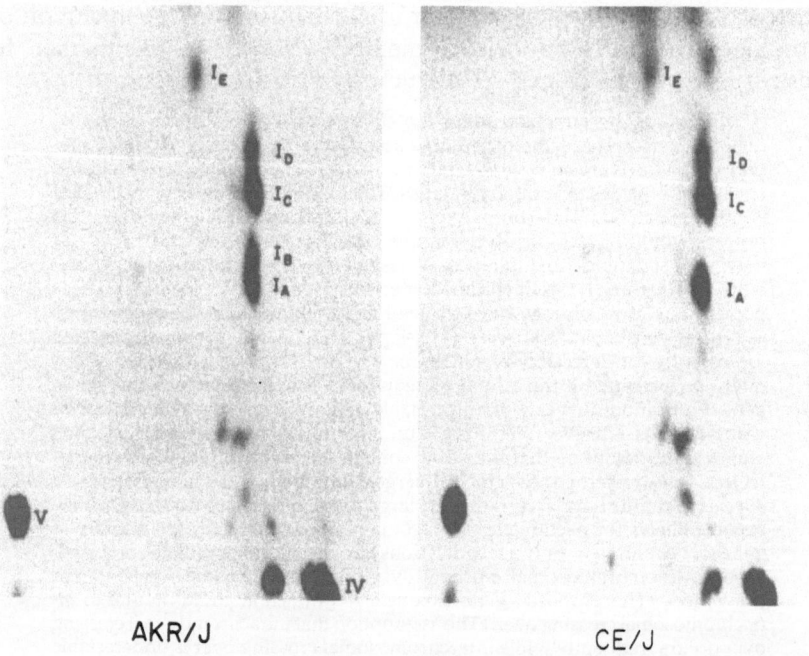

AKR/J   CE/J

Figure 5.2. Autoradiograms of peptide maps of light chains from mouse strains AKR/J and CE/J. Pooled light chains from each strain were used. Peptide I_B was not found in CE/J strain. From Cunningham *et al.* (1971).

half that of the positive parental strain. The marker showed segregation in the F_2 generation consistent with that expected for a Mendelian co-dominant trait. This marker was designated the I_B peptide. It was estimated that 5% to 10% of kappa light chains in the positive strain carried this peptide (see Fig. 5.2).

The I_B peptide was definitely a V-region marker and its detection did not depend on serologic reagents. Breeding studies showed it to be inherited in a simple Mendelian fashion. Therefore, the major objections that were raised to the group a allotypes of the rabbit could not be applied to I_B. The existence of this marker was interpreted to indicate that it was present on only one of perhaps ten different kappa V-region genes. Because of the arguments developed above for maintenance of genetic purity in large V-region gene sets and because of the difficulty in spreading a marker over a large number of genes, this I_B peptide was taken as strong proof for the existence of a small number of V-region genes in the mouse kappa system.

5.6. WAITING FOR THE ANSWER

The controversy between the proponents of the two polar theories was crucial to the development of our understanding of the genetic basis of antibody diversity. The contestants used every available bit of data that could suit their argument and they beat these into the mold predicted by their respective theory. When the data grew sparse, computerized interpretations of old data were devised to massage new life into the theories. Although there were relatively few active participants in the main arena of this controversy, almost every immunologist had a favorite theory and it was usually one or the other of the polar theories. Most would not be so rash as to commit themselves to an unambigous endorsement of either theory on paper, but rather they contented themselves with theoretical insinuations often hidden deep within the discussions of their papers.

Those not embracing a major theory were a bit more difficult to classify because there was not a clearly definable third choice. The next chapter will deal with these mavericks and their more diverse views of antibody diversity. The mavericks were not nearly as vocal as the germline or somatic mutation proponents and did not attract the disciples in large numbers as did the proponents of the polar theories.

The irony of the great controversy is that in spite of the many words and pages devoted to the polar theories, neither extreme would prove to be correct. In the final analysis, a compromise between everything in the genome and just a few genes in the genome for antibodies was necessary. This compromise, along with a few twists, some of which were predicted by the mavericks, presently provides the best explanation for antibody diversity. Therefore, those waiting for the answer could point to success or failure of either of the polar theories depending on their individual orientation.

REFERENCES AND BIBLIOGRAPHY

Brenner, S., and Milstein, C., 1966, Origin of antibody variation, *Nature (London)* **211**:242.

Cohn, M., 1970, Selection under a somatic model, *Cell. Immunol.* **1**:461.

Cohn, M., 1973, Antibody diversification: The somatic mutation model revisited, in: *The Biochemistry of Gene Expression in Higher Organisms* (J. K. Pollak and J. W. Lee, eds.), D. Reidel Publishing Co., Dordrecht, Holland, pp. 574–592.

Cunningham, B., Gottlieb, P. D., Pflumm, M. N., and Edelman, G. M., 1971, Immunolgobulin structure: Diversity, gene duplication and domains, in: *Progress in Immunology* (B. Amos, ed.), Academic Press, New York, pp. 3–24.

Edelman, G. M., and Gottlieb, P. D., 1970, A gentic marker in variable region of light chain of mouse immunoglobulins, *Proc. Nat. Acad. Sci.* **67**:1192.

Eichmann, K., and Kindt, T. J., 1971, The inheritance of individual antigenic specificities of rabbit antibodies to streptococcal carbohydrates, *J. Exp. Med.* **134**:532.

Fitch, W. M., and Margoliash, E., 1967, Construction of phylogenetic trees, *Science* **155**:279.

Hart, D. A., Pawlak, L. L., and Nisonoff, A., 1973, Nature of anti-hapten antibodies arising after immune suppression of a set of cross-reactive idiotypic specificities, *Eur. J. Immunol.* **3**:44.

Hood, L., and Talmage, D. W., 1970, Mechanism of antibody diversity: Germline basis for variability, *Science* **168**:325.

Hood, L., 1973, The genetics, evolution and expression of antibody molecules, in: *Stadler Symposium*, Volume 5, pp. 73–142.

Jerne, N. K., 1971, The somatic generation of immune recognition, *Eur. J. Immunol.* **1**:1.

Lederberg, J., 1959, Genes and antibodies, *Science* **129**:1649.

Milstein, C., 1967, Linked groups of residues in immunoglobulin kappa chains, *Nature (London)* **216**:330.

Weigert, M. G., Cesari, I. M., Yonkovich, S. J., and Cohn, M., 1970, Variability in the lambda light chain sequences of mouse antibody, *Nature (London)* **228**:371.

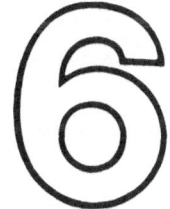

THE MAVERICK SOLUTIONS

. . . . there are many possible worlds; but the interesting one is the world that exists and has already shown itself to be at work for a long time. Science attempts to confront the possible with the actual. It is the means devised to build a representation of the world that comes ever closer to what we call reality.

—FRANCOIS JACOB

6.1. INTRODUCTION

From the mid 1960s to the late 1970s, most immunologists espoused either the germline or somatic theory to explain antibody variability. There were, however, a number of investigators who steadfastly maintained that neither theory adequately explained the structural and/or genetic data. Each proposed different solutions that we refer to here as "maverick" because they do not depend on the germline position (for every immunoglobulin V region there resides in the DNA a faithful copy) or the somatic mutation theory (that in the DNA there exists only a very few genes that somatically mutate and give rise to the great variety of antibody molecules). Although each author of a maverick solution depended on different interpretations of much of the data that has been presented so far in this volume, there were six bodies of evidence that the maverick theorists focused on that were difficult to reconcile with either the germline or somatic theories. We will first review these data and then discuss the various alternative theories that were developed that attempted to explain not only these data but also data generally used to support germline or somatic theories.

6.2. DATA DIFFICULT TO RATIONALIZE WITH EITHER GERMLINE OR SOMATIC THEORIES

6.2.1. V-Region Subgroup Distinctions Are Not Evident throughout the V Regions

The principle of subgroups was introduced in Chapter 3 with a detailed description of the so-called "linked substitutions." The impact of variable region subgroups on the germline theory (favorable) was described in Chapter 5. However, very early it was appreciated (perhaps first by Milstein in his paper describing the complete amino acid sequence of four human $V_\kappa 2$ proteins) that beyond position 86, human immunoglobulin kappa chains could not be easily classified into subgroups. Thus, the subgroup distinctions that were described in Chapter 3 that allow one on the basis of a stretch of five to ten amino acids in the amino terminal part of the variable region to classify a protein as a $V_\kappa 1$ or $V_\kappa 2$; $V_\kappa 1$ or $V_\kappa 3$; or $V_\lambda 1$ or $V_\lambda 2$ did not persist throughout the variable region. In his early paper, Milstein suggested two possibilities to explain the results: somatic recombination and separate germline genes encoding the N-terminal and C-terminal halves of immunoglobulin light chains.

In 1976, Alistair Cunningham edited a small book that had an important impact on the field. It was titled *Antibody Diversity: A New Look*. In it, a number of authors were asked to "lay bare their innermost thoughts on the subject." The book proved crucial as it gathered together different views on the diversity issue in one volume. Most of the authors took issue with the polar solutions, and articles by Cunningham, Gershon, Klinman, Baltimore, and Capra provided arguments not easily dealt with by the germline or the somatic mutation theory. For example, Capra pointed out that analysis of the available amino acid sequence data on immunoglobulin heavy chains indicated that subgroup specific residues were primarily clustered at the N-terminal end of the heavy chain V region. In comparing the N-terminal 40 residues with the C-terminal 40 residues of the heavy chain, it was pointed out that the number of invariant residues was approximately equal, but the number of subgroup-specific positions in the N-terminal 40 residues were 16 out of 40, whereas there were none in the C-terminal 40 residues. This suggested the possibility (similar to the Milstein notion for the human kappa data) that the two ends of the immunoglobulin heavy chain V region were under separate genetic control. The data on which this argument is based are illustrated in Figs. 6.1 to 6.4.

A corollary of the notion that V-region subgroups were not evident throughout the entire variable region derived from the work of Fett and

```
V_H II
                  10              20                 30                40
Daw  PCA  V T L R E S G P A L V R P T Q T L T L T C T F S G F S L S G E T M C V A W I R
Ou   PCA  V T L T E S G P A L V K P K Q P L T L T C T F S G F S L S T S R M R V S W I R
He   PCA  V T L K E N G P T L V K P T E T L T L T C T L S G L S L T D G V A V G W I R
Cor  PCA  V T L R E S G P A L V K P T Q T L T L T C T F S G F S L S S T G M C V G W I R

V_H III
Tei  Glu  V Q L V E S G G G L V Q P G G S L R L S C A A S G F T F S T S A V Y ( ) W V R
Was  Glu  V Q L L E S G G G L V Q P G G S L R L S C A A S G F S F S T D A M Y ( ) W V R
Jon  Asp  V Q L V E S G G G L V K P G G S L R L S C A A S G F T F S T A W M K ( ) W V R
Zap  Glu  V Q L V E S G G A L V Q P G G S G R L S C A A S G F T F S T T S R F ( ) W V R
Tur  Glu  V Q L L E S G G G L V Q P G G S L R L S C A A S G F T F S R V L S S ( ) W V R
```

Figure 6.1. The invariant positions in human immunoglobulin heavy chains, positions 1–40. The invariant positions in both the V_H2 and V_H3 subgroup have been enclosed. The exceptions are highlighted by circles. In this stretch of 40 amino acids, 17 positions are considered invariant. From Capra (1976).

```
V_H II
             90              100              110              120
Daw  M N T V G P G D T A T Y Y C A R S C G S Q (    ) Y F D Y W G Q G I L V T V S S
Ou   M I N V N P V D T A T Y Y C A R V V N S V M A G Y Y M D V W G K G T T V T V S S
He   M T N M D P V D T A T Y Y C V H R H P R T L (    ) A F D V W G Q G T K V A V S S
Cor  M (    ) D P V D T A T Y Y C A R I T V I P A P A G Y M D V W G R G T P V T V S S

V_H III
Tei  M L S L E P E D T A V Y Y C A R V T P A A A S L T F S A V W G Q G T L V T V S S
Was  M N R L E A E D T A V Y Y C A R F R Q P F V Q ( ) F F D V F G Q G T L V T V S S
Jon  M I S V T P E D T A V Y Y C A R V V V S T (    ) S M D V W G Q G T P V T V S S
Zap  M N T G E A E D T A V Y Y C A R T R P G G Y (  ) F S D V W G Q G T L V S V S S
Tur  M L S L Q A E D T A L L Y Y C A R L S V T A V (  ) A F D V W G Q G T K V T V S S
```

Figure 6.2. The invariant positions in human immunoglobulin heavy chains, positions 85 to 124. The invariant positions have been enclosed with the exceptions highlighted in circles. In this stretch of 40 amino acids, 21 positions are considered invariant. From Capra (1976).

```
V_H II
                  10              20                 30                40
Daw  PCA  V T L R E S G P A L V R P T Q T L T L T C T F S G F S L S G E T M C V A W I R
Ou   PCA  V T L T E S G P A L V K P K Q P L T L T C T F S G F S L S T S R M R V S W I R
He   PCA  V T L K E N G P T L V K P T E T L T L T C T L S G L S L T T D G V A V G W I R
Cor  PCA  V T L R E S G P A L V K P T Q T L T L T C T F S G F S L S S T G M C V G W I R

V_H III
Tei  Glu  V Q L V E S G G G L V Q P G G S L R L S C A A S G F T F S T S A V Y ( ) W V R
Was  Glu  V Q L L E S G G G L V Q P G G S L R L S C A A S G F S F S T D A M Y ( ) W V R
Jon  Asp  V Q L V E S G G G L V K P G G S L R L S C A A S G F T F S T A W M K ( ) W V R
Zap  Glu  V Q L V E S G G A L V Q P G G S G R L S C A A S G F T F S T T S R F ( ) W V R
Tur  Glu  V Q L L E S G G G L V Q P G G S L R L S C A A S G F T F S R V L S S ( ) W V R
```

Figure 6.3. The subgroup-specific positions in immunoglobulin heavy chains, positions 1 to 40. Subgroup-specific positions that differentiate human V_H2 from V_H3 proteins have been enclosed. Sixteen such positions exist in the N-terminal 40 residues in human immunoglobulin heavy chains. The exceptions have been highlighted by circles. From Capra (1976).

$V_H II$ 90   100   110   120

```
VHII          90            100          110          120

Daw   M N T V G P G D T A T Y Y C A R S C G S Q (    ) Y F D Y W G Q G I L V T V S S
Ou    M I N V N P V D T A T Y Y C A R V V N S V M A G Y Y M D V W G K G T T V T V S S
He    M T N M D P V D T A T Y Y C V H R H P R T L (    ) A F D V W G Q G T K V A V S S
Cor   M (    ) D P V D T A T Y Y C A R I T V I P A P A G Y M D V W G R G T P V T V S S

VHIII

Tei   M L S L E P E D T A V Y Y C A R V T P A A A S L T F S A V W G Q G T L V T V S S
Was   M N R L E A E D T A V Y Y C A R F R Q P F V Q ( ) F F D V F G Q G T L V T V S S
Jon   M I S V T P E D T A V Y Y C A R V V V S T (    ) S M D V W G Q G T P V T V S S
Zap   M N T G E A E D T A V Y Y C A R T R P G G Y (    ) F S D V W G Q G T L V S V S S
Tur   M L S L Q A E D T A L Y Y C A R L S V T A V (    ) A F D V W G Q G T K V T V S S
```

Figure 6.4. Positions 85 to 124 of human immunoglobulin heavy chains. No subgroup positions are detectable in this region of the molecule. From Capra (1976).

Deutsch (1975). These authors systematically studied human immuno-globulin lambda chains and discovered a multiplicity of isotypes that were characterized not only in human lambda Bence Jones proteins but in the serum immunoglobulin pool as well. The lambda chain C regions differed by one to five amino acid residues, and many of these variations correlated with both biochemical and serologic data that had been available for some time. Implicit in the original Dreyer-Bennet two-gene model was the notion that within a linkage group any variable region could associate with any constant region. Since it was clear from a large body of both genetic and structural data that there was but a single immuno-globulin kappa chain in man and mouse and many V-region subgroups (3 to 4 in man, 40-plus in mouse), the association of any kappa V-region subgroup with the constant region of the single kappa locus was obvious. Similarly, in the heavy chain every V-region subgroup had at one point or another been detected in association with at least two if not more heavy chain isotypes.

With the Fett and Deutsch discovery of multiple human lambda isotypes, a serologic and biochemical study of the associations of various lambda V-region subgroups with each of the lambda isotypes was undertaken. Although most of these studies indicated that the association was reasonably random, in a 1975 paper Fett and Deutsch made the crucial observation that the lambda chain C-region isotype could be predicted on the basis of the amino acid sequence between positions 101 and 106, an area of the molecule that had for ten years been considered a portion of the V region. They concluded that

> The finding of a specific correlation between V region substitutions and C region substitutions suggests that at least in lambda chains the mechanism of V-C joining is non-random in nature. Indeed, as more sequence data accumulate for all classes and types of immunoglobulin polypeptide chains,

> this nonrandomness of joining of V-region portion of its C region may well emerge as an important facet in the genetics of immunoglobulin biosynthesis.

Thus, three kinds of arguments have been presented that suggest that the variable region of immunoglobulin molecules may be under the control of more than one gene: (1) in human immunoglobulin kappa chains, V-region subgroups are not evident throughout the V region (Milstein); (2) in immunoglobulin heavy chains, the distribution of subgroup-specific residues is remarkably different in the two ends of the immunoglobulin heavy chain variable region (Capra, 1976); and (3) in the human lambda system, although there is an apparent random association of V-region subgroups with C-region isotypes, this randomness breaks down near the V-C bridge (Fett and Deutsch, 1975).

The difficulty that somatic and germline theories would have with these data should be evident. The germline theory would have to postulate that certain sections of immunoglobulin variable regions remain reasonably conserved and lack subgroup specificity whereas at the same time the remaining portion of the chain could vary significantly from duplicated gene to duplicated gene. The somatic theorists would have to propose that after V-gene duplication that generated the two V-region subgroups, repeated mutations occurred in one subline but not in the other *in particular portions of the chain*. The most parsimonious interpretation of the data, although clearly heretical, is that at least two separate groups of genes under different selective pressure encode immunoglobulin V regions.

6.2.2. The Rabbit Allotypes Are Not Evident throughout the V Regions

The rabbit V_H allotypes had always posed problems for the germline theory, and as mentioned in Chapters 3 through 5, most viewed the rabbit allotypes as supporting pauci gene (somatic) theories. The final proof that the rabbit allotypes indeed existed in the V region of the heavy chain came from the work of Mole, who isolated the Fv fragment of rabbit heavy chains derived from pooled immunoglobulins and demonstrated that this V_H fragment bore the full complement of V_H allotypes.

The full implications of the rabbit allotypic locations, however, came from primary structural analyses. First, pooled data on the N-terminus from Porter's laboratory in studies by Wilkinson (1969) and later by Mole demonstrated conclusively that the amino acids in the V_H region were distinct from allotype to allotype. More importantly, there were *several different amino acid residues* that correlated with the allotype designation of the heavy chain. Later studies using peptide map analysis demonstrated that further structural correlations could be made in the region between 75 and 85 of the rabbit heavy chain. *However, beyond position 85, no allotype correlates were evident.*

When the rabbit homogeneous antibodies became available and were subjected to amino acid sequence analysis in the laboratories of Haber, Strosberg, Jaton, Braun, and Kindt, the situation became clearer as the amino acid sequences of several rabbit heavy chains were assembled. Although it was true that with rare exceptions no single position absolutely correlated with an allotypic specificity, again, as has been noted for the human immunoglobulin heavy chains for subgroup specific residues, there were no rabbit allotype correlates beyond position 85. The location of the rabbit V_H allotypes, therefore, further pointed to the disjunction between the amino terminal (1–85) and carboxy terminal (86–120) portions of immunoglobulin V regions (see Fig. 6.5).

6.2.3. Phylogenetically Associated Residues Are Not Evident throughout the V Regions

Phylogenetically associated residues were introduced in the previous chapter and shown to favor somatic theories of diversity. Here we discuss their location and further implications. The concept of phylogenetically associated residues is complicated by the terminology as well as the theoretical construct. The original notions were first described by Hood in his studies of mouse and human immunoglobulin kappa chains. He noted that at a particular position a particular amino acid appeared in the V region of one species, but a different amino acid occurred in the same position in a second species. Since the earliest studies were done on relatively few species and with relatively few sequences, the term species-specific residue came to be applied to these positions, although it was obvious that as the immunoglobulin V regions of more species were sequenced, there were not enough amino acids to make *any* position specific to a species. More importantly for the concept, perhaps, there would likely be exceptions to every species-*specific* residue, as with subgroup-specific residues and rabbit allotypic residues, both principles of which represented an amalgamation of several amino acids. As such, Kehoe and Capra suggested the term "phylogenetically associated residue" for the principle. Examples of phylogenetically associated residues are illustrated in Figs. 6.6 and 6.7 where it is seen that in a number of human, dog, cat, mouse, rat, and guinea pig immuno-

Allotype	H chain designation	Position												
		4	7	9	11 12	14 15 16	64	66	69 70 73		84 85
	3381	GLU	GLY	ARG	VAL THR	GLY THR PRO	GLY	PHE	SER LYS THR		THR GLU
a1	3374	—	—	—	———	———	—	—	———		———
	Pool IgG	—	—	—	———	———	—	—	———		———
	K25	LYS	GLU	GLY	PHE LYS	THR ASP THR	SER	SER	THR ARG ASX		ALA GLN
a2	BS-1	LYS	GLU	GLY	PHE LYS	THR ASP THR	SER	SER	THR ARG ASX		ALA GLX
	Pool IgG	LYS	GLU	GLY	PHE LYS	THR ASP THR		SER	THR ARG		ALA ALA
a3	Pool IgG	—	—	ASP	— LYS	— ALA SER	—	—	———	—	ALA ALA
a neg	3547	—	—	GLY	— GLN	— GLY SER	MET	GLY	— ILE ASP		ASN SER

Figure 6.5. Amino acid sequence data for allotype-defined heavy chains compiled from rabbit homogeneous antibodies and immunoglobulin pools. Those residues correlating with group a allotype are shown. All residues shown are in framework regions.

		10	20	30	40
Tei (Human)	E	V Q L V E S G G G	L V Q P G G S L R L S C A	A S G F T F S T S A V Y (	) W V R
Was (Human)	E	V Q L L E S G G G	L V Q P G G S L R L S C A	A S G F S F S T D A M Y (	) W V R
Jon (Human)	D	V Q L V E S G G G	L V K P G G S L R L S C A	A S G F T F S T A W M K (	) W V R
Zap (Human)	E	V Q L V E S G G A	L V Q P G G S G R L S C A	A S G F T F S T T S R F (	) W V R
Tur (Human)	E	V Q L L E S G G G	L V Q P G G S L R L S C A	A S G F T F S R V L S S (	) W V R
Gom (Dog)	E	V Q L V E S G G D	L V K P G G S L R L S C V	A S G I T F S G Y S M Q (	) W V R
Moo (Dog)	E	V K L V E S G G D	L V K P G G S L R L S C V	A S G F T F S S N G M D (	) W V R
Di (Cat)	D	V Q L V E S G G D	L V Q P D G S L R L T C V	A S G F T F S T R H M K (	) W V R
Gr (Cat)	D	V Q L V E S G G D	L V Q P G G S L R L T C V	A S G F T F S T S K V Y (	) W V R
T15 (Mouse)	E	V K L V E S G G G	L V Q P G G S L R L S C A	T S G F T F S B F Y M E (	) W V R
S107(Mouse)	E	V K L V E S G G G	L V Q P G G S L R L S C A	T S G F T F S B F Y M E (	) W V R
M167(Mouse)	E	V K V V E S G G G	L V Q P G G S L R L S C A	T S G F T F S B F Y M E (	) W V R
21 (Mouse)	D	V Q L L E S G G G	L V Q P G G S R K L S C A	A S G F T F S S F G M H (	) W V R
173 (Mouse)	E	V K L L E S G G P	L V Q L G G S L K L S C A	A S G F D F S R Y W M S (	) W V R
IR27 (Rat)	E	V R L V E S G G G	L V Q P G R S M K L S C A	V S G F T F S D F Y M A (	) W V R
IR64 (Rat)	E	V Q L V E S G G G	L V Q P G G S L K L S C A	A S G F S F S F Y D M A (	) W V R
Guinea Pig*	E	X Q L V E S G G G	L V Q P G X S L R L S C V	A S G F T F S X X X X X (	) W I R

Figure 6.6. Phylogenetically associated residues in the V_H3 subgroup of the myeloma proteins of various mammals, positions 1–40. Six positions are noted to be phylogenetically associated: 1, 10, 19, 21, 23, and 39. The asterisk indicates the only pooled sequence utilized. The exceptions to the phylogenetically associated positions are circled. Note that in position 10, for example, with the exception of a single human myeloma protein and a single mouse myeloma protein, rodents and primates can be distinguished from all carnivores. Position 39 is an isoleucine in the guinea pig whereas in every other species studied to date valine is found at this position. From Capra (1976).

```
              90                100               110               120
Tie  (Human)  M L S L E P E D T A V Y Y C A R V T P A A A S L T F S A V W G Q G T L V T V S S
Was  (Human)  M N R L E A E D T A V Y Y C A R F R Q P F V Q ( ) F F D V F G Q G T L V T V S S
Jon  (Human)  M I S V T P E D T A V Y Y C A R V V V S T (   ) S M D V W G Q G T L V T V S S
Zap  (Human)  M N T G E A E D T A V Y Y C A R T R P G G Y ( ) F S D V W G Q G T L V T V S S
Tur  (Human)  M L S L Q A E D T A L Y Y C A R L S V T A V ( ) A F A H W G Q G T L V T V S S
Gom  (Dog)    M N S L R A E D T A V Y Y C A P W (         ) Q F E Y W G Q G T L V T V S S
Moo  (Dog)    M E D L R V E D T A V Y Y C A T E E G D L E ( ) I P R V F G Q G T I
T15  (Mouse)  M N A L R A E D T A I Y Y C A R Y Y G S S Y W ( ) Y F D V W G A G T T V T V S S
S107 (Mouse)  M N A L R A E D T A I Y Y C A R D Y Y G S S W ( ) Y F D V W G A G T T V T V S S
M167 (Mouse)  M N A L R A E D T A T Y Y C T R D A D G Y G D S ( ) Y F G Y F G A G T T V T V S S
M21  (Mouse)  M T S L R S E D T A M Y Y C A R H G N Y P W Y ( ) A M D Y W G Q G T S V T V S S
M173 (Mouse)  M S K V R S E D T A L Y Y C A R S P Y Y (     ) A M D Y W G
IR27 (Rat)    M D S L R S E D T A T Y Y C A R T V G Y P (   ) Y F G V W G Q G T L V T V S S
```

Figure 6.7. The V_H3 subgroup of various mammals, positions 85–124. No phylogenetically associated positions are noted in this region of the heavy chain. In virtually every position in which all the human proteins have a particular amino acid, with only a few exceptions, each of the other species (dog, mouse, and rat) has the same amino acid at that position. In those positions where one of the dog or mouse proteins has a different amino acid from the human, the other sequence from the same species does not share that difference. Thus, this region of the molecule is devoid of phylogenetically associated positions. From Capra (1976).

globulin (all of these are myeloma proteins with the exception of guinea pig which is a "homogeneous antibody") there are six positions that as a whole mark a particular species.

One of the important points to appreciate is that when comparing phylogenetically associated residues from one species to the next, *the same V-region subgroup must be compared*. This is because it is likely that a given V-region subgroup, when found in two different species, arose before speciation rather than through gene duplication after speciation. Therefore, it is inappropriate to compare, for example, the human $V_\kappa 2$ subgroup with the mouse $V_\kappa 2$ subgroup when the human $V_\kappa 2$ subgroup may be more like the mouse $V_\kappa 5$ subgroup. In the illustrations shown in Figs. 6.6 and 6.7, we see much the same thing as shown in Figs. 6.3 and 6.4; that is, as with the subgroup specific residues, the phylogenetically associated residues are clustered at the N-terminal 40 residues of the molecule, and there are none in the C-terminal 40 residues of the molecule.

These notions were put forth in the mid 1970s prior to the development of myelomas in strains of mice other than BALB/c and prior to the discovery of hybridomas that allowed homogeneous antibodies to be made in virtually any strain. However, the principle has remained intact. Those amino acid positions that distinguish a species or a phylogenetic group are largely clustered in the N-terminal two thirds of the heavy or light polypeptide chain variable regions, whereas the C-terminal third of these molecules, although different, cannot be directly linked to the N-terminal two thirds of the molecule.

6.2.4. Shared Idiotypes Occur in Molecules of Differing V-Region Subgroup

Immunologists appreciated early that subgroups have a structural basis and important genetic implications. They later came to understand the role of primary structure (particularly of hypervariable regions) in the constellation of determinants that are collectively termed idiotypes. A priori, one would assume that there would be a strict linkage of subgroup and idiotype. Although a large body of experimental evidence supports such as association, there are some glaring exceptions.

In 1973 Kindt *et al.* demonstrated an idiotypic cross-reaction between two different rabbit antibodies to the streptococcal group C carbohydrate that was isolated from the same rabbit serum. One antibody was allotype a3, whereas the other was y-. Serologic analysis failed to demonstrate any idiotype differences between these two antibodies. This idiotypic determinant required both heavy and light chains for its expression, and structural studies indicated that the light chains from these two antibodies were identical. Consistent with the allotypic difference, amino acid sequence data on the heavy chains showed that they differed at the amino terminus. Kindt reasoned that if a3 and y- molecules were as different as heavy chains belonging to different V-region subgroups, they would have over 30% amino acid sequence differences throughout their variable regions, presumably in the relative invariant portions of the V region that distinguish subgroups and rabbit allotypes. However, since the molecules were idiotypically identical, their hypervariable regions–antibody combining sites were similar if not identical. This was the first suggestion that the association between allotype and idiotype was not *obligatory.*

Another example of the disjunction of idiotypy and V-region subgroup came from Klinman's laboratory in 1976. An idiotypic antiserum directed against the T15 combining site and another antiserum that detected T15 framework determinants were used in the splenic focusing technique to study class-switching variants. The clonal progeny of a single precursor cell, stimulated in vitro, produced antibody of identical binding site idiotype. Strikingly, clones were identified with the T15 hypervariable region idiotype but lacking the T15 framework idiotype. Conversely, a DNP-specific clone was identified with the T15 framework idiotype but lacking the T15 hypervariable region idiotype.

Another example of the disjunction between idiotype and V-region subgroup came from Kunkel's laboratory where it was demonstrated that shared idiotypic specificities occurred among groups of human antigamma globulins. This system has been described in Chapter 2 and will be further detailed in Section 6.2.5. However, for the purposes of the discussion here, two members of the same cross-idiotype group, Lay/Pom, had on primary structural analysis immunoglobulin light chains of differing V_κ subgroups.

These results argue that there can be a disjunction between idiotype and subgroup. It is important to point out that most evidence suggested that there was a correlation between subgroup and idiotype. However, the results presented above are exceptions.

6.2.5. Identical Hypervariable Regions Occur in Proteins of Differing V-Region Subgroup

In the early 1970s, the human antigamma globulins with crossreacting idiotypes were studied in a number of laboratories in order to elucidate the structural basis of idiotypy. Capra and Kehoe (1974) and later Capra and Klapper (1976) published the complete amino acid sequences of the V regions of both the heavy and light chains of two idiotypically cross-reacting IgM human antigamma globulins. Although the sequences were important in establishing the relationship between hypervariable regions and the idiotype, another important fact emerged from the sequence data. The heavy chains belonged to the same V-region subgroup (and had a few scattered framework variations between them), but two hypervariable regions were of identical sequence (Fig. 6.8). More strikingly in the light chains (see Fig. 6.9), which belonged to *different* V-region subgroups (27 framework substitutions between the two chains), two of the three hypervariable regions were identical.

In 1975, Wu and co-workers, in a computer-aided analysis of immunoglobulin amino acid sequence data, found a human $V_\lambda 5$ protein (McG) and a human $V_\lambda 2$ protein (VIL) that had the identical sequence in all fourteen positions of their first hypervariable regions. Since these proteins belong to different V_λ subgroups (of the five described in the human), their differences (21 positions throughout the variable region) are quite significant. In the same report, an additional example of $V_\kappa 1$ proteins (Au and Ni) with identical second hypervariable regions was noted. The amino acid sequences of VIL and McG are shown in Fig. 6.10.

Although many authors struggled to interpret these data in terms of the polar solutions, it was clearly difficult to argue for either theory of antibody diversity based on these startling findings.

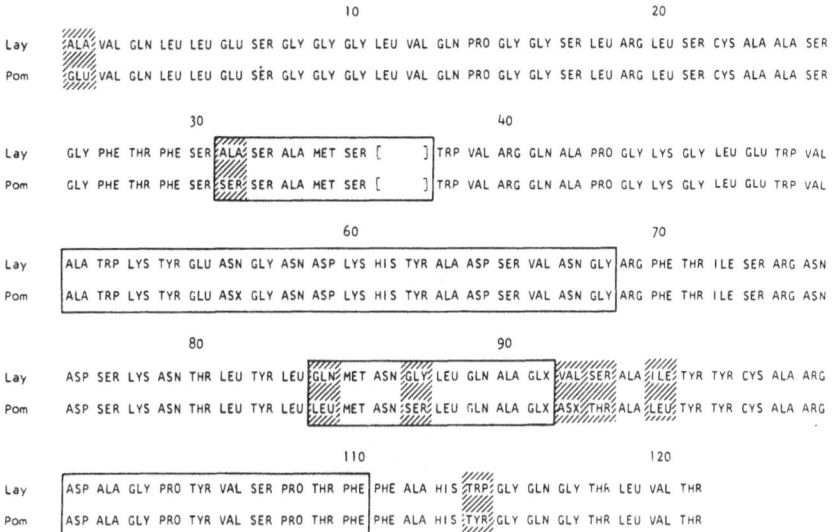

Figure 6.8. Amino acid sequences of the V_H regions of two human IgM molecules with cross-reacting idiotypes. These molecules were isolated from two unrelated individuals. The amino acid differences are shaded, and the hypervariable regions enclosed. From Capra and Kehoe (1974).

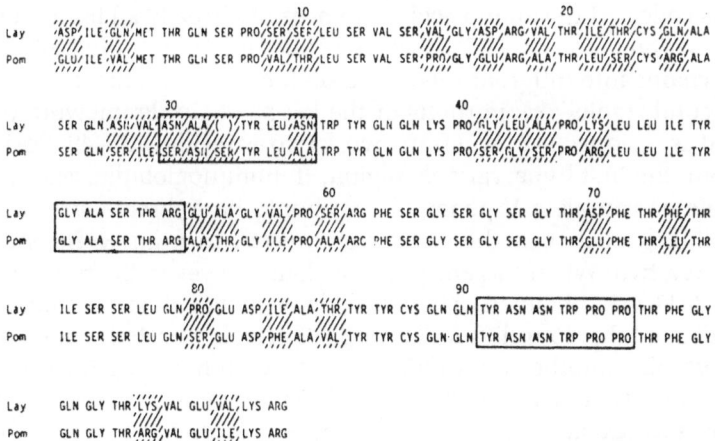

Figure 6.9. Amino acid sequences of the V_L regions of two human IgM molecules with cross-reacting idiotypes. These molecules were isolated from two unrelated individuals. The amino acid differences are shaded, and the hypervariable regions enclosed. From Capra and Klapper (1976).

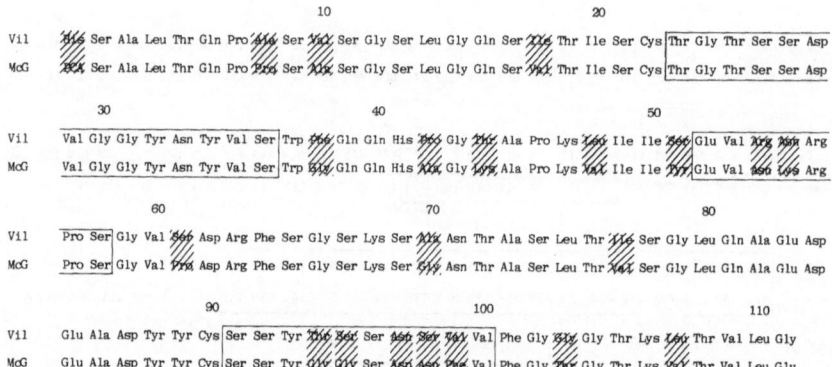

Figure 6.10. The amino acid sequence of a human $V_\lambda 5$ protein (McG) sequenced by Deutsch and a human $V_\lambda 2$ protein (ViL) sequenced by Hilschmann. The differences between the sequences are shaded, and the hypervariable regions enclosed. Adapted from Wu *et al.* (1975).

6.2.6. The Framework Portions of the V Region Do Not Occur in Absolute Linkage

This could be considered a variation of the argument proposed concerning the subgroup classifications based on the N-terminal and C-terminal portions of the V region, but is considered separately because of the sophistication of the analysis that was done. Kabat and his colleagues collected the amino acid sequences of virtually all immunoglobulin V regions, and in 1979, analyzed the data by grouping all mouse kappa chains into different sets based on identical structures in the first and second framework portions of the kappa chain. Framework one is defined as residues 1–23 and framework two as residues 35–49. Positions 24–34 are the first hypervariable region. If immunoglobulins exist in the germline as complete V genes, there should be a direct correlation or direct linkage between the structures present in framework one and framework two. When this analysis was done, however, the result shown in Fig. 6.11 was obtained. The available sequence data for framework one indicated that four different groups of proteins existed. One typified by MOPC321, another by MOPC63, and two others in which there is but one representative, MCPC603 and 2154. In framework two, a similar circumstance existed. There is a large group of proteins again typified by MOPC321, another group typified by MOPC70, and two groups that consist of only a single protein each, C101 and 7769. The predicted result based on both the germline and somatic theories is depicted by the first

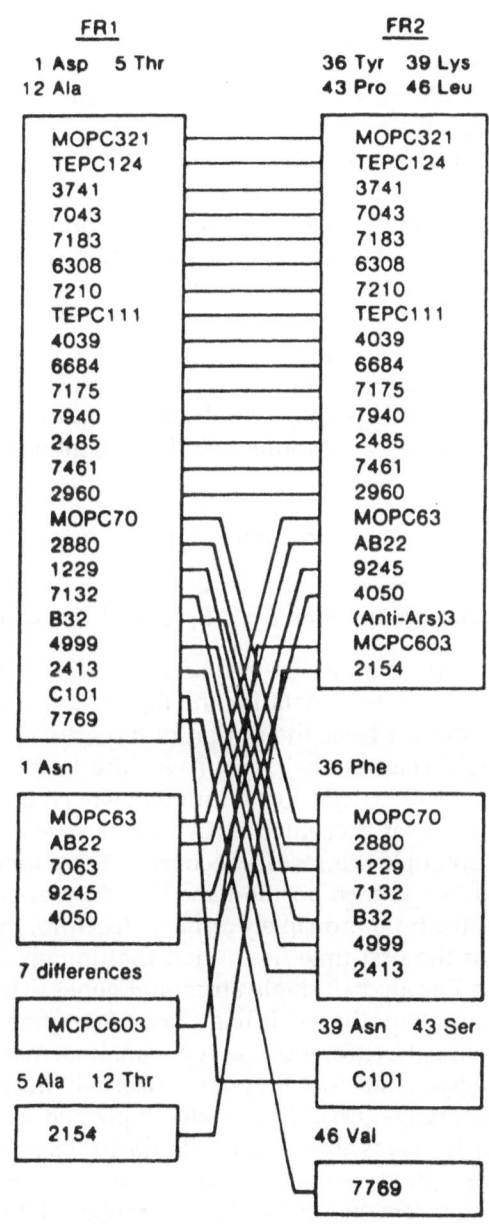

Figure 6.11. Assortment of FR1 and FR2 in mouse V_κ light chains. Each set of identical sequences is enclosed in a box. The position and the amino acid residues by which it differs from the other sets are listed above the FR1 and FR2 set with the largest number of chains. Only the positions at which differences are found are given above the other sets. From Kabat *et al.* (1979).

15 proteins; that is, from MOPC321 through 2960, in which framework one and framework two are directly linked. *What is difficult to reconcile with either of the polar solutions is that many of the proteins that are in one group in framework one are in a different group in framework two.* Thus, MOPC70, which has all the characteristics of group one framework one, has all the characteristics of group two framework two. Similarly, MOPC63, which has all the characteristics of group two framework one, has the four substitutions that put it into group one of framework two. Although one can dismiss the bottom two proteins in each grouping (MCPC603, 2154, and C101, 7769), since there is but one representative in each group, the presence of a large group of proteins in which there is a disjunction between the two framework structures implies strongly that framework one and framework two are under separate genetic control.

There are a number of examples similar to the one illustrated here, but this is perhaps the best studied that indicates the possible somatic assembly of immunoglobulin V-region segments.

6.3. THE MAVERICK SOLUTIONS

6.3.1. Kabat and Wu's Episomal Insertion-Mini-Gene Model

In 1970, Kabat and colleagues assembled the then available amino acid sequence data for the light chains of all species and put on a firm statistical basis the notion of hypervariable regions in immunoglobulin light chains. Their paper was the first compendium of amino acid sequences strictly for immunologists (Wu and Kabat, 1970). In addition, the paper presented a revolutionary solution to the antibody problem. Although the results section of the paper largely dealt with the variabilities at each position and the impact of each of the various amino acid substitutions on likely tertiary structure, the discussion section contained for the first time the notion that immunoglobulin V regions might not be encoded as single structural genes. The model proposed (as with all good hypotheses, it has since undergone considerable refinement) was that extrachromosomal (episomal) elements encoded the hypervariable regions and that they are "inserted" into a basic V-region gene during embryogenesis. The model explained a number of the then available facts. It was able to deal with the problem of the amount of DNA required for a strict germline theory, since the specificity sections were relatively short sections of DNA. The rabbit allotypes and the phylogenetically associated residues could be incorporated within the stable portion of the V-region gene as only the complementarity-determining portions would be varied from molecule to molecule. The theory was basically compatible with both the germline and somatic mutation theories since it suggested that the large bulk of DNA was, in fact, germline encoded but that the somatic process of "insertion" generated the bulk of the diversity. It was also suggested that somatic mutation might add to diversity after "insertion."

The theory faced immediate difficulty largely because it was six to seven years ahead of its time. Genes in pieces were unheard of, and the only known mechanisms of episomal insertion required long segments of DNA with recognition sequences far greater than could possibly exist in immunoglobulin light chains. These difficulties with the theory were acknowledged and freely discussed in the original paper, and as notions of exons and introns became available, the theory was refined into a "mini-gene" theory that suggested that each discrete portion of the immunoglobulin chain (the four framework sections and the three hypervariable regions) is under separate genetic control and that immunoglobulin chains can be assembled from different sets.

The theory has little difficulty explaining the issues raised in Section 6.2. The observation that subgroups are not evident throughout the V region is explained by the hypothesis that different portions of the V region are under different genetic control. The distribution of rabbit allotypes and phylogenetically associated residues is explained since they are on the portion of the immunoglobulin V region that is relatively stable and acts in evolution as if it were a single gene. Identical hypervariable regions occurring in proteins that differ in V-region subgroup are simple to explain since all that is required is that an identical episomal element insert the same piece of information into any V region. That there is no absolute linkage of framework portions of the immunoglobulin V region would, in fact, be a prediction of the "mini-gene" theory.

6.3.2. Capra and Kindt's Gene Interaction Hypothesis

Five years after Kabat and Wu's episomal insertion theory, Capra and Kindt (1975) developed a gene interaction hypothesis that proposed that at least two genes are involved in the synthesis of a single immunoglobulin V region. Starting from the position that neither the germline nor somatic mutation theories adequately explained the structural and genetic data, they proposed several different possibilities for gene interaction. Crucial observations in each of their laboratories had led them separately to suggest this possibility one or two years earlier. Kindt *et al.*, for example, suggested this in a 1973 paper that demonstrated an idiotypic cross-reaction between rabbit antibodies of different V_H allotypes as discussed in Section 6.2.4. Capra (1974) had suggested much the same thing in his papers describing identical hypervariable regions in proteins of different V-region subgroups. Capra and Kindt (1975) brought these thoughts together in the first volume of the new journal *Immunogenetics*.

In one model (shown in Fig. 6.12), it was proposed that the heavy chain from positions 1–85 is encoded separately from the section from positions 86–124. In this model, a single gene for each of the V-region subgroups encodes the region of the molecule between positions 1 and 85 (position 85 was chosen because positions 82–84 are the last subgroup specific positions in human immunoglobulin heavy chains). The region of the molecule devoid of subgroup-specific and phylogenetically associated residues (positions 86–124) is separately encoded and exists as multiple copies. The interaction of these two gene groups completes the V-region gene, which is subsequently translocated to join the C-region genes to form the completed immunoglobulin gene.

The hypervariable insertion model that is shown in Fig. 6.13 is an alternative method of providing gene interaction. The basic outline relied on the model of Wu and Kabat (1970). A difference from the Kabat and Wu model was the insistence that the "second gene" not be episomally encoded but be directly within the chromosomal DNA. This latter view took advantage of the analogy of the joining of the V- and C-region genes. In addition, the placement of the "second genes" within the germline and within the chromosome and linked to the heavy chain V

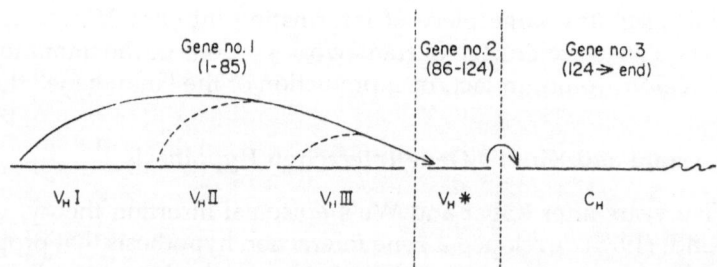

Figure 6.12. Gene interaction: the two-gene model. In this construct there is a single gene for each of the V-region subgroups that codes for the region of the molecule between positions 1 and 85. The region of the molecule devoid of subgroup-specific and phylogenetically associated residues (positions 86–124) is separately encoded and exists as multiple copies. The interaction of these two gene groups completes the V-region gene that is subsequently translocated to join the constant-region gene and form the completed immunoglobulin gene. From Capra (1976).

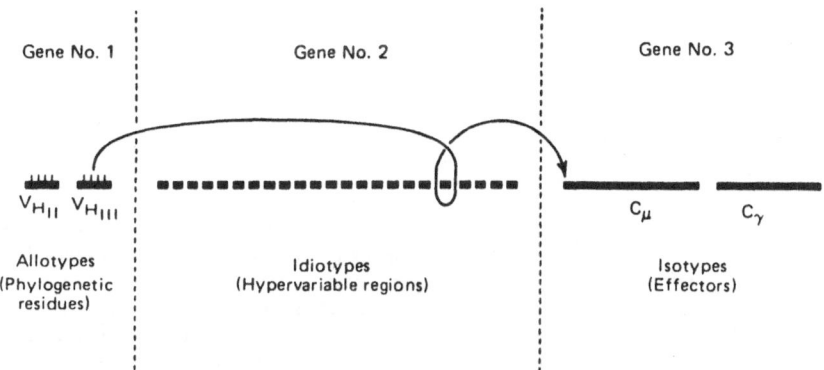

Figure 6.13. Gene interaction: the original Capra-Kindt insertion model—hypothetical genes involved in the synthesis of an immunoglobulin heavy chain. The arrow indicates selection of one gene from each group prior to the synthesis of the complete heavy chain. From Capra and Kindt (1975).

and C regions was more consistent with the inheritance and linkage of antibody idiotypes. The term episome conveys the idea of extrachromosomal (epigenetic) inheritance. Such a notion is difficult to reconcile with idiotypic inheritance.

Three years later, Kindt and Capra (1978) restated the theory (Fig. 6.14) and dealt with the arguments against gene interaction. By 1978, the major argument against gene interaction, that the molecular mechanism was too complicated, seemed trivial, as the first evidence was coming out of nonimmunoglobulin systems for the presence of introns and exons in viral and later mammalian genomes.

In addition, Kindt and Capra pointed out additional data supporting the gene interaction model and argued that there are a relatively limited number of germline V-region genes and that the second set of genes was separate from the basic framework genes. Joining the two gene segments occurs almost exclusively in a cis fashion, and there is preferential association between certain framework and hypervariable gene segments. The theory required that gene interaction take place at the DNA level. In addition, it was pointed out that the presence of hypervariable gene segments controlling idiotypes might explain the presence of idiotypes on T cells but the lack of defined immunoglobulin on T cells.

The two theories, Kabat-Wu/Capra-Kindt, draw heavily on the data presented in section 6.2 of this chapter, and virtually all these data are

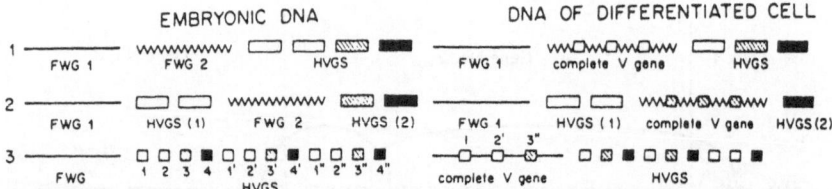

Figure 6.14. This figure is presented to aid in visualizing the concept of gene interaction. These are only some of the possible mechanisms by which insertion could take place. Model 1. In embryonic DNA the framework genes exist as one group and the hypervariable gene segments exist as a separate group. In the DNA of differentiated cells, a complete V gene is formed from one of the framework genes interacting with one of the hypervariable gene segments that has been fragmented into the three hypervariable regions. There is nothing to preclude a framework gene encoding a functional V region. Model 2. This illustrates what may be dictated by the strong linkage between framework genes and hypervariable gene segments. In this model, the hypervariable gene segments are physically closer to the framework gene with which they typically interact. In the DNA of the differentiated cell, integration occurs with one of the hypervariable gene segments producing a complete V gene. The major difference between models 1 and 2 is the closer linkage between hypervariable gene segments and framework genes in model 2. Model 3. This illustrates only a single framework gene for simplicity. In this model there are separate segments of DNA for each of the hypervariable regions, and those to be inserted in hypervariable region one are physically closer to it than those encoding the second and third hypervariable regions. In the DNA of a differentiated cell, the power of the insertion theory is seen. It allows the selection of one hypervariable gene segment from each of the three banks of hypervariable gene segments. There is no necessary linkage among the three gene segments so chosen. From Kindt and Capra (1978).

easily reconciled with either of these forms of gene interaction theory and will not be reiterated here as they were reviewed at the end of Section 6.3.1.

6.3.3. Smithies' Networks of Branched DNA Hypothesis

Smithies' (1970) DNA network hypothesis addressed two crucial issues of antibody diversity. First, the extraordinary variability of immunoglobulin V regions and second, the lack of subgroup specificity near the C terminus of both immunoglobulin light and heavy chain V regions. He assumed that DNA can exist in a branched two-dimensional network as well as the conventional one-dimensional form, and that at the branch points there were "switches" that could have alternate settings: "left" and "right." During the transcription of a chromosomal region in a differentiated cell, he envisioned that the RNA polymerase followed the pathway determined by the switch settings and that various other proteins or small molecules such as hormones could influence the switching process. Two diagrams illustrating the concept are shown in Figs. 6.15 and 6.16. Figure 6.15 represents an attempt to describe both the evolution and replication of such branch networks and Fig. 6.16 provides a hypothetical locus for an immunoglobulin heavy chain with 16 different V regions showing how identity at the N- and C-terminal portions of immunoglobulin V regions could be easily explained by a branch chain model and yet the extreme variability in the central regions maintained.

This model, which was first proposed in 1970 and re-examined in 1978, was used by Smithies to explain the variability within immunoglobulin variable regions in two specific ways. First, as can be seen from Fig. 6.16, the switch points neatly explain the V-region subgroups since, for example, V_H1 would be a branch to the left and V_H2 a branch to the right; then the sub-subgroups would then branch from each of the main branches and then as one entered the first hypervariable region, additional branch points could be envisioned. Smithies made it clear that somatic mutation would likely operate in addition to such a scheme,

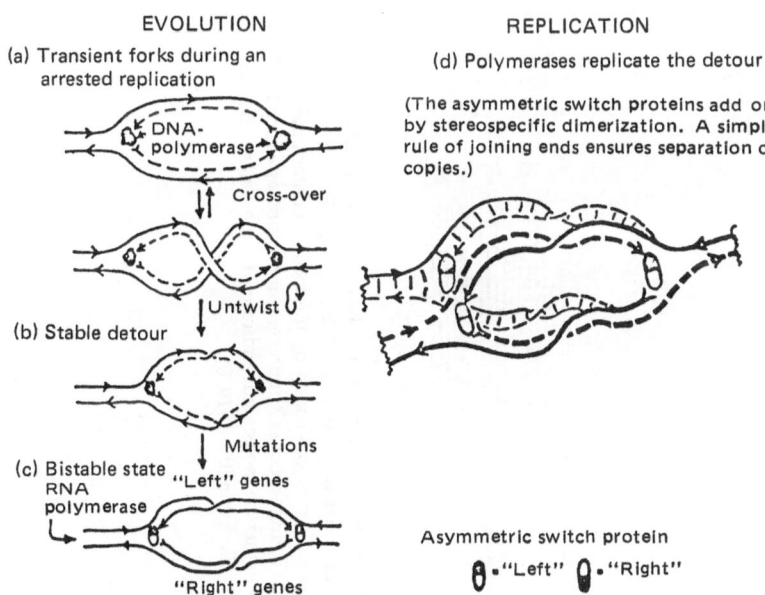

Figure 6.15. A conceptual view of the programming and replication of a DNA detour. Each line represents a DNA half helix. The cross-over appears to be a necessary prerequisite for a new "joining rule" to yield replicas that could segregate. From Smithies (1970).

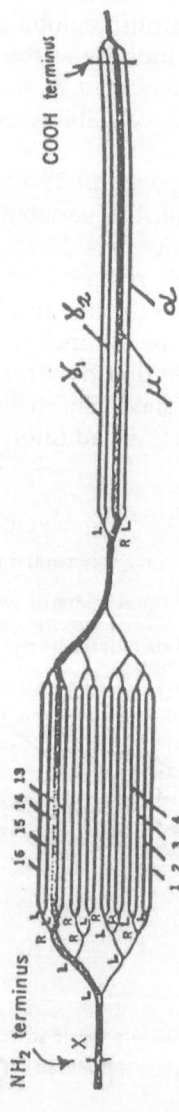

Figure 6.16. A hypothetical locus for an immunoglobulin heavy chain with 16 variable regions (V_1 to V_{16}) and four constant parts ($C_\gamma 1$, $C_\gamma 2$, C_α, C_μ). Each line represents a DNA double helix. Commitment to one of the possible proteins coded by the locus as determined by the random setting of its DNA forks in left (L) or right (R) configurations; X represents a position at which allotypic variants could easily be found. The path of an RNA polymerase molecule is indicated by the heavy line that would translate messenger RNA corresponding to V_{14}–C_μ. From Smithies (1970).

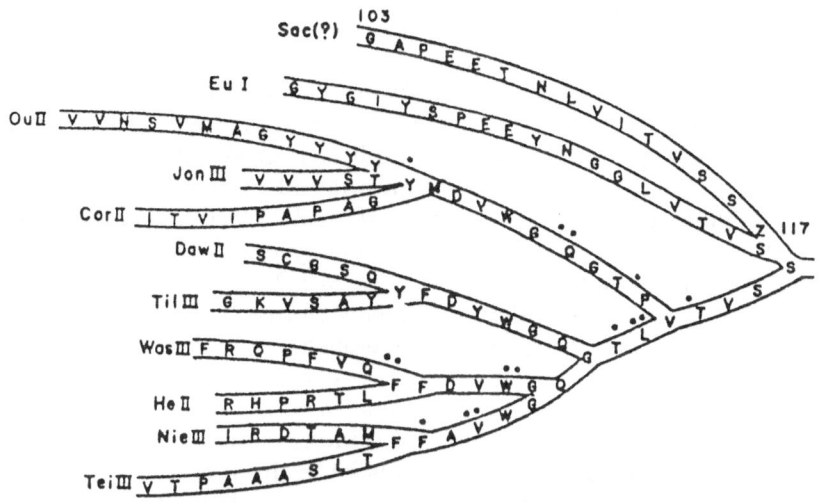

Figure 6.17. A presentation of the DNA network for human heavy chains. All sequences begin at position 99 except Sac, which begins at 103. Only elements of the network represented in sequences are shown. Dots above the network show 15 single-base-pair mutations that must be assumed to have occurred in the networks of some individuals (or plasma cell lines) but not in others in order to account for all the sequences. Roman numerals represent the designated V_H subgroup. From Smithies (1978).

and therefore, attributed the scattered variations seen in immunoglobulin sequences to this mechanism.

The second issue that was nicely dealt with in the Smithies' proposal (perhaps more so than in either of the polar solutions or the models proposed above) is the breakdown in subgroup specificity near the C-terminal ends of immunoglobulin V regions. Figure 6.17 shows Smithies' analysis of the C-terminal end of the human heavy chain. In this scheme, the existence of a "J segment," which will be discussed in detail in Chapter 7, is predicted.

6.3.4. Edelman and Gally's Somatic Recombination Model

In 1967, at a time when only two complete human immunoglobulin kappa chains and only fragmentary portions of five other human kappa variable regions had been sequenced, Edelman and Gally rejected both the germline theory and somatic mutation theory in favor of somatic recombination of duplicated genes as the mechanism of antibody diversity. Originally, they postulated that about 50 genes arose in evolution by tandem duplication. Point mutations accumulated in the duplicated genes so that each differed in at least one codon from the others. They proposed that the genes recombined at some stage of maturation of the lymphocyte by means of somatic crossing over. Crossing over would be favored by the homology of these genes, as well as by the fact that they were present in tandem duplicated arrays. A diagram indicating a single cross-over event in an array of ten tandem duplicated genes is illustrated in Fig. 6.18. Because of the close homology of the tandem genes and their similarity or equality in length, Edelman and Gally postulated that mispairing between two DNA strands might occur frequently so that nonidentical genes lie side-by-side. Crossing over at any point along these genes would generate genes with new sequences.

The somatic recombination theory is extremely powerful in that it requires a minimum amount of genetic material to be carried in the germline and yet does not require the randomness of somatic mutation. The information would already be present in the germline and the recombinant molecules selected from the basic germline information.

Gally and Edelman did not continue to write extensively on the theory of somatic recombination of a relatively limited number of germline genes. The fact that few if any amino acid sequences could be explained by recombinational processes led to the general decline of this theory in the mid 1970s. More recently, however, as will be pointed out in Chapter 8, such "recombinant" molecules have been described. The data described earlier in this chapter were not available at the time that Gally and Edelman proposed their theory so it is perhaps not fair to refer to their theory as a "maverick solution." However, for historical reasons and, as will become evident in Chapter 8, since parts of this hypothesis have proved to be correct, it is presented in this context.

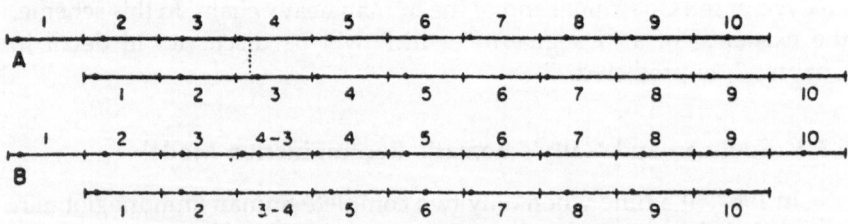

Figure 6.18. Diagram of the Edelman and Gally somatic recombination model. It shows a single crossing over (4 to 3) in a hypothetical double array of ten tandem duplicated genes. The dots indicate point mutations at different positions in each gene. (A) Before crossing over; (B) after crossing over between genes 4 and 3. From Edelman and Gally (1967).

Somatic recombination can deal with almost all of the problems raised in Section 6.2. Rapid recombination would, indeed, scramble the subgroups and could explain the maintenance of the rabbit allotypes and phylogenetically associated residues since the theory required relatively few genes. Shared idiotypes in molecules of different V-region subgroups would be explained by an occasional crossing over between subgroups. A similar mechanism could explain identical hypervariable regions in proteins of different V-region subgroup.

6.4. PRECIS

Until recently, the vast majority of immunologists subscribed to either the germline or somatic mutation theory to explain antibody variability. In this chapter, we have presented the data that were difficult to reconcile with either theory and have described four alternatives to the polar solutions. As will be seen in the next two chapters, in one of those rare occurrences in modern science, all the theories were both right and wrong, and elements of each of the maverick solutions were as important in understanding a modern synthesis of antibody diversity as were the polar solutions.

In the summer of 1977, immunologists gathered at Cold Spring Harbor for the 41st Symposium on Quantitative Biology. The title of the meeting was Origins of Lymphocyte Diversity, and on the last day of the meeting in the last session, the protagonists for many of the theories outlined in Chapters 5 and 6 presented papers. Hood had recently started to sequence NZB myeloma proteins and interpreted the data along a strict germline hypothesis, although indicating that somatic mutation may play some role. Weigert, continuing to pursue by both structure and genetic means immunoglobulin variable regions, concluded, "Although most of the V-region diversity results from a somatic mechanism, a considerable repertoire of antibodies is inherited, or germline." Clearly, the proponents of the polar solutions were hedging. Capra reviewed the data for gene interaction and pressed the case for multigene involvement in V-gene formation. However, the last speaker was Tonegawa who presented a paper entitled, "Somatic Changes in the Content and Context of Immunoglobulin Genes." He provided direct evidence for the two gene–one polypeptide chain model. More importantly, his studies ushered in the new era of direct analysis of the DNA utilizing the new powerful recombinant DNA technology. It is to the studies launched on that day that the next chapter is directed.

REFERENCES AND BIBLIOGRAPHY

Capra, J. D., 1976, The implications of phylogenetically associated residues and idiotypes on theories of antibody diversity, in: *The Generation of Antibody Diversity: A New Look* (A. J. Cunningham, ed.), Academic Press, New York, p. 65.

Capra, J. D., and Kindt, T. J., 1975, Antibody diversity: Can more than one gene encode each variable region?, editorial, *Immunogenetics* **1**:417.

Capra, J. D., and Kehoe, J. M., 1974, Structure of antibodies with shared idiotypy: The complete sequence of the heavy chain variable regions of two IsM anti-gamma globulins, *Proc. Natl. Acad. Sci. U.S.A.* **71**:4032.

Capra, J. D., and Klapper, D. G., 1976, Complete amino acid sequence of the variable domains of two human IgM anti-gamma globulins with shared idiotypic specificities, *Scand. J. Immunol.* **5**:667.

Edelman, G. M., and Gally, J. A., 1967, Somatic recombination of duplicated genes: An hypothesis on the origin of antibody diversity, *Proc. Natl. Acad. Sci. U.S.A.* **57**:353.

Fett, J. W., and Deutsch, H., 1975, A new lambda-chain gene, *Immunochemistry* **12**:643.

Gally, J. A., and Edelman, G. M., 1970, Somatic translocation of antibody genes, *Nature (London)* **227**:341.

Jacob, F., 1982, *The Possible and the Actual*, University of Washington Press/Pantheon, New York.

Kabat, E. A., Wu, T. T., and Bilofsky, H., 1979, Evidence supporting somatic assembly of the DNA segments (minigenes), coding for the framework, and complementarity-determining segments of immunoglobulin variable regions, *J. Exp. Med.* **149**:1299.

Kindt, T. J., and Capra, J. D., 1978, Gene-insertion theories of antibody diversity: A re-evaluation, *Immunogenetics* **6**:309.

Kindt, T. J., Klapper, D. G., and Waterfield, M. D., 1973, An idiotypic crossreaction between allotype A3 and allotype a negative rabbit antibodies to streptococcal carbohydrate, *J. Exp. Med.* **137**:636.

Klinman, N. R., Sigal, N. H., Metcalf, E. S., Pierce, S. K., and Gearhart, P. J., 1976, The interplay of evolution and environment in B-cell diversification, *Cold Spring Harbor Symp. Quant. Biol.* **41**:285.

Smith, G. P., 1973, *The Variation and Adaptive Expression of Antibodies*, Harvard University Press, Cambridge, Massachusetts.

Smithies, O., 1970, Pathways through networks of branched DNA, *Science* **169**:822.

Smithies, O., 1978, Immunoglobulin genes: Arranged in tandem or in parallel?, *Cold Spring Harbor Symp. Quant. Biol.*, p. 725.

Wilkinson, J. M., 1969, Variation in the N-terminal sequence of heavy chains of immunoglobulin G from rabbits of different allotype, *Biochem. J.* **112**:173.

Wu, T. T., and Kabat, E. A., 1970, An analysis of the sequences of the variable regions of Bence Jones proteins and myeloma light chains and their implications for antibody complementarity, *J. Exp. Med.* **132**:211.

Wu, T. T., Kabat, E. A., and Bilofsky, H., 1975, Similarities among hypervariable segments of immunoglobulin chains, *Proc. Natl. Acad. Sci. U.S.A.* **72**:5107.

7

THE MOLECULAR BIOLOGISTS ATTACK THE PROBLEM

> . . . le beau n'est pas dans l'analyse; mais le beau réel, celui qui ne repose pas sur les fictions de la fantaisie humaine est caché dans les résultats de l'analyse.
>
> —RENAN (L'Avenir de la Science)

7.1. INTRODUCTION

Studies on the nucleic acids involved in immunoglobulin synthesis had been underway for over a decade when the major breakthroughs came with the application of recombinant DNA technology to the antibody problem in the late 1970s. The essential groundwork for these breakthroughs had been laid by the discovery of the mouse myelomas by Potter and their adaptation to tissue culture. The new wave of discovery would be further based on the early work by Askonas, Williamson, Stavitsky, Scharff, Milstein, Mach, and others who isolated mRNA from these tumors and developed techniques for its purification and enrichment as well as assays for the synthesis in vitro of immunoglobulin polypeptide chains. The first decade of work on nucleic acids was not particularly fruitful because the powerful technologies that emerged in the mid 1970s and were immediately applied to the antibody problem had not yet been developed.

7.2. GENE COUNTING BY LIQUID HYBRIDIZATION

In 1974, using mRNA isolated from the spleens of hyperimmune mice and the technique of filter hybridization in RNA excess, Storb estimated that there were 1×10^4 V_κ genes in the mouse genome. Filter hybridization was soon replaced by liquid hybridization and measurements of reiteration frequencies using so-called Cot curves. These experiments analyzed the kinetics of hybridization of a radioactive immunoglobulin DNA or RNA "probe" with nuclear DNA in order to estimate the number of V genes per haploid genome complementary to the probe. The studies required a relatively pure mRNA preparation (or its cDNA counterpart) and excess DNA (typically isolated from liver). There were two basic experimental designs used by investigators. In one, the percent hybridization is plotted against the logarithm of the product (called Cot) of the DNA concentration (Co) and the time of incubation (t). In the second type of experiment, called "competition hybridization," increasing amounts of nonradioactive mRNA are included in a series of reaction mixtures all of which contain fixed amounts of nonradioactive DNA and radioactive mRNA and are incubated for a fixed time. The nonradioactive mRNA competes with the radioactive probe for complementary DNA strands and, thus, decreases the observed percent hybridization. By using internal controls (for example, globin genes that were assumed to have a gene number of one and ribosomal genes that were assumed to have a gene number of about 300), the data could be interpreted to indicate the reiteration frequency of immunoglobulin V-region genes.

7.2.1. Early Evidence Favors the Germline Theory

The earliest application of these hybridization techniques was by Delovitch and Baglioni, who in 1973 studied the MOPC11 mouse myeloma tumor. They translated mRNA for this kappa chain in a cell-free protein synthesis system and purified the RNA substantially. Using this product in hybridization experiments, they determined a reiteration frequency of about 40. Since they assumed that their probe only reacted with V_κ genes of the same subgroup (although there was no direct evidence for this) and since at the time the relatively few available mouse V_κ sequences indicated that there were approximately ten mouse V_κ subgroups, they concluded that there were 40×10 or approximately 400 V_κ genes. In 1973, this was interpreted as evidence in favor of the germline theory.

These studies were followed within the next two years by experiments in which Leder et al. (1974) used MOPC41 mRNA and determined that there were at most only two to three mouse C_κ genes. This demonstration provided further evidence that the two gene–one polypeptide chain hypothesis was correct. Since even the most ardent somaticist required at least ten V_κ genes in the BALB/c mouse, some form of translocation was required in order to synthesize a complete kappa chain.

Leder's work on the V_κ system at this time suggested that there were 30 to 50 genes per subgroup (a result not unlike Delovitch's and Baglioni's, 1973) and with the same assumptions used by Baglioni that the 30 to 50 represented the genes of a single subgroup, these data strongly supported the germline theory, although as the authors themselves state, "It is difficult to feel secure about these numbers." These studies were followed in the same year by those of Storb (1974) who used DNA excess solution hybridization with essentially the same probes as Leder and Baglioni to predict 2500 to 5000 V_κ genes. It was concluded that this was "probably enough to satisfy germline theories."

Finally, Williamson in a 1974 paper using "pure alpha mRNA from MOPC315" estimated that there were 5000 V_H genes and four C_α genes per haploid genome in the BALB/c mouse (Premkumar et al., 1974). Assuming a similar number of V_κ genes, there would be 5000 × 5000 or 2.5×10^7 possible H-L combinations; this seemed a sufficient repertoire to satisfy the germline theory. Figure 7.1 illustrates the method used by Williamson to arrive at these conclusions and provides a good example of a major controversy relevant to all of the early liquid hybridization experiments. The Cot curve essentially shows two regions, one with a predicted gene number of 5000 and another with a predicted gene number of four. The *assumption* by most workers at this time was that the rapidly hybridizing early peak (inflection point) represented highly reiterated genes. The heated arguments concerning these data revolved about the issue of whether these highly reiterated genes represented the variable-region genes or the 5' untranslated regions of immunoglobulins, the leader sequences, contamination in the mRNA preparations, or fragments of probe (it should be pointed out that the most commonly used technique to generate a radioactive probe was ^{125}I radioiodination, a technique known to fragment mRNA).

In spite of this technical difficulty, the results were clearly supportive of the germline theory and, as the Williamson paper ends, "The present data obviate the necessity to search for somatic generators of diversity."

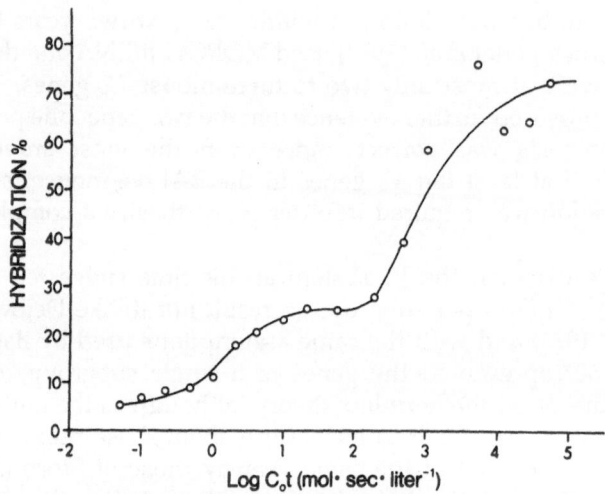

Figure 7.1. Kinetics of hybridization of mouse embryo DNA with MOPC315 H chain mRNA. Hybridization of mRNA with excess mouse DNA. The Cot curve shows two inflection points with predicted gene numbers of 5000 (left) and 4 (right). See text for details. From Premkumar *et al.* (1974).

7.2.2. Mouse V_κ Studies Favor Fewer Genes

At about the time that these three studies on mouse kappa were reported, Bernardini and Tonegawa (1974) reported evidence suggesting far fewer genes. Using MPC11, MOPC70E, and MOPC321 and 70% pure mRNA they determined (as had Leder) that there were but one or two C_κ genes and that the V region had a reiteration frequency of 230. Certain assumptions were tested in these studies. For example, light chain mRNA from other tumors was used to compete with the radioactive probe in competition hybridization experiments and from these kinds of control experiments, Tonegawa was able to ascertain the role of the "stable portion of the variable region" in hybridization kinetics. In particular, mRNA derived from tumors secreting proteins of different subgroups would not compete, whereas mRNA from those secreting proteins from within the same V-region subgroup would compete. On the basis of these studies, Tonegawa concluded that there were less than 200 V_κ genes per haploid genome encoding the MPC11 light chain and favored the conclusion that there was but one.

The next year, Rabbitts and Milstein (1975), using the MOPC21 system and both mRNA and cDNA generated by newly available procedures, obtained hybridization data showing that the MOPC21 V region was present in one or very few copies per haploid genome. They concluded that the rapidly hybridizing component was not due to V-region genes. A year later Mach (Farace *et al.*, 1976) using MOPC41 mRNA, was able to demonstrate that as the mRNA was purified, the "gene number" went from a double-peak (inflection point) Cot curve indicating either 250 V_κ genes or two to four V_κ genes, to a Cot curve with a single inflection point indicating two to four genes per haploid genome. This study concluded that there was but a single gene for each subgroup, and assuming 50 subgroups of mouse V_κ proteins, Mach suggested that there were fewer than 50 V_κ genes per haploid genome, a number obviously incompatible with the germline theory. As shown in Fig. 7.2, the highly purified mRNA fraction used by Mach effectively eliminated the first inflection point of the Cot curve that had been seen in most previous experiments and gave a curve that was much simpler to interpret.

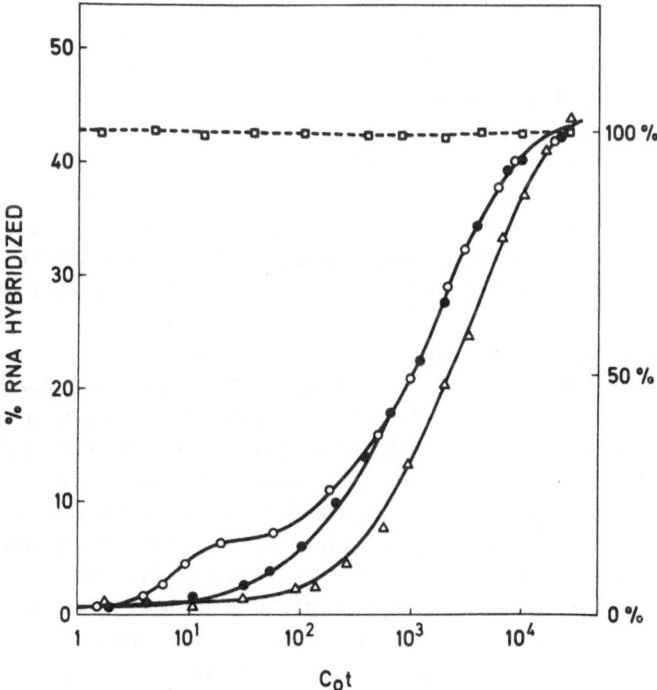

Figure 7.2. Effect of purification of mRNA on Cot curve. As the mRNA become purer, the "double" curve (left, open circles) becomes single (open triangles). From Farace *et al.* (1976).

7.2.3. Mouse V_λ Studies Favor Fewer Genes

The lambda system of BALB/c mice is ideally suited to test the germline versus somatic hypotheses. It constitutes the largest known subgroup with V-region amino acid sequences so similar to one another that their corresponding nucleotide sequences would almost certainly cross-hybridize. The amino acid sequences (described in Chapter 3) were largely done by Weigert who studied the light chains of randomly selected lambda-secreting BALB/c myelomas. Nine different BALB/c lambda V-region sequences had been described. One of them appeared in many independently arising myeloma tumors. Both the germline and somatic theories of antibody diversity agree that these were probably encoded by a germline gene that had not undergone somatic mutation, since otherwise the occurrence of the same chain in nine different tumors would have to be attributed to parallel or convergent modifications arising independently in different mice. The other eight BALB/c lambda V-region sequences were represented by a single myeloma protein each and are minor variants of the basic sequence (see Fig. 3.20). The germline theory attributes each variant to a different germline gene, whereas the somatic theory attributes the variants to somatically varied genes. A simple mathematical calculation based on the number of known mouse lambda sequences and the number of repeats of the "germline sequence" with reasonable possibility suggests that there are a minimum of 16 different mouse V_λ sequences. The germline theory predicts that by using any one of the mouse V_λ probes, approximately 16 genes should be detected, whereas the somatic theory predicts that no matter which of the lambda V-region probes is used only one V_λ gene will be found in the genome.

The experiments to test the number of V_λ genes were done almost simultaneously by Leder and by Tonegawa; they came to virtually identical conclusions. Leder used cDNA from RPC20 and determined that there were two V_λ genes per haploid genome (Leder et al., 1980). He concluded that since there were a minimum of eight known lambda variable region sequence variants, the data "rule out separate germline genes corresponding to each individual lambda-like chain variant." Tonegawa, using lambda mRNA that was greater than 90% pure, and competition hybridization experiments, also showed that there were relatively few lambda genes per haploid genome; that is, homologous (using the same lambda mRNA) and heterologous (using a different lambda mRNA) competition hybridization Cot curves were identical (Tonegawa et al., 1974). Thus, with different tumors and different techniques the same conclusion was reached. The only reservation was that lambda represents less than 5% of mouse light chains. Could these results be extrapolated to the kappa system? Might lambda be a special case?

No kappa subgroup had been studied as extensively as lambda until Weigert and Perry in 1978 decisively settled that issue using modern recombinant DNA techniques that involved liquid hybridization. The mouse $V_\kappa 21$ subgroup that has been described in Chapter 3 was chosen as a good case to test the kappa system. Over 30 $V_\kappa 21$ proteins had been sequenced and although many were identical, over 20 were different. cDNA was made from one and competition hybridization was done with mRNA from another. Elegant "protection" experiments were done that indicated the degree of cross-hybridization of the different mRNAs. They came to the same conclusion that Leder and Tonegawa had reached in the mouse lambda system and that Mach, Rabbitts, and Tonegawa (see Section 7.2.2.) had previously arrived at in the mouse kappa system that there were relatively few genes per subgroup.

7.2.4. Cautions on Interpretation of Liquid Hybridization

With the exception of some early studies indicating large numbers of V genes, the liquid hybridization experiments were in universal agreement. The data that became available in the mid 1970s showed that there were too few genes to satisfy the germline polar solution. Despite this seemingly overwhelming body of evidence for the presence of relatively few genes in the haploid genome, there were a number of important reservations that led many immunologists to continue to adhere to the germline theory. These views were probably best summarized in a paper presented at the 1977 Cold Spring Harbor Symposium by Smith. In a detailed analysis of the then-published (and many unpublished) studies, Smith criticized the basic tenets of the liquid hybridization approach and pointed out the pitfalls that existed in the technique. Smith argued that although

> . . . the results of several hybridization kinetic experiments with mouse lambda probes as well as various kappa chain probes are consistent with a small number of complementary genes in the haploid genome, when these data are analyzed more critically, they are revealed to constitute only rather weak evidence against the germline theory.

Smith's criticisms included: (1) the large, unexplained discrepancies that necessitated normalization of the data; (2) the inadequacy of the theoretical understanding of the liquid hybridization reaction itself; and (3) the absence of any direct experiments establishing the limits of certainty of the method for counting genes. Smith pointed out, for example, that there was no direct evidence that globin genes existed with copy numbers of one or ribosomal genes with copy numbers of 300, the benchmarks that were used by most investigators to establish their conditions.

All of these objections aside, the technology that was applied to the problem was not up to the task and we must digress for a time to describe recombinant DNA technology that emerged in the mid 1970s. It was the application of this technology that led to a more profound understanding of the antibody problem.

7.3. RECOMBINANT DNA METHODS

In simple terms, recombinant DNA techniques consist of joining DNA molecules in vitro and introducing them into living cells where they can replicate. The discovery of mutant *Escherichia coli* strains unable to degrade foreign DNA along with the discovery of site-specific restriction endonucleases were two of the major advances. General methods for joining DNA molecules from different sources were found. The restriction endonuclease, EcoRI, that could create self-complementary cohesive termini on DNA molecules by specific cleavage at staggered sites in two DNA strands was particularly important. By using recombinant DNA technology, a desired sequence from a complex mixture of DNA molecules (such as a eukaryotic genome) can be replicated to provide milligram quantities for biochemical study.

7.3.1. The Principle of Cloning

The incorporation of DNA fragments into DNA of bacteriophages or plasmids creates recombinant DNA that can then replicate as the phage or plasmid multiply in bacteria. The progeny of each individual organism (clone) containing a new DNA fragment will replicate that single, inserted piece along with its own genome. Many bacterial plasmids have been used as cloning vectors. For example, pBR322, a widely used plasmid for cloning DNA, has several restriction cleavage sites at which foreign DNA can be inserted. Insertions at many of these sites destroy one of the antibiotic-resistance genes of the plasmid allowing an easy test for bacterial clones containing a plasmid carrying an insert. Figure 7.3 shows pBR322. Much contemporary work is done by cloning into either the BamHI site or the PstI site. The latter has the advantage of restoring the PstI site thus aiding in the excision of foreign DNA (see Section 7.3.2). Note that each of these insertions destroys one of the antibiotic-resistance genes. Thus, foreign DNA can be inserted into this

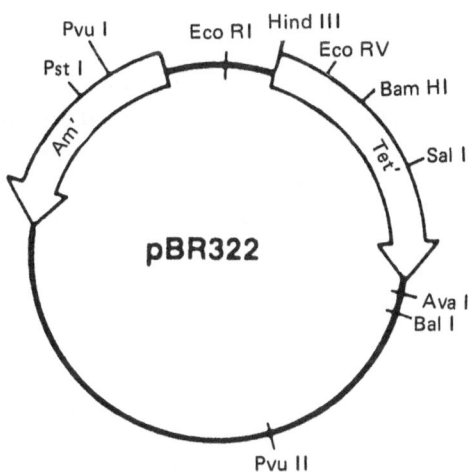

Figure 7.3. The structure of pBR322 showing the cleavage sites for some commonly used restriction endonucleases that cut the DNA only once. The arrows inside the circle show the direction of transcription of Am′ and Tet′ genes that encode resistance to ampicillin and tetracycline.

plasmid and it can be used as a vehicle for propagating the foreign DNA. One has to then transform bacteria (typically *E. coli*), isolate transformants on selective growth medium, and then screen the colonies (see Fig. 7.4). Once that is done, individual colonies can be grown up in large amounts, plasmid DNA isolated, the foreign DNA excised by restriction endonuleases, and isolated by any one of a number of techniques such as agarose gel electrophoresis or high-performance liquid chromatography.

The source of DNA for cloning could be fragments of the whole genome (thus constructing a "library") or alternatively could be complementary or cDNA that is synthesized using mRNA as the template. In this latter case, a typical procedure involves isolation of mRNA by virtue of its hybridization to columns of oligonucleotides, usually oligo dT. This is possible because mRNA molecules have a tail of poly(A) residues. The mRNA is further purified using its ability to direct the synthesis of a specific product, such as an immunoglobulin light chain, as the assay procedure. When the mRNA is enriched for the desired species, it is used to direct synthesis of cDNA using the enzyme reverse transcriptase.

The mixture of cDNA fragments representing the mRNA populations is then cloned into a suitable vector, usually a plasmid. The clones may be screened by their ability to hybridize to a known probe, or if no such probe is available they must be screened by their ability to hybridize to the specific mRNA species that direct synthesis of the product under study. This may be assayed by inhibition of the synthetic reaction or alternatively by hybridization followed by separation of the mRNA from the cDNA and testing of the eluted mRNA for its ability to direct product synthesis. The cDNA clones may be studied further by methods including DNA sequence analysis as detailed in Section 7.3.4. It is usually cloned cDNA that is used as a probe to find related genes in different cloning vectors or in the Southern blot procedure (see Section 7.3.3).

There are a number of variations in cloning procedures including variations in the use of the vector chosen. As mentioned, plasmids may be used for cloning. These are usually used when smaller fragments, especially cDNA fragments, are to be incorporated. As indicated in Fig. 7.4, the phage lambda is often used for cloning genomic DNA; typically, fragments of 10 to 20 kilobases (kb) are selected from partial enzymatic digests for cloning in lambda phage. If larger fragments are desired, vectors called cosmids are used; these have the capacity to accept foreign DNA inserts as large as 50 kb.

7.3.2. Restriction Endonucleases

The Nobel Prize in Physiology and Medicine was awarded to Arber, Nathans, and Smith in 1978 for their work on restriction endonucleases. These are enzymes that are derived from a wide variety of bacterial

---

Figure 7.4. Antibody gene is cloned by inserting fragments of mouse DNA into a bacterial virus (phage lambda), isolating a virus clone whose DNA includes the gene, and growing that virus in quantity to produce large amounts of the single gene. First, the phage DNA is cleaved with a restriction enzyme that cuts the DNA into three fragments. The middle fragment is not needed for viral growth. It can be replaced with a fragment of mouse DNA that has been cleaved with the same restriction enzyme, so that the phage and the mouse fragments have complementary terminals ("sticky ends") and bind to one another. The recombinant DNAs are packaged in new phage particles, which are incubated with E. coli, the bacteria they infect. The infected bacteria are layered onto an agar culture medium. Individual phages proliferate, killing their host and infecting neighboring cells, thus leaving clear areas called plaques in the bacterial layer; each plaque represents a phage clone. The plaque pattern is transferred to a nitrocellulose filter and the filter is incubated with a radioactively labeled probe. The probe hybridizes with any recombinant DNA incorporating a matching mouse DNA sequence, and the position of the clone having that DNA is revealed by autoradiography. Now the desired clone can be selected from culture medium and transferred to fresh bacterial host, so that pure antibody gene can be manufactured. From Leder (1982).

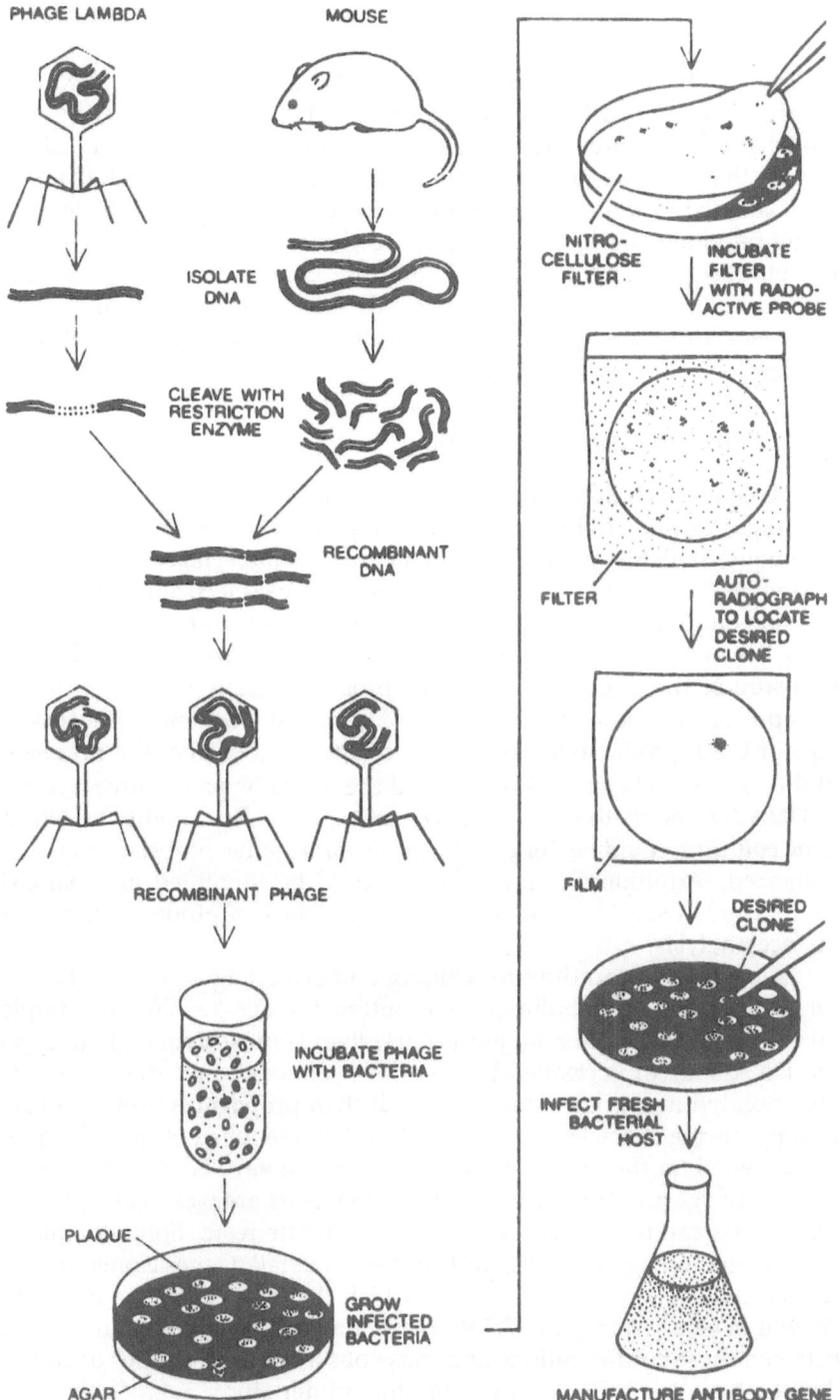

PHAGE LAMBDA

MOUSE

ISOLATE DNA

CLEAVE WITH RESTRICTION ENZYME

RECOMBINANT DNA

RECOMBINANT PHAGE

INCUBATE PHAGE WITH BACTERIA

PLAQUE

GROW INFECTED BACTERIA

AGAR

NITRO-CELLULOSE FILTER

INCUBATE FILTER WITH RADIO-ACTIVE PROBE

FILTER

AUTO-RADIOGRAPH TO LOCATE DESIRED CLONE

FILM

DESIRED CLONE

INFECT FRESH BACTERIAL HOST

MANUFACTURE ANTIBODY GENE

strains that have the capacity to specifically cleave DNA with extraordinary fidelity at particular cleavage sites. These sites typically involve stretches of from three to six bases. Almost all of the liquid hybridization studies that were described (Section 7.2) were done with DNA that had been sheared by various procedures. The restriction endonuclease technique provided the first opportunity to cleave DNA in a highly reproducible fashion, and because of this, the gene-counting experiments became more precise. More importantly, cleavage with specific endonucleases and subsequent separation of the DNA fragments allowed cloning to be done with relative ease.

7.3.3. Southern Filter Hybridization

Another technique that is used for studies of DNA exploits the technique of filter hybridization, developed by Southern in 1975. The technique, which is widely used in all areas of molecular biology at the present time, involves separation by agarose gel electrophoresis of restriction endonuclease-cleaved DNA fragments, the transfer of the DNA from the agarose gel to a sheet of nitrocellulose, and the subsequent exposure of the paper to radioactive probes typically labeled with ^{32}P. This procedure allows an estimation of gene numbers and takes advantage of the reproducibility of the endonuclease cleavage, the precision of the agarose gel electrophoresis, and the virtually quantitative transfer of DNA fragments to nitrocellulose sheets. Thus, the rapidity by which gene counting could be done with various radioactive probes was greatly enhanced. Additionally, more genes could be identified and parallel agarose gels used to isolate and clone the DNA in preparation for sequence analysis.

A complete procedure for cloning and screening a genomic library for mouse immunoglobulin genes is outlined in Fig. 7.4. In the example given, total DNA from a mouse (mouse liver is most frequently used as the DNA source) is cleaved by restriction enzymes and the fragments incorporated into phage lambda, which then propagates itself in a bacteria producing characteristic zones of lysis that are called plaques. Plaques are screened for the immunoglobulin genes that have been incorporated into the phage and those with appropriate inserts are picked and grown. The inserts can be excised using the appropriate restriction endonuclease, isolated on agarose gels, and studied in detail. Genes cloned in this manner will retain the structure in which they appear in the genome. As will be seen in Section 7.3.4, there may be considerable difference between these configurations and those observed from studies of cDNA derived from the mRNA for the product under study.

7.3.4. DNA Sequencing

Recombinant DNA technology described up to this point can provide major insights into the number and arrangements of antibody genes, but the DNA sequencing techniques that were developed by Maxam and Gilbert (1980) and by Sanger *et al.* (1977) have given precise information regarding the genes involved in the antibody problem. In particular, the sequencing technique was critical to the discovery of the boundaries between the V and J gene segments in the light chain and between the V, D, and J gene segments in the heavy chain (see Section 7.5). These sequencing techniques are so rapid that they have to a large extent supplanted the amino acid sequencing of immunoglobulin molecules.

These new techniques were discovered, introduced, and applied in molecular biology very rapidly and have been the subject of entire volumes. In immunology, the impact of these technologies was first felt around 1976, and since then most of the major advances in our understanding of the organization of immunoglobulin genes and in particular most of our insights into the antibody problem have come from this technology. We shall now return to the first applications of these procedures to the antibody problem.

7.3.5. The Antibody Question Redefined

The successful use of highly purified mRNA probes to count V-region genes in hybridization experiments was a minor triumph compared with what would happen soon after the application of recombinant DNA techniques and DNA sequence analysis to the problem of antibody diversity. The question of how many V-region genes were present in the genome had, as noted, been given a provisional answer based on data in the murine lambda and the $V_\kappa 21$ systems. It would soon be shown that these answers, although somewhat unsatisfying in terms of the major theories, were at least approximately correct. It is now known that the reason that the gene-counting answer did not yield a satisfactory solution to the problem of antibody diversity is not because the answer was wrong but because the question was inadequate! It was not sufficient for an understanding of antibody diversity to merely know how many variable region genes were encoded in genome. There were certain complexities concerning these variable region genes and mechanisms by which they were expressed that would require definition before the details of the process of antibody diversity generation could be learned. In light of these details, supplied by investigations at the DNA level, the question of antibody diversity was completely reformulated. Although the gene-counting experiments were later revisited using sophisticated new techniques, the question of how many variable region subgroups and how many variable region genes there are will be put aside for a moment and the description of the antibody genes gained by recombinant DNA techniques will be considered. Two major discoveries stand out in the early studies. One is the definitive proof of the two-gene hypothesis that included a demonstration that genes can move about in the genome. The second was the discovery of small DNA segments between the V- and C-region genes that interposed themselves in the differentiation process and thereby contributed to variable region diversity.

7.4. THE TWO-GENE HYPOTHESIS REINVESTIGATED

The first and perhaps the most exciting breakthrough using recombinant DNA technology involved a rigorous test of the Dreyer-Bennett hypothesis (see Chapter 4). There were available highly purified samples of mRNA corresponding to the kappa light chain from the mouse plasmacytoma MOPC321. It was possible to prepare fragments from this mRNA that corresonded to only the C region portion (the 3' end of the mRNA). Using the complete (that is variable and constant region) mRNA probe in conjunction with this C-terminal fragment, it was possible to isolate restriction enzyme fragments of germline DNA that corresponded to the antibody variable and constant regions. With these tools it was possible to directly answer questions concerning the relative locations of variable- and constant-region genes.

7.4.1. Gene Rearrangements

In a series of experiments first reported at the 1976 Cold Spring Harbor Symposium, Tonegawa *et al.* (1976) used such mRNA probes to examine DNA samples from embryonic tissue and from differentiated cells producing myeloma proteins. When embryonic (germline) mouse DNA was probed, it was found that the DNA segments hybridizing to variable and constant regions could be separated by electrophoresis into different fractions. As Fig. 7.5 indicates, this separation was not seen for the restriction fragments of DNA obtained from the MOPC321 cell line, where both variable and constant regions were in the same peak. Therefore, a clear difference was seen between the antibody light chain gene in the genomic (germline) form and that in the actively transcribed

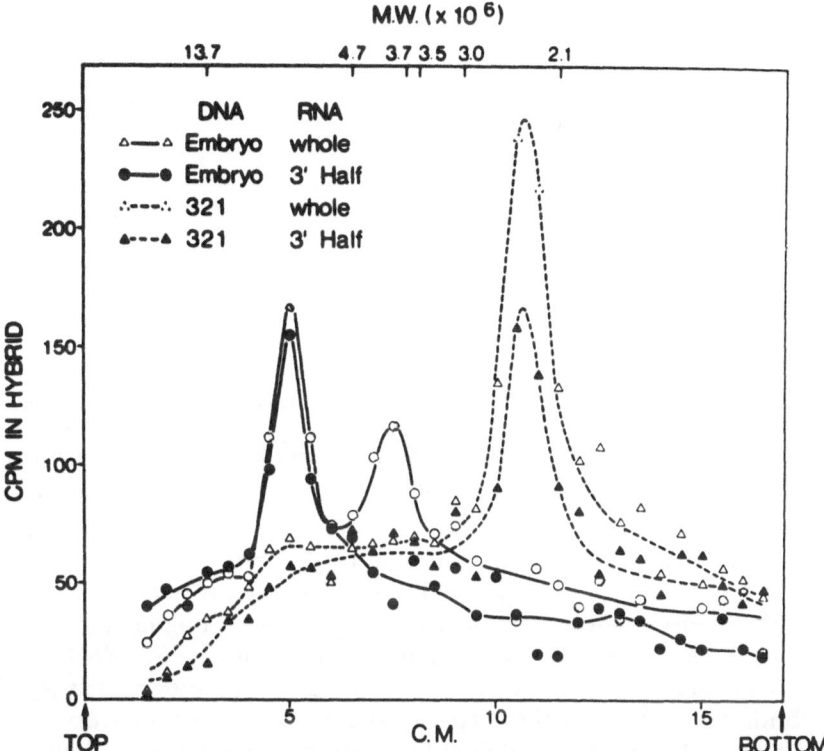

Figure 7.5. Gel electrophoresis pattern of BamHI-generated mouse DNA fragments carrying V_κ or C_κ gene sequences. Results with mouse embryo and with MOPC-321 plasmacytoma DNAs are superimposed. DNA was annealed with ^{125}I-labeled whole MOPC-321 mRNA or its 3'-end half. From Tonegawa *et al.* (1976).

form in the differentiated cell. These data gave biochemical reality to the structural, serologic, and genetic evidence that variable- and constant-region genes are separate in the genome. The Dreyer-Bennett hypothesis was now a fact; there were separate genes for the same polypeptide chain.

There was not only verification of the existence of separate variable- and constant-region genes in the original Tonegawa data, but there was also evidence that "joining" took place at the DNA level and not at any subsequent step in protein biosynthesis. Thus, the predictions put forth at the 1967 Cold Spring Harbor Meeting (Chapter 4) were experimentally verified in a report given at a meeting at Cold Spring Harbor in 1976.

The two-gene hypothesis would receive further confirmation from

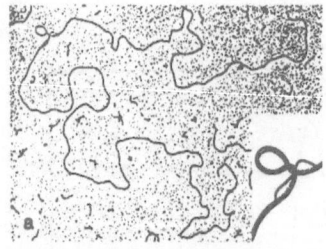

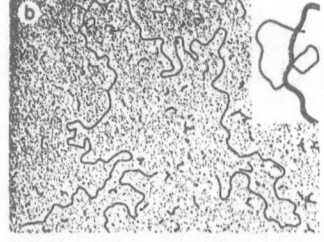

Figure 7.6. R-loop analyses between lambda chain mRNA and cloned DNA from the cell line producing the chain; interpretations are shown in the insets. The dotted lines represent RNA. From Brack and Tonegawa (1977).

numerous experimental systems. One of the most satisfying was the direct visualization of two genes by electron microscopy. A technique called "R-loop" analysis was used for this purpose. A fragment of mRNA is annealed to cloned genomic DNA under conditions where an RNA–DNA duplex is more stable than a DNA–DNA duplex. At the areas at which hybridization between these species occur, there is an interruption of the reannealment of the original DNA strand. Two types of "bubbles" or "loops" become evident in the electron micrographs. One is due to the displaced DNA strand. The other is the intron (DNA duplex) that "loops out." This technique was used to confirm separation of V- and C-region genes in myeloma DNA; that is, in the DNA of the differentiated cell, V and C genes are not contiguous—the two genes were closer than they were in the DNA derived from embryonic cells but there was still a measurable distance between them. Fig. 7.6 gives an example in which V and C genes are about 1250 bp apart. Therefore, the rearrangement or reshuffling of genes for variable and constant regions did not join them into a single light chain gene, but merely brought them closer together. More information would be needed to define totally the two-gene phenomenon and to determine how it fit into a picture of antibody biosynthesis.

7.4.2. The J Region of the Light Chain

Approximately one year after Tonegawa's demonstration of the two separate genes for V and C regions, sequences of the DNA segments including these genes were available. The excitement that greeted these first reports of DNA sequence for antibody genes was intensified by the fact that the genomic V-region sequence contained information for the amino acids only up to position 95 of the light chain, not to the end of the variable region that was assumed to be at position 108. It would soon be described by Tonegawa for the lambda chain and by Leder for the kappa chain that the light chain residues that span the region from position 96 to position 108 were encoded at a location nearer the constant-region genes but separate from *both* the V and the C-region genes. It was further shown that, depending on the system under study, there were one or several groups of genes encoding the variable–constant interface; these genes were designated J gene segments. Description of the J region allowed a complete structural picture of the genes for the light chain to be drawn. It was now possible to begin to describe the molecular events involved in light chain synthesis beginning at the embryonic DNA and ending with the light chain in its final processed form.

The experiments with J gene segments by Leder and his co-workers (Max *et al.*, 1979) in the murine kappa chain system showed that there were five coding sequences (exons) for J arranged in an evenly spaced array located to the 5' side of the C-region genes as shown in Fig. 7.7. The five sequences are repeated at intervals of approximately 300 nucleotides. The amino acids encoded in these segments with the single exception of those for J3 correspond to those previously observed by amino acid sequence analysis for BALB/c kappa chains in this region. The J3 segment contains codons for amino acids at positions 99, 103, and 108 that had not been seen in murine kappa chains, suggesting the J3 might not be a functional gene segment. It was further noted that all the J gene segments with the exception of J3 conformed to the patterns observed for intervening sequences in that each had the signal sequences necessary for RNA processing. These two observations led to the conclusion that the murine J_κ region contained four functional (J1, J2, J4, J5) and one nonfunctional (J3) gene segment. The murine J gene segments exist in their germline configuration in a position about 2.5 kb to the 5' side of the kappa constant region gene. (Note that in Fig. 7.7, the J gene segments are numbered such that J1 is closest to C_κ. In the current convention the J gene segments are numbered in the opposite order with J1 the farthest from C_κ.)

DNA sequence analysis of light chain genes cloned from cells producing light chains soon shed light on the nature of the process by which a complete V_L region was formed using these J-region gene segments. The initial step in synthesis of a light chain involves rearrangement of a given V gene segment to allow it to link up to one of the J gene segments. In the kappa system the J gene segment(s) that exist to

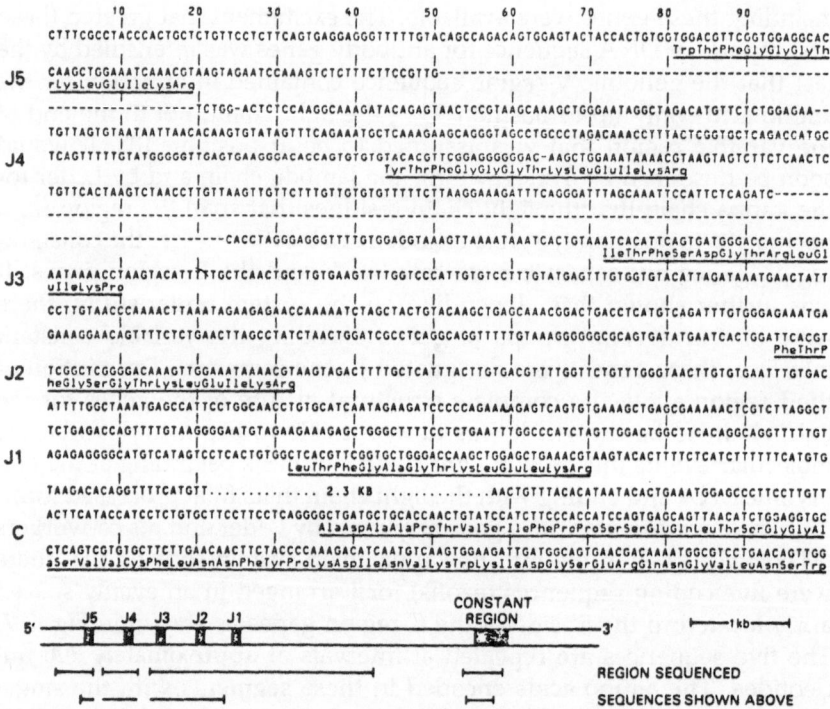

Figure 7.7. Sequence of region containing J_κ and C_κ gene segments. Coding regions of the genes are indicated by the amino acids below the nucleotide sequence. The dashes indicate undetermined nucleotides. The lengths of these unsequenced regions are estimated by restriction analysis. The diagram below indicates the extent of the sequence determined and shows which portion of the known sequence is given above. The J regions were identified by their homology with the J of the expressed MOPC-41 gene (J5). They are numbered from the J closest to the C region. From Max *et al.* (1979).

the 5' side of the one selected are excised (or possibly exchanged to the sister chromatid). Those to the 3' side remain in their original configuration(s) (Fig. 7.8). It is only after this step occurs that a complete variable-region gene exists. The V-J and C genes are then transcribed and the initial RNA product, which is termed heterogeneous nuclear RNA (hnRNA), is a faithful copy of the rearranged gene. The next step to occur is called "splicing," a process by which the mRNA to be translated is formed from the hnRNA. Now, for the first time in the process, the information for the entire light chain is assembled in one contiguous sequence (Fig. 7.9). Translation of mRNA then occurs followed by post-translational modifications that include removal of the leader sequence

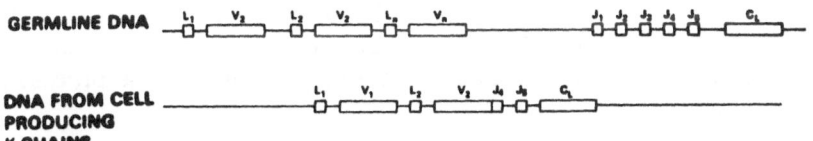

Figure 7.8. Initial step in rearrangement of genes for an idealized light chain.

at the amino terminal portion of the polypeptide chain. The completed chain is now ready for combination with a heavy chain.

The process for biosynthesis of an idealized light chain that is depicted in Figs. 7.8 and 7.9 has certain variations that are possible in different systems. As will be discussed in Section 7.5., the process for making a heavy chain is considerably more complicated in that it involves more gene segments and more steps. Similarly, the number and arrangements of J and C genes for light chains is different between the kappa and lambda system and there is good evidence that it will also be different for the kappa chains of certain other species. Notwithstanding these differences, the basic processes shown here occur in all cells that will eventually synthesize immunoglobulins.

The fact that the V gene segment may join to any of four J gene segments was immediately recognized as a possible means to generate additional diversity. It was reasoned that if there were 200 V_κ gene segments (encoding to amino acid position 95) and four functional J_κ gene segments (encoding positions 96 through 108), then 800 complete

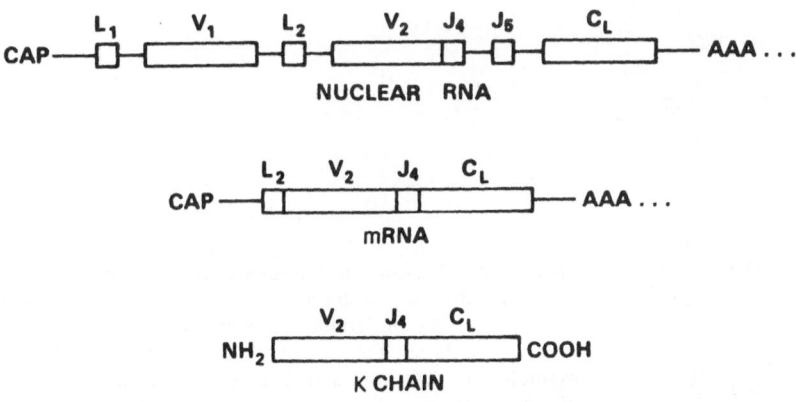

Figure 7.9. Processing of original transcript to produce mRNA and final light chain product.

light chain variable-region genes could result from their various combinations. It would soon be shown that not only was this basically correct, but that additional diversity could be generated in the process of V-J joining.

7.4.2.1. Junctional Diversity

There was a problem, however, in reconciling the four J_κ gene segment sequences with known protein sequences for the kappa chain. There was more variability in the J region positions as determined by amino acid sequence than was evident in J1, 2, 4, and 5 as determined by sequencing germline DNA. Inspection of these data revealed that the variability occurred most often at position 96 of the protein. It was then shown from DNA sequence analysis that this was the same position at which V and J gene segments connected to one another and variation at the junction point could give rise to different codons for the amino acid at the junctional position (Fig. 7.10). This so-called "junctional diversity" was detected by the sequence analysis of a pseudogene for a kappa light chain. (A pseudogene is a gene that is highly homologous to an expressed gene but is not itself expressed because of some flaw in the gene structure; see Section 7.6.4.) This phenomenon was best described in a paper by Max *et al.* (1980) in which the investigators

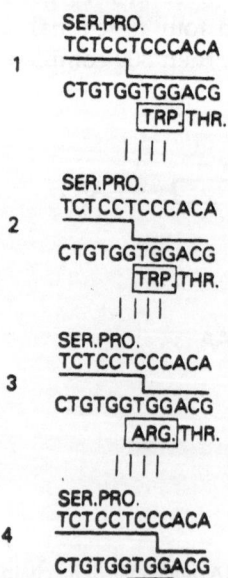

Figure 7.10. Altering the frame of somatic recombination accounts for diversity of amino acid codon 96 of murine kappa light chains. The nucleotide sequences of germline V_κ and J_κ gene segments are aligned at the V/J recombination site. The examples are $V_\kappa 41$ (top) and J5 (bottom). The cross-over point of recombination is indicated by the line under/over each sequence. The translation of the product of four cross-overs is shown. The boxed amino acid is at the cross-over point.

puzzled over the possibility that this newly discovered diversity generating mechanism could also cause "out-of-phase" rearrangements between the V and J gene segments:

> The present finding of exactly such a "forbidden recombination" suggests that such events can in fact occur, although among myelomas selected for immunoglobulin production, we would expect to detect them only as cryptic genes. In fact, until the enzymes catalyzing V-J joining can be studied in vitro such cryptic genes provide our only opportunity for assessing the broad range of recombination events which might be possible in an immunocyte. At present it is unknown what fraction of V-J recombination events in normal lymphocytes yields such "nonviable" gene products; such events may not be rare. The cost to the organism of these nonviable gene products may be outweighed by increased diversity at the recombination site, diversity which might be lost with a more rigid recombination system.

As shown in Fig. 7.10, the essence of junctional diversity lies in the generation of new codons by the joining of two DNA sequences at a variable point. In addition to generating a different amino acid at a single position, the recombined sequence may vary in the number of codons included in the recombinant thus giving rise to variations in the length of the encoded proteins. Although uncommon, such variations can result in differences in the length in the third hypervariable region of light chains. Further implications of junctional diversity will be discussed in Chapter 8.

7.4.2.2. Lambda C and J Genes Differ from Kappa

Because of analogy of the heavy and lambda to the kappa light chain, it may be expected that other loci encoding immunoglobulins would be arranged and utilized in a similar fashion. The heavy chain genes may be expected to be more complicated than those of the kappa light chain. Even before dissection of the heavy chain system with cloned DNA probes, it was apparent that there would be additional complexity in this system related to switching of the heavy chain class. Unlike the heavy chain, the lambda chain might be expected to involve a simple system (perhaps even simpler than kappa). However, analysis of the lambda system revealed that the gene arrangement may take many forms and that the lambda system was not quite as simple as predicted from the relatively low expression of this light chain type in the mouse.

Three subtypes (or isotypes) of the lambda light chain C regions had been identified by amino acid sequence analyses. The expression of the lambda subtypes is not equal but occurs in approximate ratio of 8 : 1 : 1 for the three forms lambda 1, lambda 2, and lambda 3. Detailed analysis of the DNA sequences of the lambda-region genes by Blomberg and Tonegawa (1982) and by Storb indicated, however, that there are not three C genes for lambda but rather that there are four. Furthermore, it was found that the J gene segments of lambda are not arranged in a single closely spaced array as they are in the kappa system but are interspersed among the C-region genes as indicated in Fig. 7.11. There exist two clusters of lambda genes arranged in the order, $J_\lambda 3$-$C_\lambda 3$ and $J_\lambda 1$-$C_\lambda 1$ in one and $J_\lambda 2$-$C_\lambda 2$ and $J_\lambda 4$-$C_\lambda 4$ in another.

The protein corresponding to $C_\lambda 4$ of the lambda series had not been previously observed in amino acid studies; therefore, it has been pos-

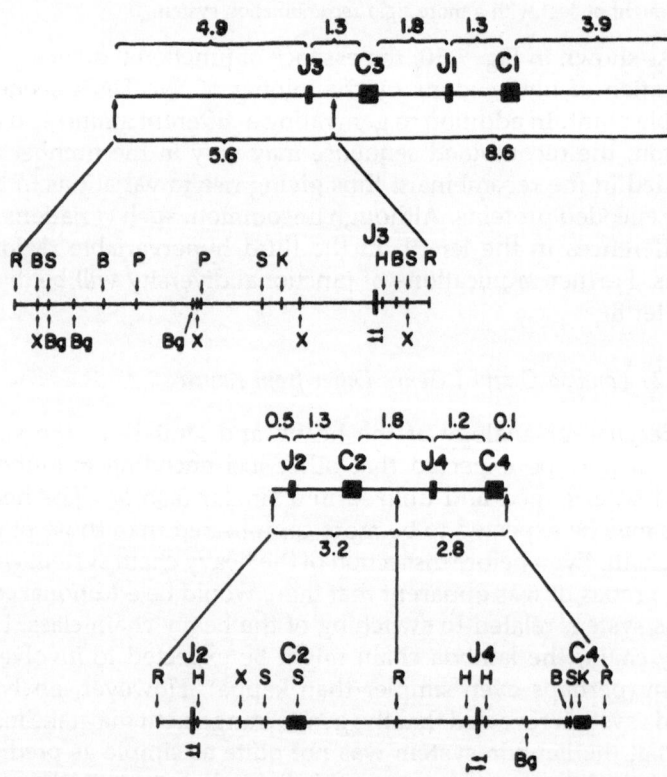

Figure 7.11. Germline configuration of mouse J_λ and C_λ gene segments and restriction endonuclease cleavage maps of EcoRI inserts containing J2, J3, and J4. Distances are in kb. Large arrows designate EcoRI cleavage sites. The distance between the two clusters is unknown although they are on the same chromosome. Each EcoRI insert was purified by electrophoresis in acrylamide and elution. Insert DNA was then digested with one or more enzymes. Horizontal arrows indicate direction and extent of sequence determination. B, BamHI; Bg, BglII; H, HindIII; K, KpnI; P, PstI; R, EcoRI; S, SacI; X, Xba I. From Blomberg and Tonegawa (1982).

tulated that this is a pseudogene. Examination of the constant region DNA sequence of $C_\lambda 4$ revealed no flaws in the sequence that would prevent expression of this gene. More detailed analysis of the $J_\lambda 4$ gene found in linkage with $C_\lambda 4$, however, revealed differences from those J gene segments carried in tandem with the expressed lambda C regions. A two base pair deletion in a signal heptamer that occurs prior to the J coding region makes it quite likely that $C_\lambda 4$ is a pseudogene because the J gene segment linked to it cannot function to form a rearranged VJ species that can be expressed.

7.5. HEAVY CHAIN GENES

There were a number of reasons to suppose that the heavy chain genes would turn out to be more complex than lambda or kappa light chain genes. Most important was the fact that the constant regions of the various different classes and subclasses use the same pool of variable regions. Furthermore, there were a number of studies showing that a single cell might make two antibodies of a different class but having identical variable regions as demonstrated by idiotypic or primary structural analysis. In fact, there was at least one good example of a cell that simultaneously synthesized antibodies of the IgD and IgM classes. The notion of maturation of the immune response involves a phenomenon that is called switching. Early, the response consists mainly of IgM antibodies, but as the response matures, mainly IgG or perhaps IgA antibodies are produced. In order to allow switching, the heavy chain rearrangement process would have to involve several steps subsequent to the formation of the complete variable region gene. The problem of simultaneous synthesis of two heavy chain classes having the same variable region introduced a further difficulty into the process. Another complicating aspect of the heavy chain was the fact that IgM and IgD as well as the IgG subclasses could exist in a membrane-bound form as well as in the secreted, circulating form. There was good evidence that these different forms of antibodies had heavy chains that vary in size indicating that these differences are in the primary structure of the antibody chain. There are additional complexities involved in heavy chain biosynthesis such as the occurrence of oligomeric forms of IgA and IgM and the additional chains that are required to join these forms, but these issues are not of primary concern for the diversity issue and will not be dealt with here.

As will be detailed in Section 7.5, studies on the heavy chain genes gave new information in several areas. The gene structure was more complex in that there were other gene segments called D, as well as J gene segments, involved in synthesis of the third hypervariable region. It was shown that additional rearrangements of V and C genes could take place and further, it was shown that several variations in the RNA processing steps could give additional options to the antibody heavy chain.

7.5.1. The VDJ Arrangement

In the course of studies on the structure of the heavy chain genes a puzzling situation arose. The genomic V_H gene segments and the genomic J_H gene segments did not account for the total sequence of the heavy chain variable region as determined by sequence analysis of the protein or the heavy chain cDNA. This situation was reminiscent of the early studies on the light chain systems except that, in the case of the heavy chains, the J gene segment had already been identified so that this could not supply the missing segment of the chain. A third gene segment called D, for diversity, was postulated.

Flanking the V and J gene segments are introns containing signals for V-J joining that consist of a nonamer and a heptamer that are spaced in intervals that are 11 or 22 base pairs (bp) apart in the genome. Joining occurs only between gene segments flanked by signals containing spacers of different lengths. For example, a V gene segment with a 22 bp spacer will only join to a J gene segment with a spacer of 11 bp and not to one with a 22 bp spacer. The length of these spacers corresponds to one (11) or two (22) turns of the DNA helix and it has been postulated that this spacing is related to enzyme recognition. This 11/22 rule appeared to be violated by the V and J pairs observed for the heavy chain in that each had a spacer of 22 bp (see Table 7.1). It was therefore apparent that the V and J genes were not contiguous in this system and that the postulated

Table 7.1. Comparison of Noncoding Nucleotides Adjacent to V and J Gene Segments

$V_{\kappa}41$	CACAGTGATACAAATCATAACATAAACC	(11)
$V_{\kappa}21$	CACAGTGCTCAGGGCTGAACAAAAACC	(10)
V_H107	CACAGTGAGGACGTCATTGTGAGCCCAGACACAAACC	(22)
$V_{\lambda}1$	CACAATGACATGTGTAGATGGGGAAGTAGATCAAGAACA	(22)
$J_{\kappa}1$	GGTTTTTGTAGAGAGGGGCATGTCATAGTCCTCACTGTG	(22)
$J_{\kappa}2$	GGTTTTTGTAAAGGGGGGCGCAGTGATATGAATCACTGTG	(23)
J_H107	AGTTTTAGTATAGGAACAGAGGCAGAACAGAGACTGTG	(21)
J_H315	GGTTTTTGTACACCCACTAAAGGGGTCTATGATAGTGTG	(22)
$J_{\lambda}1$	GGTTTTTGCATGAGTCTATATCACAGTG	(11)

germline D gene segment would require an 11 bp spacer at both ends. Several studies using D-J gene products that had been rearranged in an aberrant fashion (had a genomic segment on its 5′ side; that is, the side that would join to the V gene segment) were used to locate D genes in the genome. In the first study five D genes were found in one grouping. Furthermore, the D genes observed had the predicted spacing of 11 bp in both of their signal sequences. The number of D gene segments observed for the mouse is approximately ten, but there is evidence that there are more D gene segments than have been thus far described.

These results concerning the heavy chain showed very clearly that this larger of the two immunoglobulin chains has greater potential for diversity than did the light chain. In the third hypervariable region of the heavy chain, additional diversity can be generated by using various combinations of the V, D, and J gene segments.

7.5.2. The D Segment

The obvious importance of the D segment to the generation of the third hypervariable region of antibody V_H regions prompted a number of studies. Although these studies have not completely answered all questions concerning the number and location of D segments, there are sufficient data derived from mouse and human genes to allow certain conclusions.

The general structure of the D segment is illustrated in Table 7.2. Although there may be variation in coding sequences, the flanking se-

Table 7.2. Comparison of the Nucleotide Sequences for the Coding Regions of Ten Murine Germline D Segments[a]

SP2.3	T C T A C T A T G G T T A C G A C
SP2.4	– – – – – – – – – – – – – – – – –
SP2.5	– – – – – – – – – – – A – – T – –
SP2.6	C – – – – – – – – – – – – – – – –
SP2.7	C – – – – – – – – – A – – T – –
SP2.8	C – – – G – – – – – – A – – T – –
SP2.2	– – – – – – – – – A – – – – – –
FL16.1	T T T A T – – – – – C – – – A G T A G – T A C
FL16.2	T T C A T – – – – – C – – C – – –
Q52	– A – – – G G – A C

[a] The flanking regions of these segments (not shown) are homologous to those of human D segments. From Kurosawa and Tonegawa (1982).

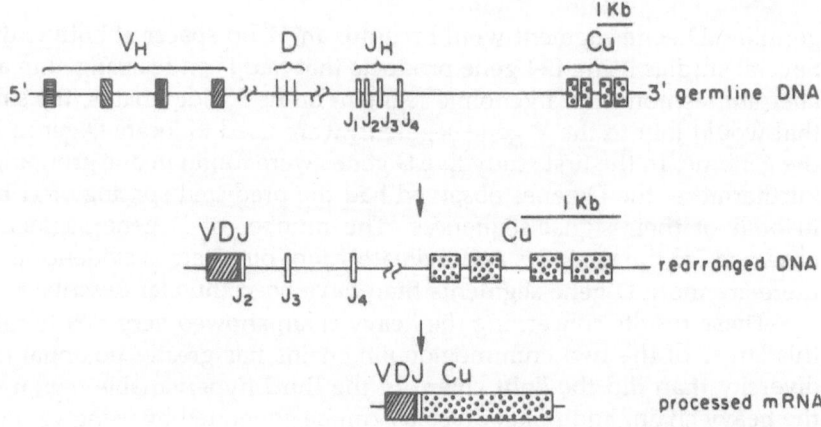

Figure 7.12. Rearrangement of heavy chain gene segments on chromosome 12 of the mouse. The scale on line one is different from that on lines two and three. The number and linkages of V genes within the V gene cluster and D genes within the D gene cluster are not known. Cμ denotes the constant gene for IgM, which is interrupted by three noncoding sequences. The joining of V, D, and J gene segments may occur by deleting the intervening DNA. From Gearhart (1982).

quences contain 12 or 13 bp spacers and recombination signal sequences that are highly conserved within a family of D gene segments. In the human, although the data are less complete, the D gene segments are contained within repeating units of about 9 kb; four of these relatively short units are in a 33 kb DNA fragment.

Similarly, in the mouse, groups of D gene segments have been observed. In this system, ten D gene segments that belong to at least three different families have been characterized (Table 7.2). As in the human D segment, there is conservation of spacing and recombination signals.

The precise location in the genome of the D segments has not been established but there is evidence suggesting that at least one of these D families in the human is located between the V and J gene segments and that it is closer to J than to V. Indeed, one D segment has been linked 5′ of J_{H_1}.

The importance of a modest number of D gene segments to the extent of antibody diversity cannot be overstated. With the implication that V, D, and J joining can occur in many combinations, an enormous number of complete variable-region genes can be generated from limited numbers of V, D, and J gene segments.

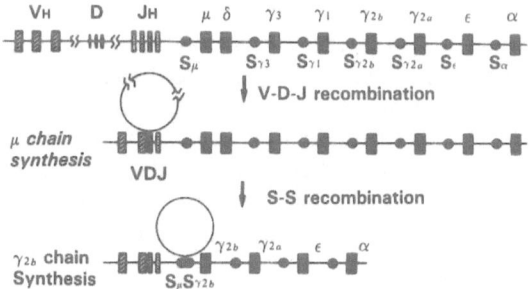

Figure 7.13. Arrangement of C region genes for the murine heavy chain (not shown to scale). Two recombinational events must occur to form a complete gene for γ2b. (Honjo, 1982).

7.6. THE V GENE SEGMENT

The data obtained in the early experiments at the DNA level clearly pointed out that merely counting V genes could not give the answer concerning the numbers of possible antibodies. Contributions of the D and J gene segments and their functional diversity introduced new and powerful multipliers for V gene numbers. However, these multipliers of diversity were concentrated on a single portion of the molecule. For both heavy and light chains, the newly found diversity involved only the third hypervariable region: the V gene segment alone contributed to the first and second hypervariable regions. Therefore, to further explore the diversity issue, it was necessary to focus on questions concerning V gene segments to determine their basic structural features and, more importantly, to count the numbers of V_L and V_H gene segments.

Two major approaches were used to study V gene segments. The first involved preparation of mRNA for the chain under study followed by preparation and characterization of cDNA clones and the subsequent preparation of V region specific probes from the cDNA. An alternative approach was possible if C region or J region probes were available. This involved searching for the rearranged V gene in genomic libraries prepared from cells producing the chain. Either the cDNA clones or rearranged genomic clones are used to prepare a V-specific probe by excision with appropriate restriction endonucleases. The probe may then be used in Southern blotting experiments to estimate numbers of V gene segments that have sufficient homology for cross hybridization. Beginning with the experiments of Tonegawa in 1978, there has been intense activity in this area, and at present it is possible to make reasonable estimates of gene numbers for several different systems.

Note that throughout this section we will be discussing the *V gene segment* as distinct from the *V-region gene,* which for our purposes is formed when the VJ or the VDJ gene segments interact. This distinction will become important in discussions (Chapter 8) of somatic mutation that appears to act only on the complete V-region gene rather than on individual V gene segments.

7.6.1. Mouse V_λ

Probably the key experiment in the modern era of molecular immunology was done by Tonegawa *et al.* (1978) who showed in the mouse that the V_λ gene segment only encoded amino acids 1 to 96. Virtually every experiment that followed was a variation on this theme. He chose the murine lambda system because of much previous work from amino acid sequence studies indicating that there were relatively few germline genes in this system (see 3.6.1). Since several myeloma (variants) were available, a direct test of the polar solutions was feasible.

As discussed earlier, murine lambda chains had been classified into two groups, $V_\lambda 1$ and $V_\lambda 2$. The $V_\lambda 1$ lambda chains studied by Weigert (see Chapter 3) were different from one another by 1 to 3 amino acids. However, since the MOPC315 lambda chain V region had 10 to 12 differences and its constant region was quite different from the other mouse lambda (by about 25 residues), MOPC315 was considered the prototype of the $V_\lambda 2$ subgroup. A $V_\lambda 1$ probe was prepared and used to screen embryonic DNA. Two and only two V_λ germline clones were identified and their sequences determined. The results confirmed that each subgroup had a counterpart in embryonic DNA. The $V_\lambda 1$ sequence from the germline was identical to the so-called lambda O (λo) pattern described by Weigert as the prototye of the $V_\lambda 1$ "nonmutated" (germline) light chains such as MOPC104E. The $V_\lambda 2$ sequence in the germline (which was detected by Tonegawa by cross-hybridization with the $V_\lambda 1$ probe), differed from germline $V_\lambda 1$ by 12 nucleotides in the coding segment that included amino acid positions 1 to 96. Of these 12 differences, ten were missense changes that encoded different amino acids at the corresponding positions in the two subgroups; the other two were silent. The germline $V_\lambda 2$ DNA sequence corresponded closely, but not exactly, to the MOPC315 sequence.

Other conclusions derived from these and similar studies on mouse V_λ seem particularly noteworthy. First, DNA coding for most of the hydrophobic leader sequence (which is important in biosynthesis and secretion of immunoglobulins) is separated from the rest of the leader and from the amino terminus of the variable region by 93 bases of noncoding sequence. Second, the J gene segment was separately encoded although very close to the C region. Third, the DNA was changed from the embryonic (germline) configuration on differentiation and plasmacytomas contained rearranged genes such that V was now contiguous with J. This "rearranged" or "active" gene represents a major step in antibody synthesis.

7.6.2. Mouse V_κ

Studies on the V_λ genes established a number of structural features that would be found for the kappa V gene segment. However, studies of lambda, as mentioned previously, were subjected to the criticism by the proponents of the germline polar solution that this light chain group contributes only a minor portion of light chains to the antibody pool of the mouse. How general the lambda solution would be was a subject of debate. As discussed in Chapter 5, the kappa chain system provides an example where there are numerous V genes as indicated by subgroup numbers and amino terminal sequence and therefore may represent a better place to observe V region diversity.

The description of variable region genes for the kappa chain must adequately explain the amino acid sequence data showing that there are large numbers of different variable-region sequences. There was no possibility after initial descriptions of the variable region structure to attribute this variability at the amino terminus to V and J gene segment joining; these differences were either encoded in the germline or alternatively they arose by an active process of somatic mutation.

Leder and his associates (Seidman et al., 1978) used a probe for the V region of the MOPC149 kappa chain gene to search a carefully fractionated EcoRI digest of DNA from this plasmacytoma. Six positive fragments were found and two of these (designated K2 and K3) were selected for cloning and DNA sequence determination. Comparison between these two genes and the protein sequence of the MOPC149 allowed several conclusions. First of all, the basic architecture of V_κ genes was similar to lambda; that is, they consisted of a leader sequence followed by the V gene segment to position 95. The comparison of the two related genes K2 and K3 to one another and to the sequence of the known portion of the expressed protein is shown in Fig. 7.14.

The K2 and K3 sequences are identical in 314 of 336 bases in the coding positions. These 22 base differences generate 11 amino acid dif-

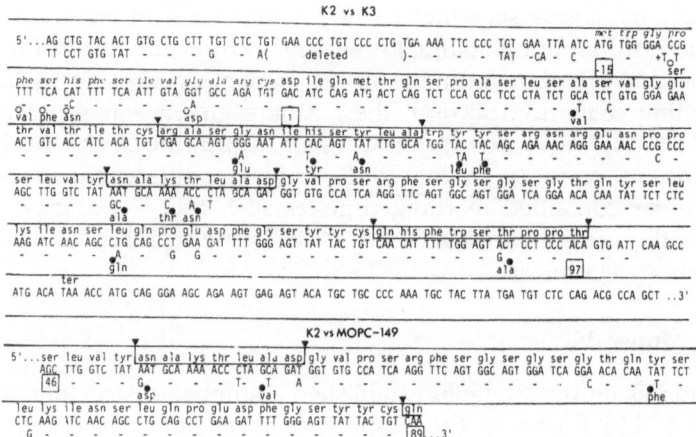

Figure 7.14. Comparison of the nucleotide sequence of the K2 variable region gene segment to the K3 and MOPC-149 sequences. K2 and K3 are germline whereas MOPC-149 is a myeloma DNA sequence. One strand (5' → 3') of the K2 gene and the amino acid sequence it encodes are shown. The predicted amino acid sequences of the K2 and K3 light chains are shown, and the putative leader sequence is indicated by italics. The amino acid residues are numbered in boxes where the first amino acid residue corresponds to the amino-terminal residue of the light chain MOPC-149. The enclosed amino acid residues correspond to the complementarity-determining segments of the light chain. The K3 and MOPC-149 sequences carry a dash where the sequence is identical to the K2 sequence, and differences in nucleotide sequence and amino acid sequence are indicated. Filled circles indicate amino acid differences in the light-chain sequence; open circles indicate differences in the putative leader sequence. Note that only amino acids codon positions 46 through 89 are compared in the K2 vs. MOPC-149 display. From Seidman *et al.* (1978).

ferences, seven of which occur within the hypervariable regions. Comparison of the two sequences to the 132 known bases (44 codons) of the expressed (MOPC149) gene revealed 125 identities with K2 and 120 with K3. The differences appeared to cluster in hypervariable regions; however, it was evident from these comparisons that neither K2 nor K3 was the source of the expressed product of plasmacytoma MOPC149. Based on these studies, a new concept of V-region subgroups emerged.

The Southern blotting experiments identified six sequences homologous to MOPC149, and of the two that were investigated thoroughly, neither could be the gene for the expressed protein. Therefore, there must exist in the BALB/c genome a minimum of three and possible six closely related germline V gene segments. This finding represented an important step in the development of ideas related to subgroup organization: variations observed *within* a subgroup were not simply somatic variants of the single gene. There could exist multiple germline genes within a single subgroup. Based on this, a subgroup had to be viewed as a family of closely related V gene segments rather than as a single germline gene. Although these data did not formally exclude somatic mutation, they were clearly supportive of germline theories. If this finding were general, each subgroup would have to be multiplied by as much as six to give the number of total V gene segments in the genome. Recall from Chapter 5 that the numbers of subgroups tended to increase with new protein sequence data; this present finding added a potential multiplier to each that had been found previously. As will be discussed in Chapter 8, somatic mutation may operate on the complete V-region genes (as opposed to nonrearranged V gene segments) to generate further changes. However, earlier models by proponents of the somatic mutation polar solution suggesting that there was but one gene per subgroup that undergoes mutation to generate all variants of that subgroup would clearly have to be modified.

7.6.3. The V_H Gene Segment

Studies on the heavy chain V gene segment lagged behind those for the light chain because of technical problems. Construction of full-length cDNA was obviously more difficult because mRNAs for heavy chains are over two times the length as that for light chain. As with the light chains, two types of analysis can be done. One can sequence either cDNA derived from myeloma or hybridoma cell lines or, alternatively, germline DNA may be studied using V_H probes made from the myeloma or hybridoma cell lines. These approaches will be discussed separately because different kinds of information derive from each type of study.

7.6.3.1. *Nucleotide Sequences of Immunoglobulin Heavy Chain Variable Regions*

Figure 7.15 is a compilation of seven murine heavy chain variable-region DNA sequences. B1-8 and S43 were derived from hybridoma DNA, whereas the others were obtained from myelomas. Since several different laboratories contributed to these studies, it may be assumed for the present purpose that these represent a random collection of V_H sequences; that is to say there was no a priori selection of these sequences. The random nature of these data is borne out by the fact that the translated protein sequences are extremely divergent.

The overall architecture of V_H is demonstrated by the sequences depicted in Fig. 7.15. The leader sequences, although not completed for

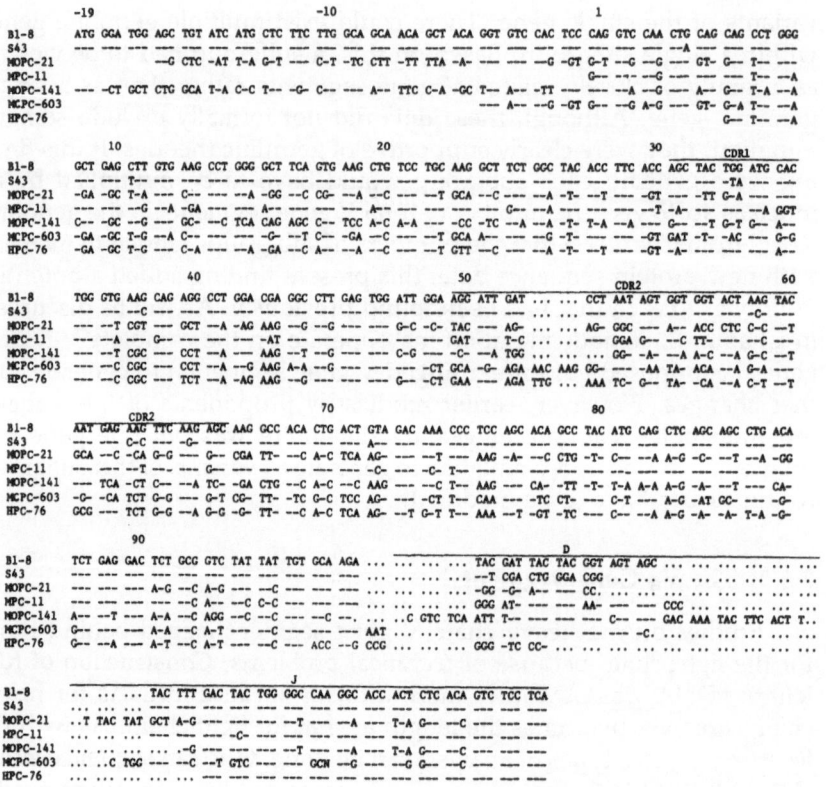

Figure 7.15. Comparison of the nucleotide sequences of immunoglobulin heavy chain variable regions. CDR1 and CDR2 are indicated as is the D and J segments. From Bothwell *et al.* (1981).

all of the molecules, show extensive differences except at the splicing site (amino acid position −4). The V gene segment begins at amino acid position 1 and ends somewhere around position 96. Most V_H gene segments end with TGT GCA AGA, although as can be seen there are exceptions to this. Also observed is variation in the length of D and in the use of different J gene segments. It is, however, not obvious from the data in Fig. 7.15 that there are clusters of variability in the hypervariable regions (designated CDR1 and CDR2). These DNA sequences do not reveal the hypervariability seen in the protein sequences in these regions (Chapter 3) nor that seen when V_H DNA sequences from a single family are compared (see Fig. 7.18).

Comparison of the sequence B1-8, which is derived from a hybridoma producing anti-NP antibodies, with that of MPC11 (a myeloma protein) in the region between amino acids 58 and 91 suggests that probes derived from either of the molecules would cross-hybridize with the other. The significance of this high degree of homology to the gene counting experiments will be discussed in Section 7.6.3.2.2.

7.6.3.2. Nucleotide Sequences of Germline V Gene Segments

There are two systems that have been studied in great detail to give information concerning V_H gene segments. Givol and his group have isolated and sequenced germline genes of the MPC11 family, whereas Bothwell has carried out similar characterizations for the NP^b (B1-8) family of V_H genes. Both studies have provided important insights into the problem of antibody diversity.

7.6.3.2.1. The MPC11 Family of V_H Gene Segments. The MPC11 heavy chain variable region was sequenced at the DNA level and a probe derived from it was used to screen a BALB/c mouse DNA library. The positive clones were screened by restriction analysis and only those that were distinct one from another were chosen for further study. The sequences of these clones are shown in Fig. 7.16 compared with the cDNA sequence of MPC11. The nucleotide sequence shows between 80% to 90% homology among these sequences and with the cDNA.

Figure 7.17 shows the sequence of the four mouse embryonic V_H genes upstream from codon 1 of the mature protein in comparison to the MPC11 cDNA sequence. The 5' noncoding and leader regions show considerable variability among the otherwise highly related and cross-hybridizing molecules. Therefore, variability between different V_H genes must extend beyond the coding region. These data further illustrate some features of the leader sequence; that is, the sequence that encodes the 19 residues that comprise the hydrophobic signal polypeptide of the precursor heavy chain. The nucleotide sequence for this region contains an intron of 83 nucleotides that begins with GT and ends with AG. There is variability in the length of the V_H leader regions, but the location of the intron within the sequence is invariant, not only among murine V_H but among human V_H, mouse V_κ, and mouse V_λ.

If one assumes that this family of V_H gene segments that show cross-hybridization to MPC11 all result in proteins belonging to the same V_H subgroup, it is obvious that the amino acid sequence of the signal peptide is not identical within the subgroup and varies about as much as the V_H-coding region itself. This variation had been observed earlier in the mRNA translation studies. There is evidence to suggest that the leader

```
                                                                                  20
     Glu Val Gln Leu Gln Gln Ser Gly Pro Glu Leu Val Lys Pro Gly Ala Ser Val Lys Ile
108A GAG GTC CAG CTT CAG CAG TCA GGA CCT GAG CTG GTG AAA CCT GGG GCC TCA GTG AAG ATA
108B --A --- --- --G --- --- --- --- --- --- --- --- --G --- --C --T --- --- --- ---
     Gln                                             Arg         Thr
104  C-- --- --- --G --- --- --T --- --- --- --- -GG --- A-T --- --- ---
     Gln                         Ala             Arg         Thr             Lys
111  C-- --- --- --G --- --- --T --- G-- --- --- --A -GG --- A-T --- --- --- -AG
     Gln                         Ala             Thr             Met
M11  C-- --- --- --G --- --- --T --- G-- --- --- --A -G- --- A-T --- --- --- --G

                             30                                              40
     Ser Cys Lys Ala Ser Gly Tyr Thr Phe Thr Asp Tyr Asn Met His Trp Val Lys Gln Ser
108A TCC TGC AAG GCT TCT GGA TAC ACA TTC ACT GAC TAC AAC ATG CAC TGG GTG AAG CAG AGC
     Thr                          Asp Ser          Gly     Ile     Asn
108B A-- --- --- --- --- --AT --- T-- --- --- -G- --- -T- --- A-- --- --- --- --- ---
                                  Leu Thr          Trp     Asn             Ter Met
104  --- --- --- --- --- --C --T --C --- CTC AC- --- TGG A-- --- --- --- T-- -TG
                                  Ala Asn          Trp Ile Gly             Arg
111  --- --- --- --- --C Ala --- G-- A-- --- --- TGG --A GGT --- --A --- --- --G
                                  Asn             Trp Ile Gly             Glu Arg
M11  --- --- --- --- --- G-- --- A-- --- --- TGG --A GGT --- --- --G-- --G
                                                                 CDR 1

                                 50                                          60
     His Gly Lys Ser Leu Glu Trp Ile Gly Tyr Ile Tyr Pro Tyr Asn Gly Gly Thr Gly Tyr
108A CAT GGA AAG AGC CTT GAG TGG ATT GGA TAT ATT TAT CCT TAC AAT GGT GGT ACT GGC TAC
                                         Gln     Asn                             Ser
108B --- --- --- --- --- --A --- --- --- G-A A-- --- --- --- --- --- --- --- --- ---
     Pro     Gln Gly                      Ala     Phe     Ala Gly     Ser     Asn
104  -C-- --- C-- G-- --- --- --- --- --- GCG --- -T- --- GCA GG- --- A--- --- AA- ---
     Pro     His Gly                      Asp             Gly Asp     Val     Asn
111  -C-- --- C-T G-- --- --- --- --- --- G-- --- --C --- GGA G-C --- -T- --- AA- ---
     Pro     His Gly                      Asp             Gly Gly     Phe     Asn
M11  -C-- --- C-T G-- --- --- --- --- --- G-- --- --C --- GGA GG- --C TT- --- AA- ---
                                                                 CDR 2

                                             70                                  80
     Asn Gln Lys Phe Lys Ser Lys Ala Thr Leu Thr Val Asp Asn Ser Ser Ser Thr Ala Tyr
108A AAC CAG AAG TTC AAG AGC AAG GCC ACA TTG ACT GTA GAC AAT TCC TCC AGC ACA GCC TAC
                             Gly                      Thr
108B --- --- --- --- --- --- G-- --- --- --- --- --- --CA --- --- --- --- --G ---
             Met     Gly                             Thr
104  --T G-- --T-- --- --- G-- --- --- --- --- --- --CA --- --- --- --- --- ---
     Glu             Gly                     Ala     Lys
111  --T G-- --- --- --- G-- --- --- C-- --- -C- --- --A --- --- --- --- --- --T
     Glu Asn         Gly                     Ala     Thr
M11  --T G-- --T --- G-- --- --- C-- --- -C- --- --CA --- --- --- ---

                             90
     Met Glu Leu Ser Ser Leu Thr Ser Glu Asp Ser Ala Val Tyr Tyr Cys Ala Arg CACAGTGTTA
108A ATG GAG CTC AGC AGC CTG ACA TCT GAG GAC TCT GCA GTC TAT TAC TGT GCA AGA CACAGTGTTA
             His                                      Leu
108B --- --- --- CA- --- --- --- --- --- --- TTG --- --- --- --- --- -----C---G
     Gln                                          Phe
104  --- C-- --A --- --- --- --- --- --- --G --- --- -T- --- --- --- ----------G
                                                 Ter
     Arg
111  --- --- --T --T --A T--- --- --- --- --- --A --- --- --- --- --- -----C---G
     Gln                                      Ile     His         Gly Ile Tyr Tyr
M11  C-- --- --- --- --- --- --- --- --C A-- --C C-- --- --- --- GGG ATT TAC TAC
                                                              ———— D ———→


108A CAAACACATC CTGAGTGTGT CAGAAACCCT GAGGTGCAGC AAGCTTCCTT GGGACTGACA AGAGTTAGAG AATAGTCGCT
108B T--C-----GG ---------- ------A-TG A--------- ---G-G---- -A-------- ---C------ --GT--A---
104  T--C------ ---------- ---------- --AGA----G -----G-AC- --------G- T--CAG-A-- -T--A--T -
111  ---C------ --------- -----C-T-- ----A----G -----G-AC- -C---G--G- T--CAG-A-- -T--A--A--


108A TGCAGACTTG CTTAGATGCA GTCATTTGAA TGGTTGTTTT GTG
108B -----GT--- ----------T --T----CG -AA------- T--
104  T--T----- --C---AATT -A----TG- AT--CCA--- A-T
111  C---A--- --C---AATT --A----CG- AT--CCA-G- A-T
```

Figure 7.16. Nucleotide sequence of the V_H gene segments and 3′ flanking regions of the four embryonic genes and MPC-11 cDNA. CDR regions are underlined. Recombination recognition signals at the 3′ end of the coding segment are boxed. From Givol *et al.* (1981).

```
                          pCh 108A   TGCTGCTTGA CCTATGAACC TTTTAAGTCC TTCCTCTCCA
                          pCh 108B   ---------- --C-A-T--- -A--C----- --------T-
                          pCh 104    (   N.D.   )---G-TG-- ---CCG---- --T-- GTT
                          pCh 111    --T---C--- ---G-T--- ----C----- ---TG--(


108A   TCTATTCTCC ATTTAGATTG GTTATTATAT ACAAAGTCCC CTGCTCATGA ATATGCAAAT TACCTAAGTC TATGGTAGTT
108B   --CC------ -G--G--C-A -A-C----G- ---------- ---------- ---------- ----GTTC-- ----T-G---
104    ---TC---A- - -GGAC-A- ---T---CC- -AG----A-- ---C------ -----A---- ----C----- -------- -
111        N.D.    )C-A- A-CC--GCTG -GT--TG-A- ---------- ---------- C--GC----- --T---C-- T

108A   AAAAACAGGG ATATCAACAC GCTGAAAACA ACATATGTCC AATGTCCTCT CCACAGACAC TGAACACACT GACTCTAACC
108B   ---------- --G------- C--------C ---------- -G---T---- ------CAC- -T-------- ----------
104    ---T---T-- --G--C---- C--------- --C----AT- -G-A------ ---T--T-T- ---------- -----A----
111    ---T---A-- --G--C---T T--------- --C--A-AT- -G-------- ------T-C- ---------- ----T-C---

       -19          -15              -10              -4
       Met Gly Trp Ser Trp Ile Phe Leu Phe Leu Leu Ser Gly Thr Ala G
108A   ATG GGA TGG AGC TGG ATC TTT CTC TTC CTC CTG TCA GGA ACT GCA G/GTAAGGGGC TCACCATTTC
       Ile Lys                 Ser
108B   --A AA- --- --- --- -C- --- --- --- --- --- --- --- - ----A---- ----A-G---
       Glu Cys         Val                         Leu
104    --- -A- --C --- --- G-- --- --- --- --- --- TT- --- --- - -------A- ------G---
       Glu             Gly Val  Ile                 Val
111    --- -A- --- --- G-- G-- --- A-- --T --- --- -T- --- --- - ---------- -C--------
                       Val  Ile                 Val
M 11 (   N.D.        ) G-- --- A-- --T --- --- -T- --- --- -

                                                                       -1
                                                           ly Val His Ser
108A   CAAATCTGAA GAAAAGAAAT GGCTTGTGAT GTCACTGACA TCCACTCTGT CTTTCTCTCC TCAG/GC GTC CAC TCT
108B   ---------- ----G----T AT-C-AA--- ----A----- ---------- ------T--- A--- -T --- --- ---
                                                                       Ile      Cys
104    A--------- ATG--A-A-AA----C--CC-- -G--AA-T-- ------G--C A--------- A--- -T A-- --- -GC
                                                                       Tyr
111    ---------- --GG-T-T-G ---C--A-GA -A--A--C-- A--------C -'C------- AT-- -T --- T-- --G
M11                                                                    -T --- --- --C
```

Figure 7.17. Nucleotide sequence of the 5' segment of four embryonic V_H gene segments including the codons for the signal peptide. The insert of MPC-11 (M11) cDNA clone begins at codon −14. From Givol *et al.* (1981).

sequence and the 5' noncoding region is part of the duplication unit that gives rise to the V-region subgroup.

Coding regions for four genes are shown in Fig. 7.16 and comparison with MPC11 demonstrates that all four genes end at position 98 with the codon for Arg. Comparison for the V_H-coding sequences illustrates that *in the genome, substitutions occur preferentially in the hypervariable regions.* Many of the substitutions in the framework result in an alternative codon that causes a conservative change of amino acids. It is likely that major alterations in framework structure would be selected against in evolution, as such changes would drastically alter the overall V domain three-dimensional structure.

Each of the V_H gene segments ends its coding region with a nearly identical sequence CACAGTG (the penultimate T may be a C) that starts immediately after the codon for Arg 98. In certain other genes, additional bases have been inserted between the Arg codon and this splicing signal.

This sequence is similar in these positions in mouse V_L and human V_H genes regardless of subgroup.

Two of the genes in this comparison, PCH104 and PCH111, contain termination codons at position 39 and 94, respectively. It is likely that these are pseudogenes and are not directly involved in V_H gene assembly; however, as discussed in Section 7.6.4 they may play a role in diversity.

We will return to the critical question of the comparison between germline V-gene sequences and those for expressed genes in Chapter 8.

7.6.3.2.2. The NP^b Family of V_H Gene Segments. The serology of the NP^b idiotype system was described in Chapter 2 (2.7.2.3). A number of hybridomas with NP specificity have been derived by Rajewsky's group, and Bothwell analyzed the DNA for the NP antibodies. First, cDNA clones derived from two of the hybridomas (one producing an IgM anti-NP antibody, the other an IgG) were isolated and sequenced. Sequence comparisons between the V_H regions showed differences in only ten nucleotide positions. A set of closely related germline V_H genes was cloned from a genomic library prepared from DNA derived from the C57BL/6 mouse strain. Seven germline genes from this family of NP-hybridizing sequences were sequenced and these are shown in Fig. 7.18.

The sequences contained in Fig. 7.18 illustrate many of the features that were evident from examination of the MPC11 system. Specifically, note that the key residues occurring prior to the beginning of the leader (-19) sequence and those after residue -4 (again of the leader sequence) and those occurring after residue 98 are virtually identical to those found for the MPC11 structures described in Section 7.6.3.2.1. The sequence listed at the top of the figure (186.2) appears to have given rise to much of the NP^b immune response. The other germline sequences are highly homologous as would be expected in this cross-hybridizing group. Sequences for 186.2, 186.1, and 145 are more closely related to one another and another group of sequences V6, 3, 102, and 23 are also closely related one to another suggesting the possibility that these comprise two gene families that may have arisen from common precursors.

It may be seen from the data in Fig. 7.18 that 70% of the variations between 186.2 and other sequences involved a second gene that has the same variation. This coincidence of variable positions rises to 80% in CDR2. There is a striking paucity of silent substitutions in these sequences with over 80% of the variations seen in the coding segments

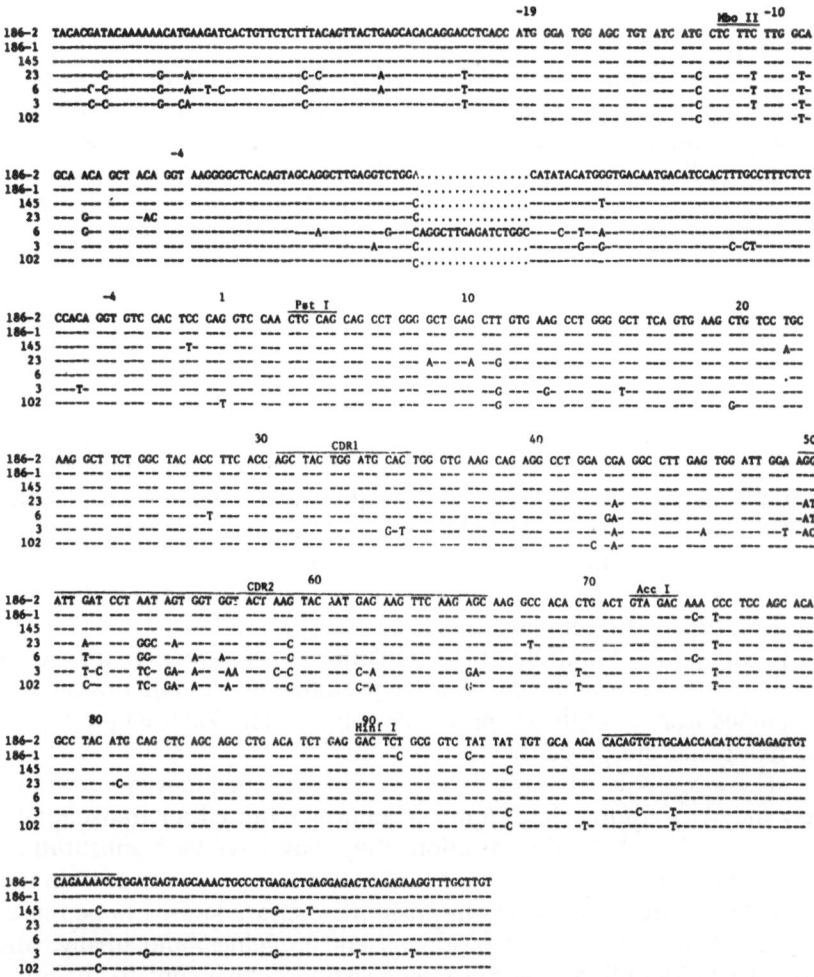

Figure 7.18. Nucleotide sequence of germline V_H sequences of the NP family. Above the sequence the amino acid codons are numbered. From Bothwell *et al.* (1981).

resulting in amino acid changes. This suggests that there is selective pressure at both the phylogenetic and ontogenetic level contributing to functional diversity.

Although it is difficult to devise an unambiguous pathway showing the duplications that gave rise to these seven genes, it is very likely that they arose by such a process. However, recombinations and/or gene conversions (discussed in Chapter 8) may well have played an important role in the evolution of this gene family.

Recently, Bothwell *et al.* (1981) has presented evidence for the physical linkage of the seven NP genes; they span approximately 100 kb. If these preliminary findings can be extrapolated to other systems, we would predict that about ten kb of DNA is used per V_H gene segment. If there are, as will be discussed (see Chapter 8) approximately 200 V_H gene segments, this would mean that about 200×10 or 2000 kb would be required for the V_H gene segments.

7.6.4. Pseudogenes

DNA sequence analyses of the gene segments of both V and J segments have revealed a surprisingly high frequency of pseudogenes. For example, of three V_κ gene segments sequenced by Bentley and Rabbitts (1983) from a human genomic library, one was a pseudogene. As mentioned above, the mouse $J_\lambda 4$-$C_\lambda 4$ structures are also pseudogenes (see Fig. 7.19). In mouse, V_H pseudogenes are also common. As shown in Fig. 7.16, two of the germline MPC11-related genes (PCH104 and PCH111) are pseudogenes. Similarly, the compilation of V_H sequences for the NP family (Fig. 7.18) contains at least one pseudogene. A more drastic sample comes from a study of the rabbit J_κ locus (Fig. 7.20) where four of the five genes are probably nonfunctional.

There are several ways in which pseudogenes may be defective: they may lack appropriate signal sequences required for transcription, splicing, or initiation of translation; they may have base substitutions that would introduce amino acids that may never have been seen in that particular position, especially in positions that are known to be highly conserved, for example, tryptophans and cysteines; and finally, and more easily identified, are those gene segments that contain chain-terminating codons within the reading frame. Examples of these are illustrated in Figs. 7.16, 7.19, and 7.20.

7.7. HEAVY CHAIN C-REGION GENES

Although questions concerning the constant-region genes of the heavy chain are not of primary concern to the issue of antibody diversity, they are worth some discussion because of the novel mechanisms in-

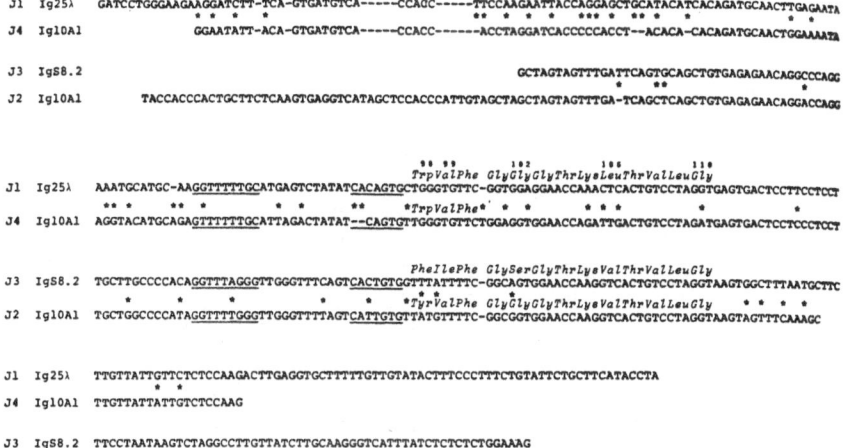

Figure 7.19. Comparison of nucleotide sequences for germline lambda J segments of the mouse. Asterisks indicate nonidentical positions in the J1-J4 and J2-J3 comparisons. Note that the substitutions in J4 are sufficient to render this gene nonfunctional and this probably precludes expression of the lambda 4 C region. Blomberg and Tonegawa (1982).

volved. In addition, results from these studies allow a more complete picture of immunoglobulin genes to be drawn. There are in addition to the features common to the synthesis of heavy and light chains, several features that uniquely concern heavy chain genes. These are related to switching of immunoglobulin class in the immune response and the possibility of simultaneous synthesis of two antibodies with identical variable regions but with different constant regions. It is these events that were found to involve mechanisms not utilized by light chain genes.

In the course of a normal immune response, the class of antibody synthesized changes from predominantly IgM in the initial phase to predominantly IgG (or another class such as IgE or IgA) after some time has elapsed or in the anamnestic secondary response. The possibility that all the early and late antibodies have different light chain and different V_H regions was precluded by earlier studies of idiotypes and V-region structures for IgM and other antibody classes. Therefore, in terms of what is now known, it must be assumed that after the VDJ composite is used to synthesize IgM, it must be again used to synthesize another class of antibody.

The arrangement of genes for C_H regions provided an immediate clue to the sequential nature of class-switching events (refer to Fig. 7.13).

```
J1   TGGGTGAGAAGGGTTTTGTACAATGAGGAGTTGTCACTGTGT   TTGACTTTTGGAGCTGGCACCAAGGTAGAAATCAAACGTGAGTA
          --*------     (15 bp)                      LeuThrPheGlyAlaGlyThrLysValGluIleLys

J2   TCAGTTTTTGTACAGGAGGAGGTTAGGAGGAACCACTGTGTATAATGCTTCGGCGGAGGGACCGAGGTGGTGGTCAAAGGTAAGTG
     *------                (23 bp)                 ------TyrAsnAlaPheGlyGlyGlyThrGluValValLys

J3   GGAGGGTTTTGTGGAGGAGAAGGTAAAGGAGGAGGCCACCGTGA   TCCACTTTCGGCCCAGGGACCAAACTGGAAATCAAACCTAAGTC
        --*------              (22 bp)                SerThrLeuGlyProGlyThrLysLeuGluIleLys *

J4   CCGCAAAGGGAGGGTTTTTGTCAGGGGTGGGATGACAGAGTGA   CTTACTTTGGCTCAGGGACCATGGTGGAGATCAAATGTAAGTG
           --**------          (14 bp)               LeuThrPheGlySerGlyThrMetValGluIleLys

J5   AGAGGTTTTGTTGAGGGAAAGCAATAAAGCTAATTCCATGA   ATCACCTTTGGCGAGGAGACCAAGCTGGAGATCAAACGTAAGTA
            **-**--             (22 bp)              IleThrPheGlyGluThrLysLeuGluIleLys


b4 cDNA pB4D5               AGTAGTAATGTTGAGAATGTTTTCGGCGGAGGGACCGAGGTGGTGGTCAAAGGTGATCC
                           SerSerAsnValGluAsnValPheGlyGlyGlyThrGluValValLysGlyAspPr

                                                   98                     108
b4 K LIGHT CHAIN J REGION   --------hv3-------PheGlyGlyGlyThrGluValValValLysGlyAspPr
```

Figure 7.20. Comparison of the 5 germline J_K sequences of a rabbit with kappa allotype b4 with cDNA and b4 light chain protein sequence. Deviations from the consensus sequence are indicated by asterisks and arrows show splice sites. Spacing of nonamer and heptamer signal elements are shown by numbers in parentheses. The only sequence observed in the approximately 24 b4 light chains reported is that of J2. From this and from the deviations in the other sequences from the consensus it was concluded that of the five J_K genes only J2 was functional. Emorine *et al.* (1983).

The IgM and IgD C regions were found in close proximity to the heavy chain J gene segment, the IgG subclasses are located to the 3' side, and IgE and IgA genes are beyond these. The entire heavy chain constant gene complex in the mouse is located within a DNA segment of approximately 200 kb. Although not shown in the diagram in Fig. 7.13, spacing between the different genes varies considerably. The distance between IgM and IgD genes is only 4.5 kb whereas the distance between IgD gene and the next C gene, IgG3, is 55 kb.

As details of the primary gene structure were elucidated, switch sites were seen in positions to the 5' side of each C-region gene. Tandem repeats of approximately 150 units, with each unit containing 10 to 40 bases occur. These (S) regions are different for the various classes and there is some controversy concerning their precise mode of action in the switching procedures. It is postulated that specific proteins may recognize and join two S regions, or alternatively the short sequences common to the S regions may allow recombination without specific enzymes.

Another point of controversy involves the fate of genes at positions between those genes that are recombined. When, for example, a cell synthesizes IgE, are the C-region genes to the 5' side of epsilon looped out and deleted? According to one model, that is exactly what happens, but there is an opposing viewpoint in which the genes are not deleted but exchanged with the opposing (sister) chromatid. In this model, the actively synthesizing cell would have one chromosome with deletions and another with duplications of the intervening genes. These models have relevance to J gene segments as well as constant-region genes in that selection of a given J gene segment may necessitate deletion of others to the 5' side (see Fig. 7.13). There is some evidence supporting the sister chromatid exchange model, but this issue is not yet settled.

The process of class switching is analogous to the V-J gene rearrangements that occur in V gene joining. The sequence of events in heavy chain class switching is dictated by the order of genes. Thus, an IgM-producing cell may switch to produce any other immunoglobulin class that is to the 3' side; an IgA-producing cell, on the other hand, may not undergo further rearrangement. The nature of the events that trigger class switching are not yet known. This system provides, however, an excellent example of a structure–function relationship.

Related to the issue of class switching is the observation that certain cells may at the same time synthesize two antibodies with identical variable regions but with different constant regions. The best-documented examples of this are cells that simultaneously produce IgD and IgM. In the same category are observations of the same antibody occurring as a secreted molecule and in its membrane-bound form. The recombinations occurring in class switching or in variable region synthesis would not easily explain these events because they are irreversible.

It has been found that multiple forms of the same antibody may be simultaneously produced using alternative RNA splicing mechanisms. The primary transcript (hnRNA) contains information for a secreted form and a membrane-bound form of IgM and IgD mRNA molecules corresponding to each type may be produced (Rogers *et al.*, 1980). Similarly a transcript may contain both IgM and IgD constant regions and this would allow simultaneous production of these two classes each having the same variable region. No loss of information such as may occur in class switching (as described in Fig. 7.8) would be involved in this use of the same hnRNA to produce two mRNA transcripts.

7.8. ALLELIC EXCLUSION

As discussed in Chapter 4, it has been recognized for a number of years that immunoglobulin-producing cells synthesize only one of the possible allelic products. This was surprising because allelic exclusion had not been observed for any other products of autosomal genes. The sole precedent was the exclusion observed in the cells of females where one of the two X chromosomes was inactivated in early embryonic development. The exclusion phenomenon for antibodies was further complicated by the fact that the two loci for light chains were involved in the exclusion. Thus, it remained to be explained how the antibody-producing cell chose one of the two heavy chain loci and one of the four possible light chain loci to the exclusion of all the others.

Data showing that gene rearrangements occur prior to transcription lead to a rational experimental test for allelic exclusion. It was known that joining of a light chain V gene segment to a J gene segment was one of the steps occurring prior to transcription of that gene. Therefore, it could be asked whether all light chain genes rearranged or only those that were expressed. This experiment was facilitated by the Southern blot technique that allowed easy demonstration of rearrangement by shifts in the molecular weights of restriction enzyme fragments carrying the kappa or lambda genes.

In a series of experiments using malignant lymphoid cells (Hieter *et al.*, 1981) it was shown that there was a hierarchy of rearrangement and that once a successful gene rearrangement occurred, the cell produces that chain and does not continue along the sequential rearrangement pathway. However, if the rearrangement is abortive for some reason and leads to the production of a nonusable gene, the rearrangements could continue. In Fig. 7.21 are summarized the experiments and the conclusions concerning the order of light chain rearrangement and synthesis; with this information, allelic exclusion involving multiple loci was no longer a complete mystery. It is not known whether the order of rearrangement is "predetermined" or "statistical."

The order of events in the example shown (Fig. 7.21) would favor the production of kappa chains because these are first rearranged to their active configuration. However, the possibility of a nonfunctional gene resulting from the process appears to be rather high. When this occurs the process is repeated for the next gene, which would be the other (allelic) kappa, and then the lambda genes are used. This could be clearly shown because the rearranged genes migrate to new positions that are easily identified on the Southern blot. The human leukemic cells used for this demonstration provided examples of B cells that produced either kappa or lambda chains.

7.9. MAPPING THE IMMUNOGLOBULIN GENES

Application of classical genetic methodology in the early 1960s gave information concerning the linkage of genes for the immunoglobulin chains (see Chapter 2). It was ascertained that the genes for immunoglobulins, in all species studies, were in three unlinked loci. In some cases, other markers were found to be linked to immunoglobulins allowing the genes to be placed within defined linkage groups. In most instances there was no information available concerning the chromosomal locations of the genes.

Somatic cell genetics allowed further information concerning the immunoglobulin genes to be obtained. The basic technique involved the use of interspecies hybrid cells. The karyotype of those cells producing a product of interest was studied to identify the chromosomes remaining. This was possible because hybrid cells quickly eliminate chromosomes in a more or less selective fashion. For example, if hybrids of human splenic B cells and mouse L cells are produced, the human chromosomes will be preferentially eliminated. A large number of hybrids are studied for concordance between product synthesis and chromosome complement. Although these methods are extremely useful for many different genes, especially those without known polymorphisms, they did not serve well in the immunoglobulin system because of com-

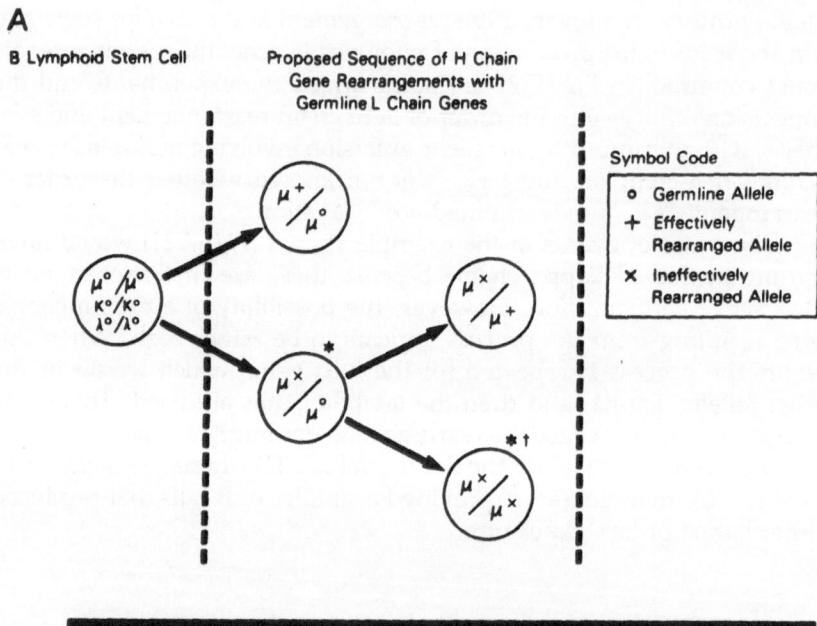

A

B Lymphoid Stem Cell   Proposed Sequence of H Chain
                               Gene Rearrangements with
                               Germline L Chain Genes

Symbol Code

○ Germline Allele
+ Effectively
   Rearranged Allele
× Ineffectively
   Rearranged Allele

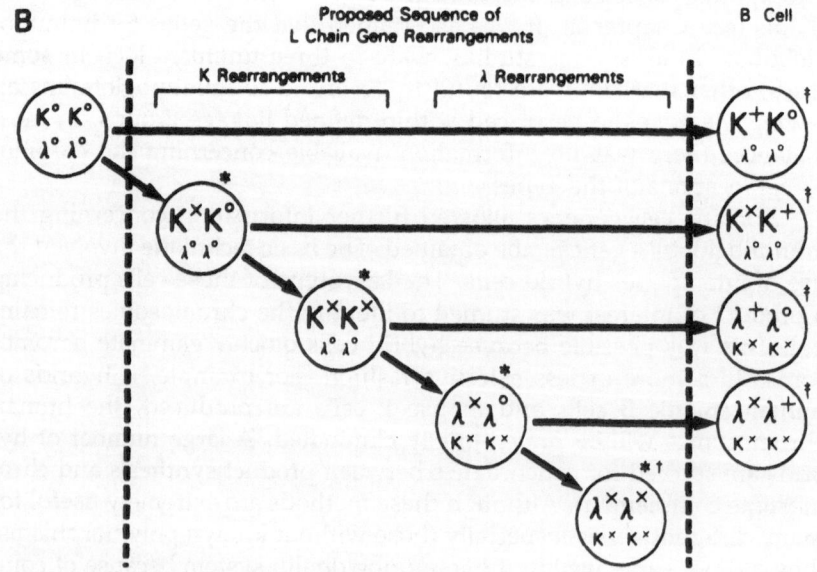

B   Proposed Sequence of   B Cell
                   L Chain Gene Rearrangements

            K Rearrangements   λ Rearrangements

plications inherent in this system. For example, it is possible to have inactive genes that are the result of aberrant rearrangements. In addition, heavy chains are usually not secreted in the absence of light chains.

The answer to the location of the genes came from a combination of Southern blotting, *in situ* hybridization, and somatic cell genetics. The presence or absence of the immunoglobulin genes was established for a number of hybrid cells that were then karyotyped. Positive identification of the immunoglobulin genes was based not only on hybridization to an appropriate probe but also on the molecular weight of the hybridizing DNA fragment. In this way any interspecific cross-hybridization could be controlled because the corresponding genes would be on different-sized fragments for the two species of which the hybrid is composed.

These studies have allowed assignments for human and mouse immunoglobulin genes for heavy, kappa, and lambda chains. In the human the locations are chromosomes 14, 2, and 22 for heavy, kappa, and lambda, respectively. In the mouse, heavy, kappa, and lambda are found on chromosomes 12, 2, and 16, respectively. These studies have also confirmed that variable- and constant-region genes are located on the same chromosome.

7.10. CONCLUSIONS

Many of the questions concerning antibodies and the genes that encode them were resolved by molecular biologic experiments. The phenomena that had set antibodies apart from other systems could now be

Figure 7.21. (A) Proposed sequence of H chain gene rearrangements within B-cell precursors. A B-lymphoid stem cell uncommitted at the Ig gene level would have its heavy chains (μ) and light chains (κ and λ) in the germ-line form. Gene rearrangement would begin with the H chain genes, and if effective, this cell (μ^+) would be capable of μ chain production and further maturation. Included here is a hypothetical set of cells trapped within the B-cell precursor series (†) because they have no remaining germ-line J_H or D_H segments with which to assemble an effective gene. (B) Proposed sequence of light-chain gene rearrangements within B-cell precursors with rearranged heavy-chain genes. In general, light chain rearrangement would begin with the κ genes, and if ineffective (X), λ rearrangements could follow. Cells with effectively rearranged kappa or lambda genes could be mature B cells (†) if prior heavy chain rearrangements were effective, whereas the cells with only ineffectively rearranged light chain genes (*) would lack light chain production and would be B-cell precursors. A theoretical population of cells might exist which had exhausted all light chain recombinational opportunities (†).

more fully described and in many cases explained in terms of underlying genetic mechanisms. This was particularly true for the two gene hypothesis and for allelic exclusion in antibody-producing cells. Separate variable- and constant-region genes were irrefutably demonstrated, and it was further shown that there were additional coding sequences that interposed themselves between the variable and constant region genes when they joined. These demonstrations gave credence to some of the gene interaction theories that had been proposed by the maverick theorists. The allelic exclusion data were supported by a demonstration that V-J rearrangements took place in an ordered sequence and that this comprised the signal to preclude further arrangements and further synthesis of other allelic or nonallelic products. The three-locus model for immunoglobulins was given direct proof by in situ hybridization experiments that used the techniques of somatic cell genetics to pinpoint the chromosomal locations of the heavy, kappa, and lambda loci.

The question of how many variable-region genes existed in the genome, a question that had been the focal point of over ten years of theoretical debate, was not the sole issue of debate in this new era. The discovery of the J and D gene segments and the discovery that additional diversity could be generated at interfaces between the gene segments gave new multipliers for the number of antibody variable regions. The question of how many variable genes were present in the genome was no longer a complete question. It was necessary to state the question concerning antibody diversity in an entirely new format. The question of how many variable region genes would now be given in terms of how many V, J, and D gene segments exist. The frequent observation of pseudogenes further made it necessary to determine if all of the observed V gene segments could be expressed in antibody molecules. These data led to a new synthesis of the antibody diversity problem. This new synthesis and some of the answers that can be derived from it are given in the final chapter.

REFERENCES AND BIBLIOGRAPHY

Askonas, B. A., and Williamson, A. R., 1967, Biosynthesis and assembly of immunoglobulin G, *Cold Spring Harbor Symp. Quant. Biol.* **32**:223.

Bentley, D. L., and Rabbitts, T. H., 1983, Evolution of immunoglobulin V genes: Evidence indicating that recently duplicated human V_κ sequences have diverged by gene conversion, *Cell* **32**:181.

Blomberg, B., and Tonegawa, S., 1982, DNA sequences of the joining regions of mouse λ light chain immunoglobulin genes, *Proc. Natl. Acad. Sci. U.S.A.* **79**:530.

Bothwell, A. L. M., Paskind, M., Reth, M., Imanishi-Kari, T., Rajewsky, K., and Baltimore, D., 1981, Heavy chain variable region contribution to the NP^b family of antibodies: Somatic mutations evident in a γ2a variable region, *Cell* **24**:625.

Brack, C., and Tonegawa, S., 1977, Variable and constant parts of the immunoglobulin light chain gene of a mouse myeloma cell are 1250 nontranslated bases apart, *Proc. Natl. Acad. Sci. U.S.A.* **74**:5652.

Delovitch, T. L., and Baglioni, C., 1973, Estimation of light-chain gene reiteration of mouse immunoglobulin by DNA-RNA hybridization, *Proc. Natl. Acad. Sci. U.S.A.* **70**:173.

Early, P., Huang, H., Davis, J., Calame, K., and Hood, L., 1980, An immunoglobulin heavy chain variable region gene is generated from three segments of DNA:V$_H$, D and J$_H$, *Cell* **19**:981.

Early, P., Rogers, J., Davis, M., Calame, K., Bond, M., Wall, R., and Hood, L., 1980, Two mRNAs can be produced from a single immunoglobulin gene by alternative RNA processing pathways, *Cell* **20**:313.

Emorine, L., Dreher, K., Kindt, T. J., and Max, E. E., 1983, Rabbit immunoglobulin kappa genes: Structure of a germline b4 allotype J-C locus and evidence for several b4-related sequences in the rabbit genome, *Proc. Natl. Acad. Sci. USA* **80**:5709.

Farace, M.-G., Aellen, M.-F., Briand, P.-A., Faust, C. H., Vassali, P., and Mach, B., 1976, No detectable reiteration of genes coding for mouse MOPC41 immunoglobulin light-chain mRNA, *Proc. Natl. Acad. Sci. U.S.A.* **73**:727.

Gearhart, P. J., 1982, Generation of immunoglobulin variable gene diversity, *Immunol. Today* **3**:107.

Givol, D., Zakut, R., Effron, K., Rechavi, G., Ram, D., and Cohen, J. B., 1981, Diversity of germ-line immunoglobulin V$_H$ genes, *Nature (London)* **292**:426.

Hieter, P. A., Korsmeyer, S. J., Waldmann, T. A., and Leder, P., 1981, Human immunoglobulin light-chain genes are deleted or rearranged in λ-producing B cells, *Nature (London)* **290**:368.

Honjo, T., 1982, The molecular mechanism of immunoglobulin class switch, *Immunol. Today* **3**:214.

Knapp, M. R., Liu, C.-P., Newell, N., Ward, R. B., Tucker, P. W., Strober, S., and Blattner, F., 1982, Simultaneous expression of immunoglobulin μ and δ heavy chains by a cloned B-cell lymphoma: A single copy of the V$_H$ gene is shared by two adjacent C$_H$ genes, *Proc. Natl. Acad. Sci. U.S.A.* **79**:2996.

Korsmeyer, S. J., Arnold, A., Bakhshi, A., Ravetch, J. V., Siebenlist, U., Hieter, P. A., Sharrow, S. O., LeBien, T. W., Kersey, J. H., Poplack, D. G., Leder, P., and Waldmann, T. A., 1983, Immunoglobulin gene rearrangement and cell surface antigen expression in acute lymphocytic leukemias of T cell and B cell precursor origins, *J. Clin. Invest.* **71**:301.

Kurosawa, Y., and Tonegawa, S., 1982, Organization, structure, and assembly of immunoglobulin heavy chain diversity DNA segments, *J. Exp. Med.* **155**:201.

Leder, P., 1982, The genetics of antibody diversity, *Sci. Am.* **246**:108.

Leder, P., Honjo, T., Swan, D., Packman, S., and Norman, B., 1974, The organization and diversity of immunoglobulin genes, *Proc. Natl. Acad. Sci. U.S.A.* **71**:5109.

Leder, P., Max, E. E., and Seidman, J. G., 1980, The organization of immunoglobulin genes and the origin of their diversity, in: *Fourth International Congress of Immunology, Immunology 80*, Volume 2, (M. Fougereau and J. Daussets, eds.), Academic Press, London, pp. 34–50.

Max, E. E., Seidman, J. G., and Leder, P., 1979, The sequences of five potential recombination sites encoded close to an immunoglobulin kappa constant region gene, *Proc. Natl. Acad. Sci. U.S.A.* **76**:3450.

Max, E. E., Seidman, J. G., Miller, H., and Leder, P., 1980, Variation in the crossover point of kappa immunoglobulin gene V-J recombination: Evidence from a cryptic gene, *Cell* **21**:793.

Maxam, A. M., and Gilbert, W., 1980, Sequencing end-labeled DNA with base-specific chemical cleavages, *Meth. Enzymol.* **65**:499.

McBride, O. W., Hieter, P. A., Hollis, G. F., Swan, D., Otey, M. C., and Leder, P., 1982, Chromosomal location of human kappa and lambda immunoglobulin light chain constant region genes, *J. Exp. Med.* **155**:1480.

Potter, M., and Lieberman, R., 1967, Genetics of immunoglobulins in mice, *Adv. Immunol.* **7**:92.

Premkumar, E., Shoyab, M., and Williamson, A. R., 1974, Germline basis for antibody diversity: Immunoglobulin V_H and C_H-gene frequencies measured by DNA-RNA hybridization, *Proc. Natl. Acad. Sci. U.S.A.* **71**:99.

Rabbitts, T., and Milstein, C., 1975, Mouse immunoglobulin genes: Studies on the reiteration frequency of light-chain genes by hybridization procedures, *Eur. J. Biochem.* **52**:125.

Rechavi, G., Bienz, B., Ram, D., Ben-Neriah, Y., Cohen, J. B., Zakut, R., and Givol, D., 1982, Organization and evolution of immunoglobulin V_H gene subgroup, *Proc. Natl. Acad. Sci. U.S.A.* **79**:4405.

Reth, M., Imanishi-Kari, T., and Rajewsky, K., 1979, Analysis of the repertoire of anti (4-hydroxy-3-nitro-phenyl) acetyl (NP) antibodies in C57BL/6 mice by cell fusion, *Eur. J. Immunol.* **9**:1004.

Rogers, J., Early, P., Carter, C., Calame, K., Bond, M., Hood, L., and Wall, R., 1980, Two mRNAs with different 3' ends encode membrane-bound and secreted forms of immunoglobulin chain, *Cell* **20**:303.

Sanger, F., Nicklen, S., and Coulson, A. R., 1977, DNA sequencing with chain-terminating inhibitors, *Proc. Natl. Acad. Sci. U.S.A.* **74**:5463.

Seidman, J. G., Leder, A., Edgell, M. H., Polsky, F., Tilghman, S. M., Tiemeier, D. C., and Leder, P., 1978, Multiple related immunoglobulin variable-region genes identified by cloning and sequence analysis, *Proc. Natl. Acad. Sci. U.S.A.* **75**:3881.

Selsing, E., Miller, J., Wilson, R., and Storb, U., 1982, Evolution of mouse immunoglobulin λ genes, *Proc. Natl. Acad. Sci. U.S.A.* **79**:4681.

Sheppard, H. W., and Gutman, G. A., 1982, Rat kappa-chain J-segment genes: Two recent gene duplications separate rat and mouse, *Cell* **29**:121.

Siebenlist, U., Ravetch, J. V., Korsmeyer, S., Waldmann, T., and Leder, P., 1981, Human immunoglobulin D segments encoded in tandem multigenic families, *Nature* **294**:631.

Shimizu, A., Takahashi, N., Yaoita, Y., and Honjo, T., 1982, Organization of the constant-region gene family of the mouse immunoglobulin heavy chain, *Cell* **28**:499.

Smith, G. P., 1977, The significance of hybridization kinetic experiements for theories of antibody diversity, *Cold Spring Harbor Symp. Quant. Biol.* **41**:863.

Southern, E. M., 1975, Detection of specific DNA sequences among DNA fragments separated by gel electrophoresis, *J. Mol. Biol.* **98**:503.

Storb, U., 1974, Evidence for multiple immunoglobulin genes, *Biochem. Biophy. Res. Comm.* **57**:31.

Tonegawa, S., Bernardini, A., Weimann, B. J., and Steinberg, C., 1974, Reiteration frequency of antibody genes. Studies with κ chain mRNA. *F.E.B.S. Lett.* **40**:92.

Tonegawa, S., Hozumi, N., Matthyssens, G., and Schuller, R., 1976, Somatic changes in the content and context of immunoglobulin genes, *Cold Spring Harbor Symp. Quant. Biol.* **41**:877.

Tonegawa, S., Maxam, A. M., Tizard, R., Bernard, O., and Gilbert, W., 1978, Sequence of a mouse germ-line gene for a variable region of an immunoglobulin light chain, *Proc. Natl. Acad. Sci. U.S.A.* **75:**1485.

Valbuena, O., Marcu, K. B., Weigert, M., and Perry, R. P., 1978, Multiplicity of germline genes specifying a group of related mouse κ chains with implications for the generation of immunoglobulin diversity, *Nature* **276:**780.

Van Ness, B. G., Coleclough, C., Perry, R. P., and Weigert, M., 1982, DNA between variable and joining gene segments of immunoglobulin κ light chain is frequently retained in cells that rearrange the κ locus, *Proc. Natl. Acad. Sci. U.S.A.* **79:**262.

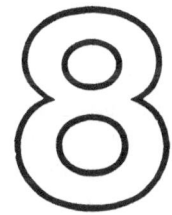

ANTIBODY DIVERSITY:
A CONTEMPORARY
SOLUTION

I think that there is only one way to science—or to philosophy, for that matter: to meet a problem, to see its beauty and fall in love with it; to get married to it, and to live with it happily, till death do ye part—unless you should meet another and even more fascinating problem, or unless, indeed, you should obtain a solution. But even if you do obtain a solution, you may then discover, to your delight, the existence of a whole family of enchanting though perhaps difficult problem children for whose welfare you may work, with a purpose, to the end of your days.

—KARL POPPER

8.1. INTRODUCTION

As stressed from the beginning of this book, for over three decades immunologists have appreciated that over a million different antibody specificities are likely extant in each vertebrate organism. Gradually over the past twenty years, immunologists came to espouse one of two major theories to explain the origin of this potential diversity. Many adhered to the germline theory; that is, for every antibody variable region structure there was a corresponding gene in germline DNA. A consequence of this model is that the genome must contain thousands if not millions of genes encoding antibody variable regions. Other immunologists adhered to the somatic diversification theory that postulated that a few inherited genes undergo extensive somatic alteration to generate the thousands of genes that give rise to the myriad of antibodies. In addition to the two major theories were the maverick solutions that suggested that antibody diversity might be due to new and radically different mechanisms; for example, that two or more genes could interact to form an immunoglobulin variable region. Over the past five years, data have accumulated indicating that all of these theories are correct, at least in part. There are multiple germline genes but not as many as anticipated by the germline theory. There is, indeed, somatic mutation of V-region (and J and D region) gene segments but this operates on a greater number of germline genes than was anticipated by the somatic theory. Finally, although gene rearrangement and interaction play a major role in the generation of diversity, it is only one part.

Up to this point, we have discussed several of the common systems used in immunology, especially the mouse and the human, and have shown what was learned in studies at the serologic level, the protein level, and the DNA level in each system. In this chapter, we will attempt to assimilate much of this information into a contemporary solution to the antibody problem.

8.2. THERE ARE A MODEST NUMBER OF GERMLINE GENES

8.2.1. V Gene Segments

The first point to clarify in the contemporary solution is the answer to the perennial question "How many germline V genes are there in the genome?" Realizing that this is no longer the only issue, it remains, nonetheless, a key question in any model. The answers vary for different systems so a number of these will be discussed.

8.2.1.1. There Are Approximately 200 Mouse V_κ Gene Segments

This estimate is based on two kinds of experiments both of which depend on protein structural information, but which take advantage of DNA analysis. The first type of DNA analysis was described at the beginning of Chapter 7; that is, liquid hybridization analysis. Most of these studies concluded that there were relatively few genes per subgroup (between one and four). The second type of study uses Southern blot analysis (also described in Chapter 7), which tends to give somewhat higher numbers when virtually identical types of experiments are done. Although there has not been a systematic study of each of the approximately 30 mouse subgroups that have been defined in the V_κ system by protein sequence analysis, enough is known so that it is clear that the number of genes per subgroup can very considerably. In some sit-

uations (MOPC 167) when a cDNA probe is made, only a single gene
is detected in the BALB/c genome by Southern blot analysis (Fig. 8.1—
left). In other circumstances (like the $V_\kappa 21$ group), seven restriction fragments (genes) can be detected (Fig. 8.1—right). An average figure that
may be derived from a number of different studies is that there are
approximately five V_κ gene segments in the genome for each subgroup.
Assuming that the number of subgroups in the mouse has not yet pla-
teaued, but will do so around 40, we may conclude that there are approximately 5 × 40 or 200 mouse V_κ gene segments. It is unlikely that
this number is off by more than a factor of two so we may tentatively
conclude that the number of mouse V_κ gene segments is between one
and four hundred.

The two examples illustrated in Fig. 8.1 show the close correlation

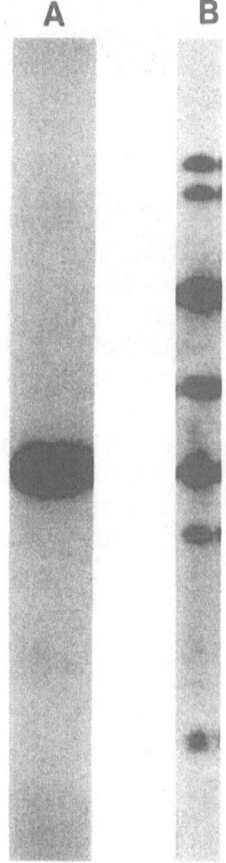

Figure 8.1. Southern filter hybridization with two different cloned
murine V_κ probes on BALB/c germline DNA illustrating one (left)
and several (right) hybridizing restriction fragments (related V_κ
gene segments). From Selsing and Storb, 1981 (left) and Weigert,
unpublished (right).

that emerged between the protein data and the DNA data. Thus, for example, referring to Fig. 3.20 and the discussion in Section 3.6.2, it was concluded that the $V_\kappa 21$ group could be divided into approximately seven or eight subgroups which were each likely encoded by separate germline genes. Figure 8.1—right shows that when a DNA probe is made from a member of one of these subgroups, all members of the group are detected by Southern filter hybridization, and the number of restriction fragments (genes) detected is very close, if not exactly the number predicted from the protein data. See Section 8.5.2 for a further discussion of Fig. 8.1—left.

8.2.1.2. There Are Approximately 50 Human V_κ Gene Segments

The most extensive study of the human V_κ system was done by Rabbitts who prepared cDNA clones representing two different human V_κ subgroups, $V_\kappa 1$ and $V_\kappa 3$. Together these two V_κ subgroups (both serologically and by amino acid sequence analysis) represent approximately 75% of all the human kappa proteins. When the two cloned V_κ genes were studied by Southern filter hybridization against human genomic DNA, each detected approximately 15 to 20 genes (Fig. 8.2). Over half of these genes were the same (thus a total of perhaps 25 to 30 unique restriction fragments). These data suggest that there is extensive cross-hybridization between $V_\kappa 1$ and $V_\kappa 3$ in humans (there are whole stretches of both the protein and the DNA sequences of these two subgroups that are identical). Since these represent approximately 75% of human V_κ sequences, it is anticipated that they represent a very substantial part of the total V_κ gene pool. Since the cloned probes are unable to distinguish the different subgroups, it is likely that in the human there are less than 50 germline V_κ gene segments.

Recently, Bentley (1984) has added further evidence that this number is reasonably correct. In an elegant experiment using a cloned C kappa probe, and cloned $V_\kappa 1$ and $V_\kappa 3$ probes (basically the same system shown in Fig. 8.2), he quantitated the amount of kappa mRNA in human spleen and/or peripheral blood lymphocytes. The C_κ probe was used to measure total kappa messenger RNA. He found that the $V_\kappa 1$ family accounted for over 50% of the kappa mRNA in human spleen or peripheral blood lymphocytes. Since previous arguments (noted above) suggested that approximately 25 germline V_κ genes could be detected with this probe and that this family of genes encodes over 50% of kappa messenger RNA in human lymphocytes, the data provide additional evidence that the total number of V_κ genes in the human germline is 50 or fewer.

V_k3 V_k1

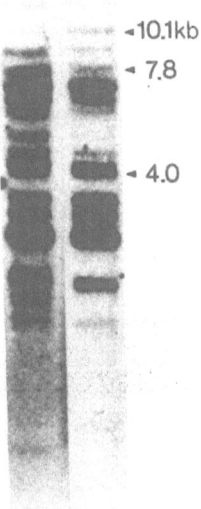

◄10.1kb

◄ 7.8

◄ 4.0

Figure 8.2. Southern filter hybridization of human $V_\kappa 1$ and $V_\kappa 3$ probes to human placental DNA. From Bentley and Rabbitts (1981).

8.2.1.3. There Are Two Mouse V_λ Gene Segments

Early studies by Tonegawa demonstrated the presence in the germline of $V_\lambda 1$ and $V_\lambda 2$ sequences by relating these two DNA sequences to the known protein sequences of the lambda light chains that had been reported by others. In fact, as mentioned earlier, these data represented some of the earliest and strongest arguments against the germline theory. Extensive analysis largely by Tonegawa's group has shown that there are no additional mouse V_λ genes and it is likely that the entire mouse lambda repertoire (approximately 5% of mouse immunoglobulins) derives from these two V_λ gene segments.

8.2.1.4. There Are Approximately 25 Human V_λ Gene Segments

The human V_λ gene segments have not attracted a great deal of attention at the present time, although some studies have been reported. The results are not significantly different than those reported in mouse V_κ that indicate approximately five genes per subgroup. Since there are five human V_λ subgroups defined by serology and protein sequence analysis, this suggests that there are approximately 5×5 or 25 human V_λ gene segments. Recall that in the human, approximately 40% of immunoglobulin molecules contain lambda light chains (Fig. 4.14).

8.2.1.5. There Are Approximately 200 Mouse V_H Gene Segments

This estimate is based on studies that are essentially identical to the studies done in the mouse V_κ system. cDNA copies of the variable regions from myeloma proteins belonging to particular mouse V_H subgroups were constructed (or alternatively, DNA probes were con-

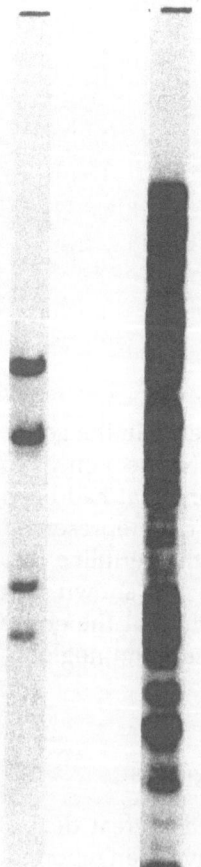

Figure 8.3. Southern filter hybridization of BALB/c DNA illustrating the number of hybridizing bands detected with V_H gene segment probes. From 4 to 35 are shown. From Riblet, unpublished data.

structed from the cloned rearranged expressed gene) and hybridized to restriction digests of mouse embryonic DNA. As few as one and as many as 30 restriction fragments are seen by Southern filter hybridization analysis, although the average seems closer to ten (Fig. 8.3). Extensive amino acid sequencing of mouse V_H regions indicates that the number of V_H subgroups will plateau at about 20. Thus, with an average of ten genes per subgroup and 20 subgroups, there are probably approximately 200 mouse V_H gene segments.

8.2.1.6. There Are Approximately 100 Human V_H Gene Segments

Extensive amino acid sequence analysis indicates that human V_H genes like human V_κ genes seem to cluster into fewer subgroups than the mouse. Thus, in humans there are approximately five V_H subgroups rather than the approximately 20 in the mouse. Using a cloned probe for the human $V_H III$ subgroup, Rabbitts detected 20 restriction fragments in human placental DNA. Extrapolation of these results to the other four subgroups indicates that there are approximately 5×20 or 100 human V_H gene segments.

8.2.2. J and D Gene Segments

Perhaps the pivotal insight provided by DNA analysis was that immunoglobulin V regions were the result of the interaction of V-J or V-D-J gene segments. In the human and mouse, we have a precise knowledge of the number of J gene segments (between four and six depending on the species and system) and a fair approximation of the number of D gene segments. Since the numbers vary in different systems, they will be covered separately.

8.2.2.1. There Are Four to Six J_κ Gene Segments Depending on the Species

By DNA analysis, the mouse appears to have five J_κ gene segments, although as detailed in Chapter 7, one of these is not utilized. In the human, there are five functional J_κ gene segments; in the rat there are six.

8.2.2.2. There Are Four to Six J_λ Gene Segments Depending on the Species

In the mouse, there are four J_λ gene segments but one is a pseudogene (see Chapter 7 and Section 8.6.2.). Humans have at least six J_λ gene segments. As has been described, the arrangement of J and C in both lambda and kappa differs in different species.

8.2.2.3. The Number of J_H Gene Segments Varies from Four to Six Depending on the Species

Mouse J_H segments have been determined by DNA analysis to be four. In humans, this number is six. Unlike the situation in J_κ and J_λ, the *length* of J_H in both mouse and man varies considerably. This can drastically change the contour of the third complementarity determining hypervariable region and undoubtedly impacts on antibody specificity.

8.2.2.4. There Are a Modest Number of D Segments, but the Exact Number is Unknown at Present

The D segment of both mouse and human represents the least understood region of the human and mouse genomes at the present time. The extent of variation and the number of D segments cannot be precisely quantitated because the D segment is so small that accurate counting by Southern filter hybridization is virtually impossible. By sequence analysis, approximately 10 to 20 D segments have been detected in human and mouse by different investigators. Since the number of D segments remains to be elucidated, the number of D segments will be estimated at ten for the present dicussion but it is appreciated that this represents the lower limit.

8.3. COMBINATORIAL JOINING OF V/J AND V, D, AND J GENE SEGMENTS

Shortly after the discovery of the V and J gene segments in mouse lambda, Weigert's group reanalyzed the protein sequences of the $V_\kappa 21$ subgroup of mouse light chains and proposed that combinatorial joining of V gene segments and J gene segments partially explained antibody variability. Since that time, the principal of combinatorial joining of V/J and V, D, and J gene segments has been more fully appreciated and is seen to be one of the major mechanisms that amplifies the limited amount of genetic material. This is obviously a somatic mechanism and, indeed, is a form of gene interaction that was described in Chapter 6. The discussion immediately following will consider the potential for diversity based on combinatorial joining of V with J (light chain) or V with D and J (heavy chain) gene segments. The following section (8.4) will describe the further amplification of diversity found in the junctional positions between these segments.

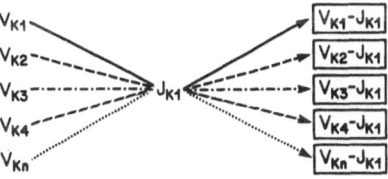

Figure 8.4. Several V_κ gene segments can combine with a single J_κ gene segment.

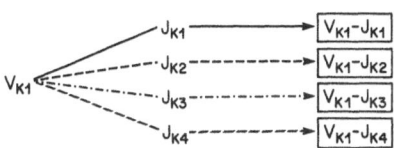

Figure 8.5. A single V_κ gene segment can combine with any of four J_κ gene segments (in mouse; in the human there are *five* J_κ gene segments).

8.3.1. Mouse V_κ

The mouse V_κ system provides an excellent example of how V and J gene segments can join in a combinatorial fashion to further generate antibody diversity. We have discussed the fact that there are approximately 200 mouse V_κ gene segments, perhaps 50 of which are pseudogenes (see Section 8.6.2), leaving about 150 mouse V_κ gene segments. Of the five mouse J_κ gene segments, one is a pseudogene, leaving four functional mouse J_κ gene segments. Since the evidence suggests that any of the V_κ gene segments may combine with any of the J_κ gene segments, this provides $150 \times 4 = 600$ different complete V_κ genes that can be generated from this limited amount of information (see Figs. 8.4 and 8.5).

8.3.2. Mouse V_H

Of the approximately 200 mouse V_H gene segments, approximately 50 are pseudogenes providing approximately 150 functional mouse V_H gene segments (see Table 8.1). (For data on humans see Table 8.2.) There are four mouse J_H gene segments and approximately ten mouse D segments. The evidence is not complete on this particular issue, but it appears that many V_H gene segments can be found in association with different J_H gene segments, and certainly the evidence is overwhelming that many different V_H gene segments can combine with the same J gene segment. This combination of V, D, and J provides another measure of variation and provides approximately $150 \times 10 \times 4$, or 6000 V_H genes from this limited amount of germline information.

There is no conclusive evidence that every one of these combinations can occur. Clearly in certain immune responses, certain V gene segments

Table 8.1. The Number of Germline Genes in the Mouse

	V	D	J
V_κ	200 (150)[a]	0	5 (4)
V_λ	2 (2)	0	4 (3)
V_H	200 (150)	10	4 (4)

[a]Figures in parentheses reflect approximate (V_κ, V_H) or exact (J_κ, J_λ, J_H, V_λ) number of gene segments which are *not* pseudogenes.

combine preferentially with particular J gene segments [for example, the light chains of the arsonate system (see Fig. 3.21)]. However, as in the $V_\kappa 21$ system, different V_κ gene segments can combine with different J_κ gene segments greatly amplifying the diversity (see Fig. 3.20). Thus, although there are clear preferences, the evidence seems reasonable that most combinations can and do occur with a reasonable randomness.

A specific example of V-D-J combinatorial joining is illustrated in Fig. 8.6. This example is taken from the arsonate system and illustrates a series of hybridomas (seven have been chosen, although many more could have been included) all of which bind p-azophenylarsonate, although with varying degrees of affinity. Two different V_H gene segments are utilized; these are designated V_H5 and V_H6 in Fig. 8.6. All utilize the FL16.1 D segment but three different J segments, J_H1, J_H2, and J_H4 are associated with different hybridomas. Most hybridomas in the A/J strain utilize V_H5 and J_H2 and, indeed, in this combination (at least in the limited number studied), this combination results in antibodies with the highest affinity for the hapten. Antibodies with lower binding activity, such as 101F11 use the same V_H and D gene segments but, instead, use J_H4. However, antibodies with good affinity can be generated utilizing the V_H6 gene segment in combination with J_H1 or J_H4. All of these hy-

Table 8.2. The Number of Germline Genes in Humans

	V	D	J
V_κ	50 (35)[a]	0	5 (5)
V_λ	25 (20)	0	6 (?)
V_H	100 (75)	10	6 (6)

[a]Figures in parentheses reflect approximate (V_κ, V_λ, V_H) or exact (J_κ, J_H) number of gene segments which are *not* pseudogenes.

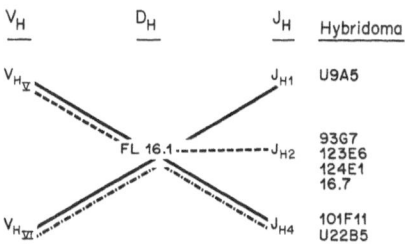

Figure 8.6. A specific example of combinatorial diversity. Gene segments used in the construction of the heavy chain variable region of several anti-arsonate hybridomas. Details are given in the text. (From Meek, K., Urbain, J., and Capra, J.D., unpublished observations.)

bridomas utilize the same or an equivalent light chain with only a few amino acid differences among them (see Fig. 3.21).

8.4. JUNCTIONAL DIVERSITY IS CREATED BY ALTERNATE FRAMES OF RECOMBINATION BETWEEN GERMLINE V, D, AND J GENE SEGMENTS

The extent of junctional diversity has best been described in the mouse V_κ system, although studies in mouse V_H are nearly as complete. As mentioned in the previous chapter, the basic mechanism involved in junctional diversity involves the notion that recombinational flexibility can amplify antibody diversity by changing the point at which the V and J sequences recombine. Since this can vary over a range of several nucleotides, it can give rise to several different nucleotide sequences in the active gene. The result in the light chain, for example, is that the codon for position 96 can vary dramatically. This high variability at position 96 was evident a decade earlier in the first analysis of immunoglobulin light chain protein sequences by Wu and Kabat who noted that position 96 was the most variable position in immunoglobulin chains. Since this is a region of the molecule that makes up part of the antibody-combining site and the idiotypic determinants, variability in this region is surely important for the function of antibody molecules, but the precise extent to which this position contributes to functional antibody diversity remains a matter of speculation. If one studies a large number of V_κ gene segments and J_κ gene segments, it is observed that for every combination, it is theoretically possible to generate four different amino acids by the flexibility of recombination. (In practice, this may be closer to three.) In the thorough analysis done by Leder, most of the predicted sequences are seen (see Fig. 7.10).

In the heavy chain this junctional diversity operates both at the V_H-D as well as the D-J_H junction. Therefore, heavy chain diversity is increased by a factor of 4×4, or 16.

Figure 8.7. Chain recombination between two hybridomas with different hapten binding activities and idiotypes. The light chains differ at only position 96 the V/J joint, and, therefore, the impact of junctional diversity is directly testable (see text for details). (From Jeske, D., Milstein, C., and Capra, J.D., unpublished observations.)

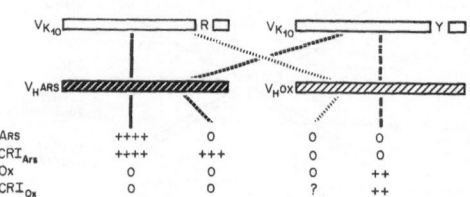

ARS	++++	0	0	0
CRI$_{Ars}$	++++	+++	0	0
Ox	0	0	0	++
CRI$_{Ox}$	0	0	?	++

Different systems utilize flexible recombination in different ways. For example, as noted in Chapter 3, the light chain genes of antiarsonate antibodies from both A/J and BALB/c always generate an arginine at position 96 that is present in neither the germline V_κ nor the germline J_κ genes. Thus, flexible recombination in this system always generates the same amino acid: an amino acid that is not present in any germline gene segment.

Figure 8.7 illustrates a recent experiment that documents that junctional diversity can be essential to antibody function. In this experiment, an anti-arsonate hybridoma which bore the cross-reacting idiotype and was shown not to bind another hapten, phenyloxazolone, or bear the oxazolone idiotype, was found to have a light chain sequence that was extremely similar to a hybridoma that bore the oxazolone idiotype, bound oxazolone, and of course, did not bear the arsonate idiotype or bind arsonate. These two light chains differed by a single amino acid, an arginine/tyrosine interchange at position 96, precisely the V-J junctional position. The heavy chains in this system were totally different. As has been pointed out previously, the arginine in the arsonate system is the result of a V-J recombinational event (an example of junctional diversity) whereas the tyrosine in the phenyloxazolone light chain represents the germline amino acid in the first position of the J_κ gene segment. Thus, it was possible to test the effect of substitutions at this particular position on the binding activity and the idiotype in the two systems. As is evident in the figure (vertical solid lines and vertical dashed lines), a chain recombination experiment between the parent molecules produced the expected result with the homologous recombinants being positive in their respective binding and idiotypic systems. The heterologous recombinants are illustrated by the set of criss-crossed dashed lines and illustrate that when the oxazolone light chain (top right) was recombined with the arsonate heavy chain (bottom left), binding activity to arsonate was abolished, although the arsonate idiotype was restored. In the reverse experiment, when the arsonate light chain (top left) was recombined with the oxazolone heavy chain (bottom right), the molecule did not bind phenyloxazolone. This experiment illustrates that a single amino acid at the junctional position can determine whether or not a molecule will bind one of two haptens and illustrates that at least in this case junctional diversity is essential to antibody function.

The arsonate heavy chains display significant variability at the D-J junctional position (see Fig. 8.8). Three amino acids (aspartic acid, serine, and tyrosine) have been found in the first five molecules sequenced.

The theoretical diversity that can be generated by this mechanism, then, represents an additional factor of 4 in the light chain; thus, $600 \times 4 = 2400$ complete V_κ genes and 16 in the heavy chain, thus, $6000 \times 16 = 96,000$ complete V_H genes (see Section 8.2). Thus, we see how a limited number of germline genes can generate 100,000 different active genes by combinatorial and junctional diversity. Although this is likely enough to account for the required diversity seen in the immune system, it clearly does not explain all of the data since there are three hypervariable regions in each chain, not one (note that the recombination at position 96 and at the V, D, and J junctions only contribute to the variability at one or two positions in the third hypervariable region of each chain). In order to account for variability in the first and second hypervariable regions as well as in the framework, we must turn to additional mechanisms. This latter variability is unlikely to be encoded in the germline since there are enough proteins sequenced through the first hypervariable region of both the heavy and light chain to indicate that there is not enough germline information to account for the observed variability.

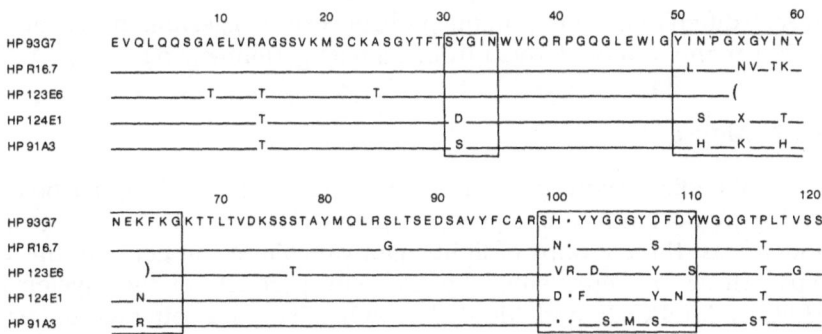

Figure 8.8. The amino acid sequence of five antiarsonate antibodies. The sequences are compared with 93G7, the first completely sequenced antiarsonate heavy chain. The hypervariable regions are boxed. (•) represents a deletion which has been added to align the sequences. Note that with few exceptions, a different amino acid occurs at the V-D and D-J boundaries in each immunoglobulin heavy chain. From Slaughter and Capra (1983).

8.5. SOMATIC MUTATION IN ALL GENE SEGMENTS LEADS TO FURTHER DIVERSITY

8.5.1. Mouse V_λ

The myelomas and hybridomas derived from inbred mice were the essential starting points for understanding that somatic mutation in all gene segments leads to further diversity. Studies in the human were not definitive because rarely was an opportunity available to study both the myeloma protein and germline DNA sequence from the same individual, and thus the problems of genetic complexity of the human population precluded definitive studies. In the mouse, however, it was possible to analyze either sperm or liver DNA from any member of an inbred strain and extrapolate to hybridoma and myeloma DNA from other members of the same strain. In this way, the most definitive information concerning actual alterations in DNA sequence were uncovered and analyzed and generalizations developed.

The earliest direct evidence proving that somatic mutation operated came from the mouse lambda system when Tonegawa demonstrated the presence of a single lambda variable-region gene for each of the two lambda V-region subgroups. Since one $V_\lambda 2$ and nine different $V_\lambda 1$ proteins had been reported by amino acid sequence analysis, a direct comparison of protein and DNA indicated that somatic mutation must have occurred to give rise to the eight variant $V_\lambda 1$ proteins. This suggests that each germline gene can give rise to a minimum of eight somatic variants; thus eight V_λ regions could derive from a single germline gene. However, considering the number of lambda proteins that had been sequenced, statistical analysis suggested that (at the 90% confidence limits) over 20 different lambda variants probably exist suggesting that as many as 20 variants can be derived from a single germline gene.

8.5.2. Mouse V_κ

Antibodies involved in the immune response to phosphylcholine in BALB/c mice utilize one group of heavy chain variable-region genes and at least three groups of light chain variable-region genes of the V_κ type. These are represented by the gene products of the myelomas TEPC15, MOPC603 and MOPC167/MOPC511. This latter group was studied extensively independently by Weissman and by Storb and similar conclusions were reached. Since the MOPC167/MOPC511 protein sequences were known and differed by six amino acids, a direct test of somatic mutation was available when it was discovered that probes for the coding sequence of this myeloma kappa chain variable region detected but a single restriction fragment by Southern filter hybridization of germline DNA (see Fig. 8.1, left). This germline gene was isolated and its sequence corresponded to *neither* the amino acid sequence of MOPC167 nor MOPC511; on the contrary, four base pair changes were needed to generate the V_κ 167 sequence and five base pair changes were needed to generate the V_κ 511 sequence. Since neither the MOPC511 nor MOPC167 genes were detected in the germline, they must have been generated somatically from the available gene that has become known as the V_κ 167 germline gene. These studies have been extended by Gearhart's (1983) laboratory and will be discussed in Section 8.11.

8.5.3. Mouse V_H

Working in the heavy chain system, Hood's group analyzed in detail the immune response to phosphorylcholine at both the protein and nucleic acid level. Amino acid sequence analysis of the heavy chain variable regions of 19 hybridoma and myeloma immunoglobulins were available. Ten of these were identical to the prototype T15 and nine were distinct variants differing by one to eight residues. A cDNA probe was constructed for the T15 heavy chain. Using the T15 V_H DNA probe, they were able to isolate four closely related members of the T15 V_H gene family including one that encoded the T15 V_H sequence itself (Fig. 8.9—top). A comparison of the germline gene sequence with the protein sequences (Fig. 8.9—bottom) indicated that the entire immune response to phosphorylcholine derived from a single T15 germline gene. The somatic variation that they detected in the expressed genes was extensive in and around the coding regions of the two variant V_H genes and it was also found in flanking as well as coding sequences. Many of the substitutions were silent. These data provided firm evidence that somatic mutation occurred in the V_H gene segment.

Similar studies have been done in the arsonate system where it has been established that a single germline V_H gene gives rise to the entire repertoire of arsonate antibodies that bear the cross-reacting idiotype. Over 35 of these molecules have been sequenced and essentially all are different. Since they derive from a single germline gene, upwards of 35 variants are possible.

It is likely that the extent of the amino acid sequence diversity that results from somatic mutation is even higher than the three figures calculated from presently available data: eight for V_λ, nine for T15, and 35 for arsonate. It should be emphasized that none of the systems have reached a plateau. A conservative estimate, however, would be that each germline V gene segment can give rise to a minimum of ten variants. This allows a further permutation of the numbers developed in Section

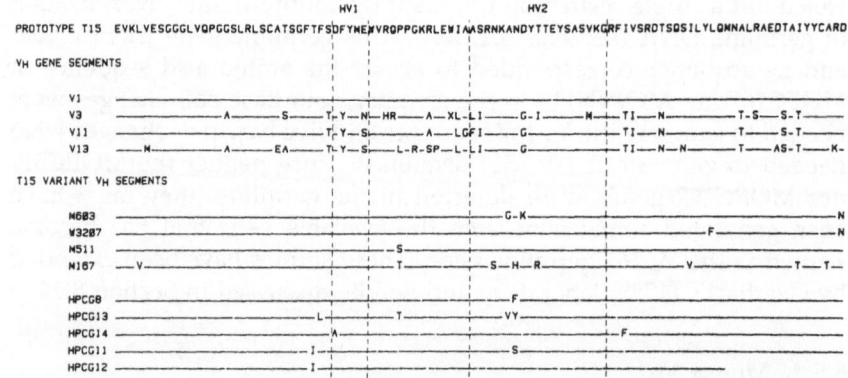

Figure 8.9. Comparison of the V_H gene segments of the T15 V_H gene family and the T15 variant V_H segments. The four gene segments of the T15 V_H gene family have been translated to protein sequences and compared with the sequences of the somatic variants. From Crews *et al.* (1981).

8.3 to suggest that the mouse V_κ system can generate $2400 \times 10 = 24{,}000$ or 2.4×10^4 complete V_κ regions, and in the heavy chain, $96{,}000 \times 10 = 9.6 \times 10^5$ complete V_H regions are possible.

Observation of the arsonate heavy chain J segments sequenced indicates that variations are relatively common (see Fig. 8.8). These data indicate that J segment somatic mutations are relatively common. Because other systems studied do not seem quite this variable, estimates of diversity based on this mechanism will not be considered in our computation. It is likely, however, that this leads to further diversity.

The important role of the J segment in antibody diversity was shown by Scharff and co-workers (Cook and Scharff, 1977) who isolated variants of the S107 myeloma protein and showed that variations in the J gene segment could lead to an alteration of binding activity for phosphorylcholine. Similar observations have been made in the arsonate system, where it has been found that when a J_H gene segment other than J_H2 is used, there is a decreased affinity for the arsonate hapten (see Fig. 8.6).

8.6. THE NUMBER OF C-REGION GENES IS LIMITED AND VARIES CONSIDERABLY AMONG THE SPECIES

8.6.1. Human and Mouse Kappa

These represent the simplest systems under study as there is now extensive evidence that there is but a single mouse kappa C-region gene and a single human kappa C-region gene. Every other system studied is far more complicated. The known allelic variations in human C_κ have been clearly delineated by DNA analysis and confirm protein chemical analysis that suggested that there were relatively few amino acid differences in the allelic forms.

8.6.2. Mouse Lambda

The organization of the mouse lambda C region provided the first insights into extensive complexity in C-region gene organization. As shown in Fig. 7.11, the entire organization of V, J, and C lambda that has been worked out independently by Tonegawa's group and Storb's group is unorthodox; that is, J segments are placed in juxtaposition to C segments. Thus, the known associations between V segments and C segments that had been studied at the protein level a decade ago are confirmed at the DNA level by these data. One of the four mouse C_λ genes has been shown to be a pseudogene (see Section 8.7.2). This form of gene organization lends itself to extensive speculation concerning regulation.

8.6.3. Human Lambda

Even more complex than mouse lambda is the human C_λ locus where a minimum of six C_λ genes have been detected to date. The organization of the J gene segments in relationship to these has not been worked out, but it is likely to be similar to mouse lambda based on the Fett and Deutsch work of a decade previously.

8.6.4. Mouse C_H

All the mouse C_H genes have now been sequenced and mapped to the 12th chromosome. Their organization is shown in Fig. 8.10. Details of the movement of variable region from mu through alpha, although not the subject of this book, are of tremendous contemporary interest and have obvious relevance to the original Dreyer-Bennett hypothesis.

8.6.5. Human C_H

The organization of the human C_H is similar to but not identical to the organization of mouse C_H. Humans have two alpha genes and two or three epsilon genes, at least one of which is a pseudogene. In addition, the organization of the gamma system is somewhat different, although relatively similar to that of the mouse.

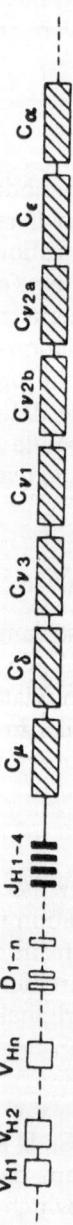

Figure 8.10. The arrangement in germline cells of the gene segments for antibody heavy chains in the mouse. The distances are not drawn to scale as the distances between the C-region genes varies considerably and V_H and D_H have not been formally linked.

8.7. FURTHER CONSIDERATIONS FOR ANTIBODY DIVERSITY

8.7.1. Gene Conversion May Account for Additional Antibody Diversity

Gene conversion is a mechanism whereby two closely related genes interact in such a way that all or part of the DNA sequence of one becomes identical to that of the other. Conversion can occur between genes on the same chromosome, homologous chromosomes, or non-homologous chromosomes. Gene conversion has been described in yeast and evidence suggests that it occurs among mammalian genes. It may be important particularly in the maintenance of homology between members of a multigene family. In relation to immunoglobulins, aspects of gene conversion may be involved in both the variable- and constant-region genes. As shown in Fig. 8.11, gene conversion has been invoked to explain amino acid sequence differences among phosphorylcholine antibodies. It is important to point out that gene conversion can occur somatically or it can occur among germline genes because the process can occur at either meiosis or mitosis. It is possible that gene conversion may account for the conservation of immunoglobulin framework regions across different subgroups and different species. It may further explain some of the still inexplicable recurrences of identical sequences within otherwise different V regions such as the Lay/Pom light chains (Chapter 6). The fact that families of closely related V genes can be maintained over long periods of time by this process makes it particularly attractive.

Gene conversion may add interesting facets to the diversity exhibited by the multigene immunoglobulin family. If the process occurs during differentiation, structural diversity can be generated by the production of "hybrid" molecules expressing segments encoded by several related genes. It is important to point out that the extent to which this adds to antibody diversity has not been determined at the present time. Thus, in our final calculations in this chapter, we will not add a factor for gene conversion, although considering that if it operates it has the potential to dramatically increase the extent of diversity.

8.7.2. Pseudogenes

Pseudogenes were described in detail in Chapter 7 (Section 7.6.4). As was indicated, approximately one third of the germline genes that have been sequenced to date appear to be pseudogenes, and thus estimates of the number of functional V, D, J, and even C gene segments based on Southern hybridization analysis are probably inflated. Only

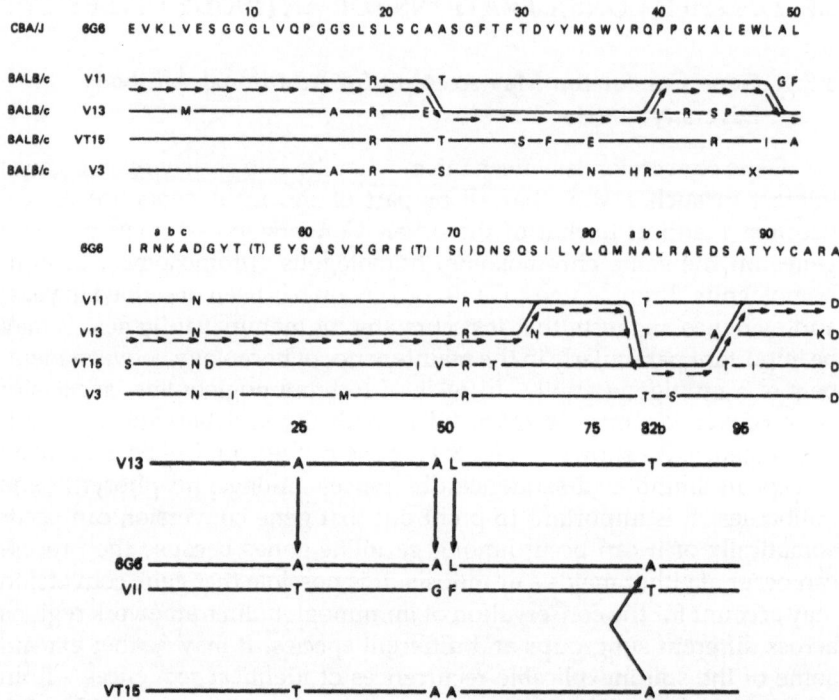

Figure 8.11. A comparison of a CBA/J antiphosphorylcholine antibody variable region with the amino acid sequences of four different BALB/c anti-PC antibody V_H regions. Arrows represent one of several possible pathways required for the assembly of the CBA sequence by multiple somatic recombination events. In the right hand portion of the figure is a schematic representation of gene conversion events occurring during the generation of the 6G6 (CBA) sequence. At four of the positions, 24, 49, 50, and 82B where differences were observed between 6G6 and V11, the substituted amino acid was found to be encoded by other members of the PCV$_H$ family as indicated by vertical arrows representing postulated conversion events. From Clarke *et al.* (1982).

when the DNA sequence of the relevant gene segments has been accomplished and/or independent evidence for expression (for example, the construction of cDNA libraries) is obtained can an accurate assessment be made of the actual number of functional genes in the immunoglobulin system. Most authors argue that pseudogenes bear on the diversity issue largely by *decreasing* the number of gene segments involved. However, it is possible that pseudogenes are actively involved in the generation of diversity by mechanisms that at this point can only be theoretical. For example, it is quite possible that pseudogenes can act in recombination events and thus increase the extent of the repertoire, although the genes themselves may be nonfunctional. In addition, it is possible that through gene conversion events, elements of pseudogenes can be introduced into "functional" genes and thereby increase diversity. There are many other mechanisms whereby pseudogenes could play a major role in antibody diversity but they are beyond the scope of our discussion.

8.7.3. V_H/D and D/J_H Recombination May Generate Additional Diversity through a Novel Mechanism

There is some evidence that V_H/D and D/J_H recombination is not wholly responsible for the diversity seen in the third complementarity-determining hypervariable region of immunoglobulin heavy chains. However, until all mouse D gene segments have been isolated and sequenced, it will be impossible to totally define alternative mechanisms. Abelson murine leukemia virus transformed cell lines contain a number of abortive D/J_H fusions and fragments containing the fusion have been cloned and sequenced. These abortive D/J_H fusions have provided evidence that joined D and J_H may undergo deletion of terminal coding sequences during recombination and that extra nucleotides may be inserted between D and J_H as part of the joining process. The enzyme terminal deoxynucleotidyltransferase may be involved in D/J_H (and probably V_H/D) joints. These additional bases added to existing germline information during or after recombination may represent a new element of heavy chain gene structure. The D/J_H region for this reason has been termed the N region and the mechanism for its generation is illustrated in Fig. 8.12.

A specific example of the postulated role of the N segment in V_H/D junctional diversity is illustrated in Figs. 8.13 and 8.14. Figure 8.13 compares D segment amino acid sequences of five anti-arsonate hybridomas (see Fig. 8.8) to the BALB/c FL16.1 germline D segment. Note that each of the anti-arsonate hybridomas has a glycine instead of a serine in position 5. Thus, it is likely that the A/J FL16.1 counterpart is polymorphic at this position. Note that each of the anti-arsonate hybridoma D segments requires an "amino-terminal extension" and in all instances a serine residue occurs in the amino-terminal position of the D segment. Figure 8.14 illustrates a hypothetical mode of recombination to generate one of the hybridoma sequences between Cys 96 and the second residue of the J segment, Phe. The V_H germline gene for arsonate has been sequenced by Gefter's group and the cDNA sequence of 93G7 is available from the work of Sims *et al.* (1981). It is likely that the first

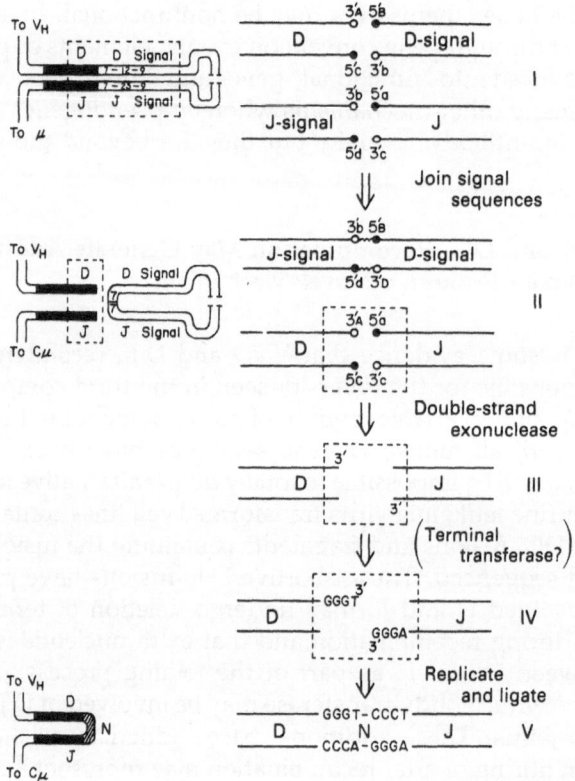

Figure 8.12. Model for the D/J$_H$ recombination reaction: generation of DNA element N. From Alt and Baltimore (1982).

three amino acids, Cys-Ala-Arg, are derived from the V segment. The core segment of all of the molecules shown in Fig. 8.13, Tyr-Tyr-Gly-Gly-Ser-Tyr, likely derives from the germline D segment. Note, however, that Ser-His which are present in the 93G7 hybridoma have no coun-

D$_{FL16.1}$	Y Y Y G S S Y
HP 93G7	S H____G__
HP R16.7	S N____G__
HP 123E6	S V R_D_G__
HP 124E1	S D F____G__
HP 91A3	S__S G M__

Figure 8.13. Relationship of anti-arsonate hybridoma D$_H$ segments to a germline D$_H$ segment gene. Comparison of amino acid sequences of D$_H$ segments with the sequence encoded by the DFL16.1 gene of BALB/c. (----) Identical residues.

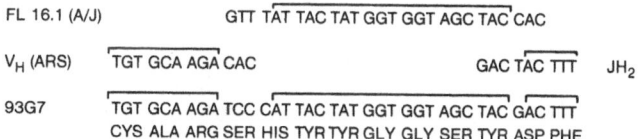

FL 16.1 (A/J)   GTT TAT TAC TAT GGT GGT AGC TAC CAC

V_H (ARS)   TGT GCA AGA CAC   GAC TAC TTT   JH_2

93G7   TGT GCA AGA TCC CAT TAC TAT GGT GGT AGC TAC GAC TTT
                 CYS ALA ARG SER HIS TYR TYR GLY GLY SER TYR ASP PHE

Figure 8.14. Hypothetical mode for the generation of the third complementarity determining hypervariable region of an anti-arsonate hybridoma, 93G7. In this example, with the exception of the germline A/J FL16.1 counterpart, all of the information presented above is available at the DNA level. The brackets illustrate how V, D, and J gene segments are used to construct the immunoglobulin V region gene. Four nucleotides between the V_H-D joint are postulated to result from the action of an unknown enzyme, possibly terminal transferase (see text for details).

terpart in the germline and, indeed, although the histidine likely derives from the second two bases of the tyrosine triplet TAT, the origin of the serine triplet, TCC, is not obvious. It is postulated that the four nucleotides, TCCC, are generated by the novel mechanism described above (Fig. 8.12). *It has not been ruled out* that an additional "mini-gene" or "novel D segment" exists in the germline to encode this region of the molecule, although this seems unlikely at the present time.

It should be pointed out that different antibodies appear to utilize N segment diversity at the V-D joint while others introduce N segment diversity at the D-J joint. Still other systems utilize N segment diversity at both junctional points.

8.7.4. Combinatorial Pairing of Heavy and Light Chains Further Amplifies Diversity

As has been mentioned in several places in this book, there is no formal evidence that every light chain can pair with every heavy chain. However, the large bulk of experimental data suggests that some form of random combinatorial pairing of heavy and light chains can be utilized to amplify antibody diversity. There is abundant evidence that different light chains, for example, can combine with the same heavy chain. This is particularly evident in the antiphosphorylcholine antibodies of the BALB/c mouse where the same T15 gene is used to generate the heavy chains, but three distinct light chain genes are used to generate three different families of anti-PC antibodies. Thus, in this example, three light chains can recombine with the same heavy chain. In other systems, multiple heavy chains have been found in association with the same light chain. Using the extreme of the argument (as has been pointed out earlier), the random association of 1000 light chains and 1000 heavy

Table 8.3. Contributions of Germline, Somatic, and Interactional Processes to Murine Antibody Diversity

	Germline		Combinatorial	Junctional (X4)/Junction	Somatic mutation (X10)
V_κ	$150V_\kappa$	$4J_\kappa$	600	2,400	2.4×10^4
V_H	$150V_H$ $10D_H$ $4J_H$		6,000	96,000	9.6×10^5

chains would produce 10^6 different antibodies. Referring to Table 8.3, the random association of 2.4×10^4 light chains and 9.6×10^5 heavy chains (leaving aside lambda chain contributions) could generate over 1×10^{10} antibodies in the mouse.

8.8. GENE FAMILIES AND SPECIFICITY

It is important to stress that counting genes by Southern filter hybridization simply provides an estimate of the number of genes in the genome that are sufficiently related in structure to cross-hybridize with a given probe. When one attempts to relate this to specificity, only modest correlations can be made. Thus, for example, most antibody responses to even simple haptens are composed of antibodies that generally fall into families of structures with similar V_H and V_L regions. For example, in the arsonate system, an analysis of a large number of hybridomas indicates that three-gene families are utilized. cDNA probes from one of the families (Ars-A) detects 20 germline restriction fragments. Although only one of these genes is used in the idiotype-positive immune response to arsonate (see Chapter 7), the other 19 may be pseudogenes or more likely are used in the immune response to other antigens.

8.9. V-REGION POLYMORPHISM

The notion that an inherited idiotype may reflect a V-region polymorphism has been considered for a number of years. It was not, however, until protein and DNA analysis had been accomplished on a number of idiotypic systems that it became clear that this was, indeed, the case. For example, in both the NP, arsonate, and phosphorylcholine systems that have been described in considerable detail, it was shown that the entire immune response of molecules bearing the idiotypic determinants arose from single germline V_H gene segments, and that by

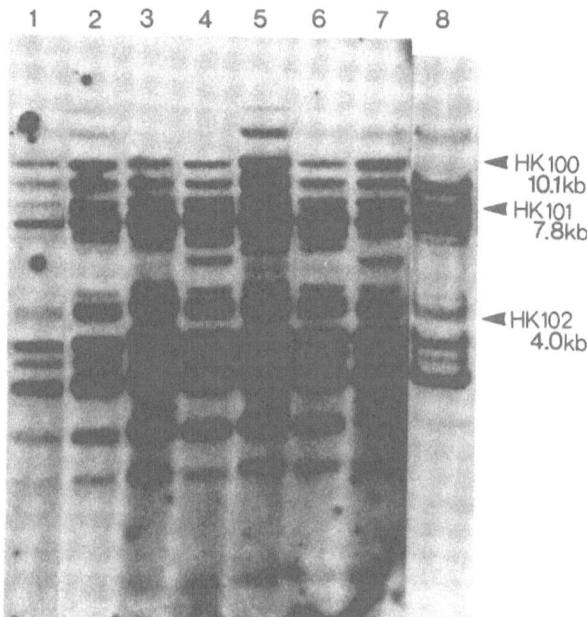

Figure 8.15. Southern filter hybridization patterns of V_κ genes from eight unrelated individuals. DNAs were digested with Bgl II, although similar results were obtained with other enzymes. From Bentley and Rabbitts (1981).

and large these germline genes existed in some (often one) inbred strain but not other strains. Thus, the concept of an inherited idiotype that was first appreciated serologically, and later extended to the protein level, could now be defined at the gene level. Once cloned gene segments were available, the genomes of different inbred strains and, indeed, different species could be compared by the technique of Southern filter hybridization or even by comparison of DNA sequences to elucidate the extent of V-region polymorphisms both between inbred mouse strains and in the human between unrelated individuals.

Figure 8.15 shows Southern filter hybridization patterns of V_κ genes from eight unrelated individuals. The surprising result is that the vast majority of hybridization bands (at least 14) are shared by all eight individuals tested. The same results were obtained when a different restriction enzyme was used. These results suggest that there is relatively little polymorphism in restriction sites flanking V_κ genes of the human population sampled, which includes people of different races.

Somewhat different results have been obtained in the mouse using both V_κ and V_H probes. For example, as shown in Figs. 8.16 and 8.17,

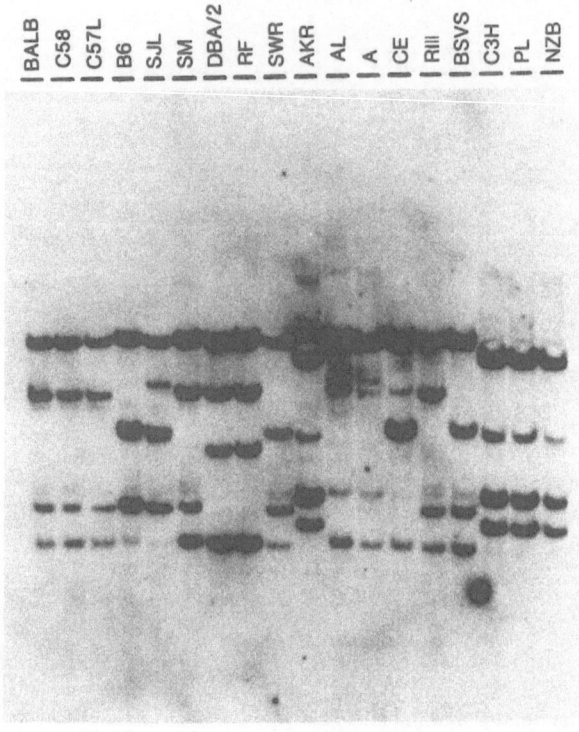

Eco R1   VhS107

Figure 8.16. Southern filter hybridization of genomic DNA from different inbred mouse strains. This illustrates the smallest family of related germline V_H segments, the S107 family. From Riblet, unpublished data.

restriction enzyme patterns of several different inbred mouse strains probed with the DNA probe (S107, Fig. 8.16; Ars-A, Fig. 8.17) indicate that there are several different restriction endonuclease digestion patterns. Analysis of 18 inbred strains demonstrates that certain strains share similar V_H patterns that are different from other strains.

These very elegant studies that have been pursued primarily by Riblet's group have established that in the inbred mouse there are in the order of six or seven different patterns that can be obtained in an inbred strain using various V_H probes. Beyond that, additional V_H probes give patterns extremely similar to one of the pre-existing six or seven patterns. Using recombinant inbred strains, Riblet has been able to establish the order of these "gene families" within the V_H locus as J606,

J558, S107, Q52, and PC7183. Additional gene families have been detected using probes for the Ars-C genes and it is likely that additional gene families will be uncovered as probes are constructed from additional hybridomas, particularly those with "blocked" heavy chains, since these have not been systematically studied. We might anticipate that the 200 mouse V_H genes might be arranged into approximately ten gene

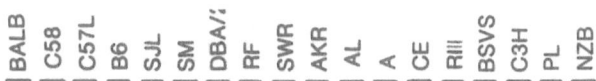

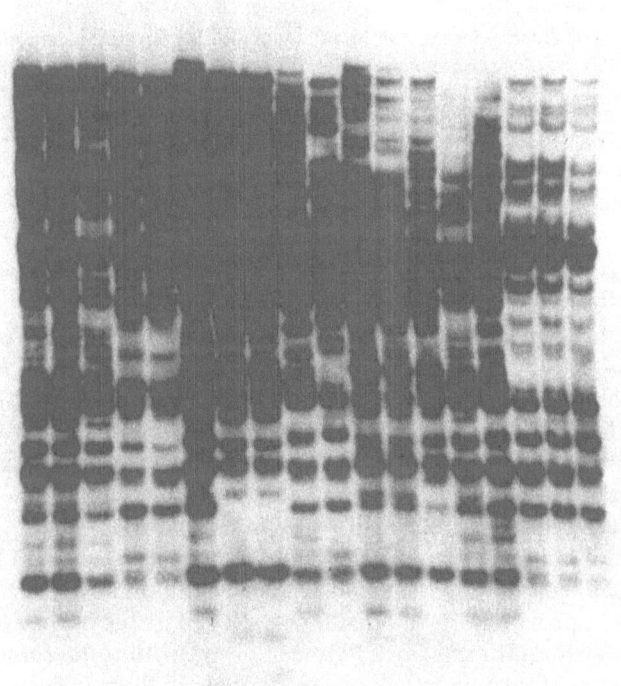

Eco R1   VhARS

Figure 8.17. Southern filter hybridization of genomic DNA from different inbred mouse strains. This illustrates probably the largest family of related germline V_H segments, the J558 family. In this illustration, the V_{ARS} probe was used, but similar results would have been obtained with V_H J558, V_H DEX, and V_H NP^b. From Riblet, unpublished data.

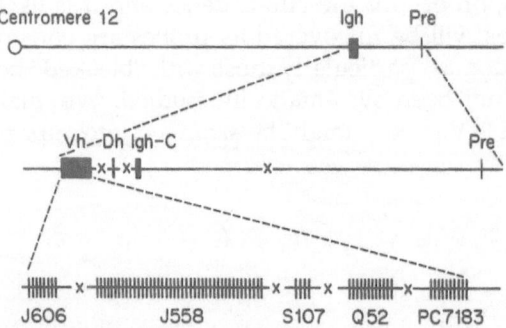

Figure 8.18. A schematic view of the immunoglobulin loci on murine chromosome 12. The Xs indicate points of recombination that have been detected using DNA probes. PRE is the prealbumin locus. The five gene families are named after the original five probes that were used to detect them, although overlap has been extensively noted. For example, the Ars-A cDNA probe (Fig. 8.13) overlaps extensively with the J558 probe. Adapted from Riblet, unpublished data.

families and the families may vary in size from four (S107) to 35 (J558). This is illustrated schematically in Fig. 8.18.

Studies of this kind coupled with the present linkage analysis of V_H genes allow an approximation of the amount of DNA involved at the immunoglobulin V_H locus. Studies from three different laboratories have now provided evidence that the approximate distance between V_H genes is between 10 and 50 kb. Since our present estimate is that there are approximately 200 murine V_H gene segments, this would suggest that approximately 2000 to 10,000 kb of DNA encompasses the V_H locus. Although the majority of recombinations observed have been between gene families, some have occurred within gene families. This suggests that at first approximation the distance between genes in different families is greater than the distance between genes within the same family. It also suggests that in recombination, gene conversion events within gene families will be favored over events between families.

8.10. EVOLUTION OF V AND J GENE SEGMENTS

The subject of V-region polymorphism is intimately related to that of V and J gene segment evolution. The majority of the issues that can now be addressed at the DNA level have been previously investigated at the level of serology or protein sequence. Now with DNA sequence analysis, a more precise understanding of the evolution of immuno-globulin genes can be developed.

The unusual arrangement of V_λ, J_λ, and C_λ genes in the BALB/c mouse has been detailed in Chapter 7. Storb postulated that a V_λ-JC_λ x-JC_λ y underwent gene duplication to generate V_λ 1-JC_λ 3-JC_λ 1 and V_λ 2-JC_λ 2-JC_λ 4. This hypothesis is based on the frequency of replacement site changes within the entire V and C_λ gene cluster. Alternatively, a recent gene conversion event might have acted upon $V_\lambda 1$ and $V_\lambda 2$ genes that might have eliminated any divergence between the V_λ genes that had accumulated. The duplication, however, of an original V_λ-J_λ x-J λ y cluster into two separate expression units possibly could explain the preferential association of $V_\lambda 1$ with $C_\lambda 1$ and $C_\lambda 3$, and $V_\lambda 2$ with $C_\lambda 2$ on the basis of physical organization in the genome.

Figure 8.19 illustrates the possible evolution of the human and murine J_κ gene segment. As mentioned previously, although the mouse germline contains five J_κ segment genes, one is a pseudogene (J3); additional sequence analysis showed the existence of a remnant of a J region (see Fig. 8.19) designated rem 5. The human J segments are five in number, all of which appear functional. Leder's group has postulated the evolution of J from an ancestral gene containing five functional J segments based on extensive sequence analysis of the entire J gene cluster in both species. It is suggested that the ancestral species common to mouse and human contained five functional J segment genes within the kappa constant locus. Relatively soon after divergence of the two species, the mouse J5 sequence was inactivated by a mutational event, subjecting it to random genetic drift and subsequent cumulative loss of homology to J-region coding segments. In addition, an equal crossing over event in the mouse between J4 and J3 on homologous chromosomes (step 2, Fig. 8.19) gave rise to a chromosome that became fixed in the population with five functional J gene segments and a remnant gene. The chronological order of these first two events is not known. Finally, a recent mutational event inactivated mouse J3. The resultant unexpressed J3 gene then drifted to the limited extent observed at this point in evolutionary time. Further analysis of J gene clusters in other species including related rodents and primates will undoubtedly provide a more precise understanding of these evolutionary events. The rabbit J region expressed with the b4 kappa chain, for example, contains five J gene segments only one of which appears to be functional.

As discussed earlier in this chapter (see Tables 8.1 and 8.2, for example) the number of germline genes encoding "subgroups" differs dramatically among species. The human V_H3 gene segment subgroup has been mapped 3' to the V_H2 gene segment subgroup based on deletion of V_H gene segments after V-D-J rearrangement. Additional studies com-

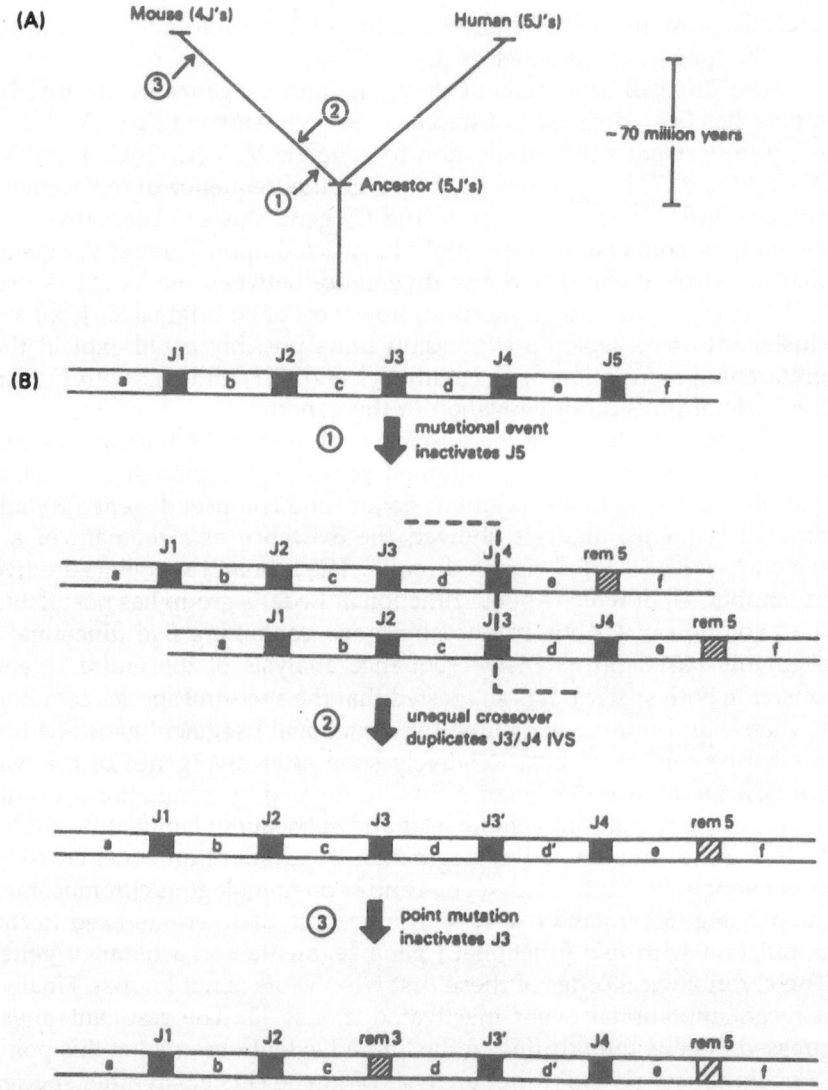

Figure 8.19. A model to account for the evolution of human and mouse J_κ gene segments after divergence of the species. A. An evolutionary tree of mouse and human J gene segments. Three hypothetical evolutionary events are indicated that are thought to have occurred in the mouse after the divergence of the species. B. A diagrammatic representation of the evolutionary events indicated above. J_κ gene coding segments are represented as solid boxes. Hatched boxes represent J genes that have been inactivated by a mutational event and subjected to sequence mutation in the absence of selection. The degree of hatching represents the extent of nucleotide sequence homology to active J gene segments. From Heiter *et al.* (1982).

paring mouse and human germline DNA with the same V gene segment probes indicate that the human V_H3 gene subgroups underwent a significant gene expansion compared with the mouse V_H3 subgroup. As has been discussed previously, amino acid sequence data indicate that human V_H3 genes correspond to only a small subset of mouse V_H3 genes. Human V_H3 genes contain a shorter intron and are two codons shorter than most BALB/c mouse V_H3 gene segments. The nature of nucleotide substitutions between V_H gene segments within a species (human) is similar to that between genes of different species (human/mouse). Both contain approximately 50% silent mutations. Figure 8.20 illustrates some of these points in comparing human and mouse V_H3 gene sequences.

8.11. SOMATIC MUTATION REVISITED

Throughout this book we have dealt with the concept of somatic mutation from its earliest inception as a hypothetical mechanism to gen-

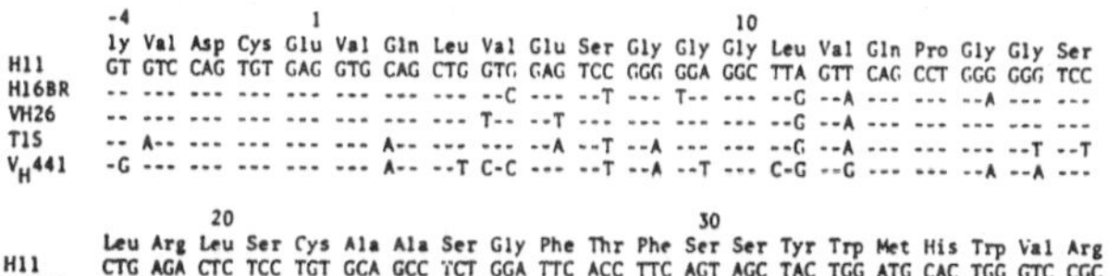

Figure 8.20. Comparison of human and mouse V_H3 gene sequences. Human genes are H11, H16BR, and VH26. Mouse genes are T15 and VH441. Only the coding strand is shown and the predicted amino acids are given of H11 above the line. Hypervariable regions HV1 and HV2 are underlined. Recombination signals at the end of V_H are boxed. From Rechavi *et al.* (1982).

erate antibody diversity to a relatively precise description of the actual somatic alterations seen in the DNA. We must now concern ourselves with a more detailed analysis of somatic mutation with specific reference to mechanisms, temporal sequence of events in ontogeny, and the question of whether only certain regions are mutated while others remain conserved.

Perhaps the most extensive analysis of the impact of somatic mutation was done by Gearhart and Hood who sequenced a series of IgG, IgA, and IgM heavy and light chains from phosphorylcholine-binding myelomas and hybridomas (see Figs. 8.21 and 8.22). These data indicate that the V_H regions from 11 IgM hybridomas do not show any diversity in their N terminal 36 residues. In contrast, the corresponding positions of the V_H regions from IgG hybridomas vary in six of the nine examples studied. The same pattern is seen in the corresponding V_L region. Of the twelve light chains from IgM antibodies, 11 are identical in sequence to the prototype sequence of their respective groups, whereas five of nine V_L regions from IgG antibodies vary. Thus, eight of the nine IgG antibodies vary from the V subgroup prototype sequences in either V_H or V_L regions, whereas only one of the 12 IgM antibodies varies. These

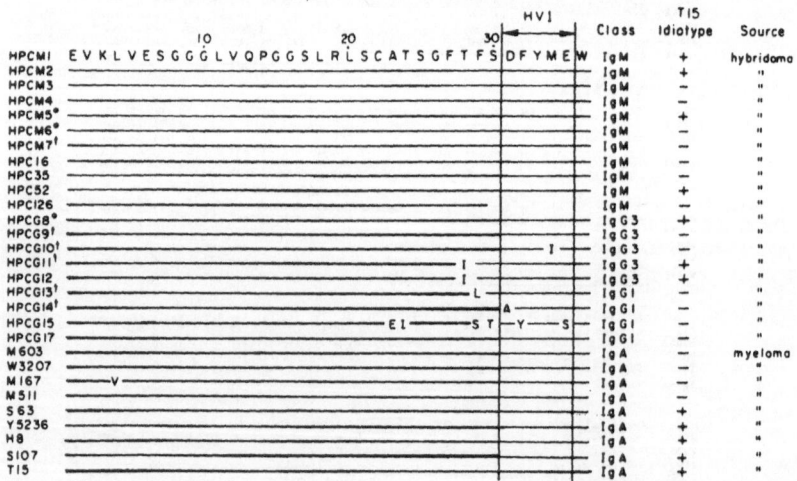

Figure 8.21. V_L regions of antiphosphorylcholine antibodies (36 residues). The proteins are grouped as shown on the right based on class and subclass and the presence or absence of the T15 idiotype. Note that the light chains derived from IgM antibodies are identical to each other, whereas the majority of the IgG antibodies differ one from the other. From Gearhart *et al.* (1981).

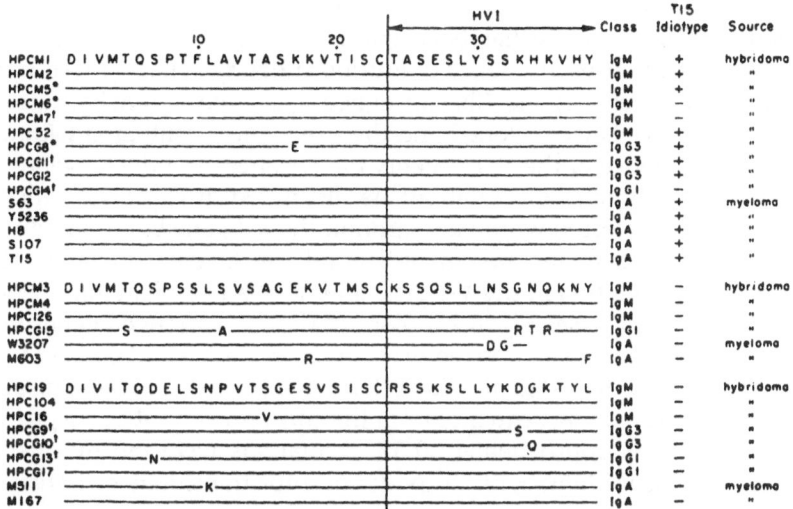

Figure 8.22. The V_H regions of antiphosphorylcholine antibodies (38 residues). Again the molecules are grouped based on immunoglobulin class and presence or absence of the T15 idiotype. From Gearhart *et al.* (1981).

authors suggested, therefore, that the actual class-switching mechanism may be involved in the generation of diversity. These studies would suggest that the maturation of the immune response, which has been known for nearly 50 years (that is, that antibodies isolated after secondary immunization have higher affinities than early in immunization), might be due to somatic mutation and selection. But what of the mechanism itself?

One issue that has been addressed by several authors is whether only the rearranged or also the germline gene is subject to somatic mutation. Thus, as has been described, during the course of B-cell maturation, a V gene segment from one allele joins a J gene segment in a cis fashion. If this is a productive rearrangement, the opposite allele is "excluded." Since somatic mutation has been detected in the rearranged gene in many systems, one might ask "what of the unrearranged allelic gene?" Several studies have now demonstrated that the unrearranged gene generally appears in the germline configuration suggesting that *somatic mutation operates only on the rearranged gene.* These findings imply that the rearrangement process itself rather than class switching may be instrumental in generating the diversity or at least in triggering the somatic mutation.

In a recent study from Gearhart's laboratory (Gearhart and Bogenhagen, 1983), this issue has been studied in detail by examining the nucleotide sequences of a series of murine antibody genes derived from one kappa light chain gene. Six rearranged $V_\kappa 167$ genes from hybridoma and myeloma cells were cloned and their sequences compared with the germline sequence of the $V_\kappa 167$ gene, the J_κ genes, and the C_κ genes in order to identify sites of mutation. As illustrated in Fig. 8.23, somatic mutation was detected within and around the V-J gene but not midway between V-J and C and not in or around the C gene segment. The frequency of mutation in the V-J gene and its 5' and 3' flanking regions approximates 0.4% (see Fig. 8.23). Four of the six rearranged genes had extensive mutation that occurred exclusively in a one kb region of DNA centered around the V-J gene. No mutations were found at more distant sites in the intervening sequence or in the constant gene. The frequency of mutation was approximately 0.5%. Mutations were mostly due to nucleotide substitutions with no preference for transitions or transversions. The location of mutations within each gene indicates that they occur in clusters at random sites. The frequency of mutation indicates that they do not occur randomly either within the V-J gene segment or the 3' and 5' flanking regions, but rather occur in clusters. Such clusters are most easily explained by a mechanism of error-prone repair that occurs during several cycles of cell division.

Thus, somatic mutation occurs in the rearranged gene and occurs in clusters and is probably due to some form of error-prone repair mechanism. The relative importance of somatic mutation to function is still unknown. It may simply represent "mutational noise" that is not selected for or against either in evolution, or during the immune response.

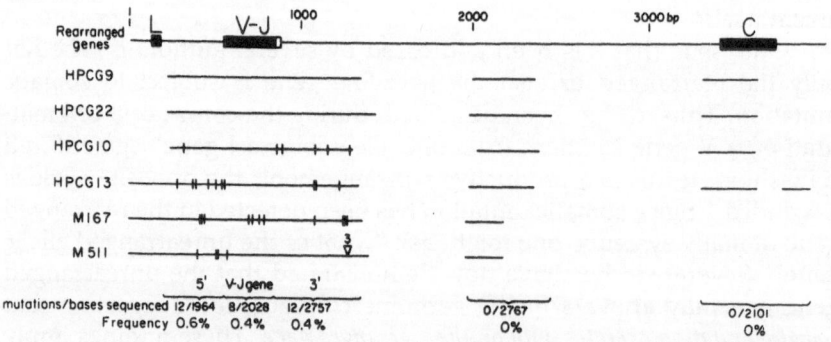

Figure 8.23. Mutations are localized to the V-J gene. The horizontal lines for hybridoma and myeloma genes indicate identity to the germline sequence shown at the top. Vertical lines represent single nucleotide substitutions and the inverted triangle a deletion of three bases. An open box next to the V gene segments represents the J gene segment. From Gearhart and Bogenhagen (1983).

8.12. WHY DO WE HAVE CERTAIN GERMLINE GENES?

The immune response to phosphorylcholine has been detailed in great depth throughout this book as one of the prototypic immune responses. It is important to appreciate that the immune response to phosphorylcholine has survival value since naturally occurring and hybridoma IgM and IgG anti-PC antibodies protect mice from fatal infections with virulent *Streptococcus pneumoniae*. Because of the protective effects of anti-PC antibodies against pneumococcal infections, Briles *et al.* (1982) postulated that the genes encoding anti-PC V_H and V_L regions might exist in the genome to produce protective antibodies reactive with PC containing techoic acids. If this were the case, one would expect the T15 anti-PC antibody to be more protective than anti-PC antibody made after extensive somatic mutation. The data indicate that this is, indeed, the case as even single amino acid substitutions in anti-PC hybridoma and myeloma antibody variable regions significantly decrease protection against fatal pneumococcal infection. Thus, there appears to be a close association between protection against *S. pneumoniae* and the presence of particular V_H and V_L chains. In all studies, the T15 antibody provided optimal protection suggesting that the germline V_H and V_L genes may have evolved to provide antibody directed against one or another common antigen or pathogen. Phosphorylcholine, for example, has been found on many microorganisms including species of fungi, nematodes, and gram-negative and -positive bacteria. The pre-existence of germline genes for antibody to common antigens might allow for a more rapid initial antibody response. Antibodies to antigens either not associated with or less commonly associated with pathogens would be expected in general to require somatic mutation of the V-region genes to produce suitable antibody-binding sites.

Another interpretation for the presence or absence of certain germline genes involves the idiotype network as a necessity of evolution. Since most germline genes are probably not used during the lifetime of one individual, how can the system evolve in anticipation of future needs? Selection pressure due to external antigens would probably be insufficient over the short term; thus, most immunoglobulins, rather than being preserved in the germline as antibodies to pathogens, might be preserved in the germline as antiidiotypic antibodies recognizing other immunoglobulins. These constructs, of course, revolve around the use of the antibody in the regulatory circuit of the immune system with internal selection pressure allowing the conservation of a large number of germline genes. This would involve a parallel evolution of germline genes for the preservation of the species on the one hand (having the genes encode the crucial information to protect against pathogens), and on the other hand, the evolution of antiidiotypic antibodies to regulate these genes.

8.13. HORIZONS

It is, of course, very risky to play the role of prophet for areas moving as fast as those covered in the last two chapters of this volume. However, it seems worthwhile to mention two recent groups of papers that give evidence that the antibody enigma will continue to provide an exciting arena of research for the foreseeable future. The introduction of cloned immunoglobulin genes into nonimmunoglobulin-producing cells with the subsequent expression of antibodies has now been accomplished in several laboratories. Both heavy and light polypeptide chains have been introduced either alone or together into various cell lines resulting in the actual production of limited amounts of immunoglobulin. By site-specific mutagenesis, investigators will soon be able to modify the genes before they are introduced into cells and thereby open up an entire new era, not only in the immunochemistry of the antibody-combining site and the idiotype, but a new era in our understanding of the mechanisms whereby immunoglobulin genes are regulated. Within reach is an understanding of the precise mechanisms whereby somatic mutation operates.

Some of the issues raised in Chapter 6 concerning the maverick solutions to the antibody enigma involve the movement of genetic information not only within chromosomes but between chromosomes. Early evidence for the transposition of genetic elements was provided in maize, bacteria, yeast, and *Drosophila*. Later movement of genes and gene segments became the rule rather than the exception in immunoglobulin gene expression. More recently it has been demonstrated that immunoglobulin genes can be found on chromosomes in addition to their customary location. In many of these situations, the "inserted" gene appears to have been a processed gene (one with a leader sequencer and/or lacking introns). Recent studies both in murine and human malignant lines indicate that not only have immunoglobulin genes been translocated but, in addition, may be involved in the large-scale production of an oncogenic substance.

For example, studies of both murine plasmacytoma and human Burkitt lymphoma cell lines provide evidence that a somatically rearranged segment of immunoglobulin gene encodes the specific oncogene, c-myc (the murine cellular analogue of an avian viral transforming gene). This mouse c-myc sequence was used to show that human c-myc is located at the precise site on chromosome 8 from which the Burkitt lymphoma translocation originates. In many Burkitt lymphoma lines, the c-myc gene region fragment has undergone a somatic rearrangement. In some situations, the c-myc and immunoglobulin sequences were on the same DNA restriction fragments, suggesting that this segment included the cross-over point for the translocation from chromosome 8 to 14. The discovery of these translocations that move a seemingly unrelated genetic message to a locus that normally undergoes a recombination event as a process of differentiation has opened up a particularly provocative question. As Leder has pointed out, "Might not the same diversity-generating mechanism that has proved so powerful for the expression of immunoglobulin genes be used in other systems?" Thus, the very mechanisms that have been described in these last two chapters that seem to be involved in the normal differentiation process of B lymphocytes as they assemble genetic information from diverse portions of the genome to produce an immunoglobulin molecule might provide important insights into the malignant process itself.

8.14. PRECIS

Thus, an uneasy consensus is being reached concerning the enigma of antibody diversity. This consensus includes elements of both the original "germline" and "somatic" models. A limited number of germline genes through the processes of combinatorial joining of various gene segments, junctional diversity at the points where gene segments recombine, somatic mutation, potentially gene conversion, and finally the combinatorial pairing of heavy and light chains that can generate an enormous amount of diversity in antibodies. The available evidence argues strongly that all of these processes contribute significantly to antibody diversity and that antibody specificities, hypervariable regions, and idiotypes can be generated from a limited amount of genetic material by a whole assortment of mechanisms that the immune system utilizes to store, manipulate, and retrieve genetic information. Despite vexing questions that remain, it is fair to say that the enigma of antibody diversity has been penetrated. It is further reasonable to expect that recent experimental advances will clear the way for future elucidation of this fascinating riddle.

REFERENCES AND BIBLIOGRAPHY

Alt, F. W., and Baltimore, D., 1982, Joining of immunoglobulin heavy chain gene segments: Implications from a chromosome with evidence of three D-J$_H$ fusions, *Proc. Natl. Acad. Sci. U.S.A.* **79**:4118.

Ben-Neriah, Y., Cohen, J. B., Rechavi, G., Zakut, R., and Givol, D., 1981, Polymorphism of germline immunoglobulin V_H genes correlates with allotype and idiotype markers, *Eur. J. Immunol.* **11**:1017.

Bentley, D. L., 1984, Most kappa immunoglobulin mRNA in human lymphocytes is homologous to a small family of germline V genes, *Nature* **307**:77.

Bentley, D. L., and Rabbitts, T. H., 1981, Human V_H immunoglobulin gene number: Implications for the origin of antibody diversity. *Cell* **24**:613.

Briles, D. E., Forman, C., Hudak, S., and Claflin, J. L., 1982, Anti-phosphorylcholine antibodies of the T15 idiotype are optimally protective against *Streptococcus pneumoniae*, *J. Exp. Med.* **156**:1177.

Clarke, S. H., Claflin, J. L., and Rudikoff, S., 1982, Polymorphisms in immunoglobulin heavy chains suggesting gene conversion, *Proc. Natl. Acad. Sci. U.S.A.* **79**:3280.

Cook, W. D., and Scharff, M. D., 1972, Antigen-binding mutants of mouse myeloma cells, *Proc. Natl. Acad. Sci. U.S.A.* **74**:5687.

Crews, S., Griffin, J., Huang, H., Calame, K., and Hood, L., 1981, A single V_H gene segment encodes the immune response to phosphorylcholine: Somatic mutation is correlated with the class of the antibody, *Cell* **25**:59.

Gearhart, P, Johnson, N. D., Douglas, R., and Hood, L., 1981, IgG antibodies to phosphorylcholine exhibit more diversity than their IgM counterparts, *Nature (London)* **291**:29.

Gearhart, P. J., and Bogenhagen, D. F., 1983, Clusters of point mutations are found exclusively around rearranged antibody variable genes, *Proc. Natl Acad. Sci. U.S.A.* **80**:3439.

Gershenfeld, H. K., Tsukamoto, A., Weissman, I. L., and Joho, R., 1981, Somatic diversification is required to generate the V_K genes of MOPC511 and MOPC167 myeloma proteins, *Proc. Natl. Acad. Sci. U.S.A.* **78**:7674.

Heiter, P. A., Maizel, C. V., and Leder, P., 1982, Evolution of human immunoglobulin kappa J region genes, *J. Biol. Chem.* **257**:1516.

Leder, P., 1983, Genetic control of immunoglobulin production, *Hosp. Pract.* **18**:73.

Pech, M., Hochtl, J., Schnell, H., and Zachau, H. G., 1981, Differences between germline and rearranged immunoglobulin V_K coding sequences suggest a localized mutation mechanism, *Nature (London)* **291**:668.

Popper, K., 1983, *Logic of Scientific Discovery*, Hutchinson, Rowmon, and Littlefield.

Rechavi, G., Bienz, B., Ram, D., Ben-Neriah, Y., Cohen, J. B., Zakut, R., and Givol, D., 1982, Organization and evolution of immunoglobulin V_H gene subgroups, *Proc. Natl. Acad. Sci. U.S.A.* **79**:4405.

Rice, D., and Baltimore, D., 1982, Regulated expression of an immunoglobulin kappa gene introduced into a mouse lymphoid cell line, *Proc. Natl. Acad. Sci. U.S.A.* **79**: 7862.

Schilling, J., Clevinger, B., Davie, J. M., and Hood, L., 1980, Amino acid sequence of homogeneous antibodies to dextran and DNA rearrangements in heavy chain V-region gene segments, *Nature (London)* **283**:35.

Selsing, E., and Storb, U., 1981, Somatic mutation of immunoglobulin light-chain variable-region genes, *Cell* **25**:47.

Selsing, E., Miller, J., Wilson, R., and Storb, U., 1982, Evolution of mouse immunoglobulin lambda genes, *Proc. Natl. Acad. Sci. U.S.A.* **79**:4681.

Sims, J., Rabbitts, T. H., Estess, P., Slaughter, C., Tucker, P. W., and Capra, J. D., 1982, Somatic mutation in genes for the variable portion of the immunoglobulin heavy chain, *Science* **216**:309.

Slaughter, C. A., and Capra, J. D., 1983, Amino acid sequence diversity within the family of antibodies bearing the major antiarsonate cross-reactive idiotype of the A strain mouse, *J. Exp. Med.* **158**:1615.

Takemori, T., Tesch, H., Reth, M., and Rajewsky, K., 1982, The immune response against anti-idiotope antibodies. I. Induction of idiotope-bearing antibodies and analysis of the idiotope repertoire, *Eur. J. Immunol.* **12**:1040.

Urbain, J., and Wuilmart, C., 1982, Some thoughts on idiotypic networks and immunoregulation, *Immunol. Today* **3**:88.

Weigert, M., Gatmaitan, L., Loh, E., Schilling, J., and Hood, L., 1978, Rearrangement of genetic information may produce immunoglobulin diversity, *Nature* **276**:785.

INDEX